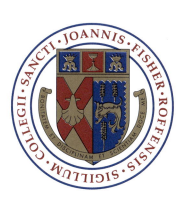

HELPING ADOLESCENTS AT RISK

Helping Adolescents at Risk

Prevention of Multiple Problem Behaviors

ANTHONY BIGLAN
PATRICIA A. BRENNAN
SHARON L. FOSTER
HAROLD D. HOLDER

with

Ted R. Miller

and

Phillippe Cunningham, James H. Derzon, Dennis D. Embry,
Diana H. Fishbein, Brian R. Flay, Nick E. Goeders,
Steven H. Kelder, Donald Kenkel, Roger Meyer, and Robert A. Zucker

THE GUILFORD PRESS
NEW YORK   LONDON

© 2004 The Guilford Press
A Division of Guilford Publications, Inc.
72 Spring Street, New York, NY 10012
www.guilford.com

Printed in the United States of America

This book is printed on acid-free paper.

Last digit is print number: 9 8 7 6 5 4 3 2 1

Library of Congress Cataloging-in-Publication Data

Helping adolescents at risk : prevention of multiple problem behaviors /
Anthony Biglan ... [et al.].
    p. cm.
Includes bibliographical references and index.
  ISBN 1-57230-973-3 (hardcover : alk. paper)
  1. Conduct disorders in adolescence. 2. Conduct disorders in
children. I. Biglan, Anthony.
  RJ506.C65H44 2004
  616.89′00835—dc22

                                       2003020510

About the Authors

Anthony Biglan, PhD, is Senior Scientist at Oregon Research Institute, where he conducts research on the prevention of child and adolescent problem behavior and on the childrearing practices that affect child and adolescent development. His current work focuses on contextual analyses of childrearing practices in communities. Dr. Biglan served on the Epidemiology and Prevention Review Committee for the National Institute on Drug Abuse and on review committees for the National Institutes of Health. He is on the editorial boards of four national journals and consults with the Office of National Drug Control Policy. Author of the book *Changing Cultural Practices: A Contextualist Framework for Intervention Research,* Dr. Biglan is president-elect of the Society of Prevention Research and cochairs its Prevention Science Advocacy Committee.

Patricia A. Brennan, PhD, is on the faculty of the Department of Psychology at Emory University. She received her BS in Psychology from the University of Massachusetts, Amherst, in 1986, and her PhD in Psychology from the University of Southern California in 1992. Her research interests include the study of etiological factors of aggression and violence from a biological perspective, and parental psychopathology (depression/ schizophrenia) and its effect on child diagnostic, neurological, and behavioral outcomes.

Sharon L. Foster, PhD, is Professor in the California School of Professional Psychology at Alliant International University. She received her PhD in Psychology from the State University of New York at Stony

Brook, after completing a clinical internship at the University of Washington Medical School. She also taught at West Virginia University. Dr. Foster has served as an associate editor for the journals *Behavioral Assessment* and the *Journal of Consulting and Clinical Psychology*, and was a Fellow at the Center for Advanced Study in the Behavioral Sciences from 2000 to 2001. She is the author of three books as well as numerous articles and book chapters on children's peer relations, assessment and treatment of parent–adolescent conflict, and research methodology.

Harold D. Holder, PhD, is Director and Senior Research Scientist of the Prevention Research Center, one of 14 federally funded centers sponsored by the National Institute on Alcohol Abuse and Alcoholism of the National Institutes of Health. In his research, he has explored two major areas: prevention of alcohol problems and cost and benefits of alcoholism treatment. In addition, he is part of a core group of researchers and scholars involved in an international alcohol public policy project, directed by the journal *Addiction*. Dr. Holder was appointed to the National Advisory Council on Alcohol Abuse and Alcoholism in 1998 and is the 1995 recipient of the Jellinek Memorial Award for his research on social and economic factors of alcohol consumption and the impact of changes in alcohol availability on alcohol problems. Dr. Holder has published more than 150 scientific papers in refereed journals and collected volumes and is an assistant editor of *Addiction*.

Contributors

Phillippe Cunningham, PhD, Department of Psychiatry and Behavioral Sciences, Medical University of South Carolina, Charleston, South Carolina

James H. Derzon, PhD, Pacific Institute for Research and Evaluation, Calverton, Maryland

Dennis D. Embry, PhD, PAXIS Institute, Tucson, Arizona

Diana H. Fishbein, PhD, Transdisciplinary Behavioral Science Program, Research Triangle Institute, Rockville, Maryland

Brian R. Flay, PhD, FAAHB, Health Research and Policy Centers, University of Illinois at Chicago, Chicago, Illinois

Nick E. Goeders, PhD, Departments of Pharmacology and Therapeutics and Psychiatry, Louisiana State University Health Sciences Center, Shreveport, Louisiana

Steven H. Kelder, PhD, MPH, Center for Health Promotion and Prevention Research, School of Public Health, University of Texas Health Science Center at Houston, Houston, Texas

Donald Kenkel, PhD, Department of Policy Analysis and Management, Cornell University, Ithaca, New York

Roger Meyer, MD, Association of American Medical Colleges, Washington, DC

Ted R. Miller, PhD, Pacific Institute for Research and Evaluation, Calverton, Maryland

Robert A. Zucker, PhD, Addiction Research Center, University of Michigan, Ann Arbor, Michigan

Acknowledgments

This unique book is the outgrowth of the work of a transdisciplinary team of clinical, developmental, physiological, and prevention psychologists, sociologists, economists, physicians, and public health researchers who came together to articulate what we know and where we need to go to improve the well-being of adolescents. Four scientists (Biglan, Brennan, Foster, and Holder) were Fellows at the Center for Advanced Study in the Behavioral Sciences (CASBS) for the 2000–2001 academic year. During the year, other scientists visited the Center to work with us for periods ranging from a few days to several weeks. Many helped write the book. Several who were not coauthors were nonetheless important in shaping our thinking and encouraging our efforts. We thank Steven Hayes, Shepard Kellam, and Roger Meyer. Herb Walberg was particularly helpful in shaping the general thrust of the project and organizing the products that would result, although other commitments kept him from participating as an on-site member of the project.

Our group opted to focus on four important problems that typically appear during the adolescent years—drug and alcohol misuse, smoking, serious antisocial behavior, and risky sexual behavior—and, in particular, on adolescents who display more than one of these problems. Besides reviewing what is known about the overlap, economic costs, development, prevention, and reduction of these problem behaviors in adolescence, we wanted to articulate what is needed to translate existing knowledge into widespread benefit. To do this, a small group of us wrote a draft of our thoughts about this topic and asked numerous people working on "science to practice" issues to join us for a 2-day brainstorming meeting. The following people participated in this meeting: Lynda Anderson, Judith Auerbach, Cathy Backinger, Virginia Cain, Richard F. Catalano Jr., Lucy Davidson, Dennis Embry, Brian Flay, Cornelius Hogan, Jan Howard, Carol Metzler, Patricia Mrazek, David Racine, Liz Robertson, Sonja Schoenwald, and Richard Spoth. Pat Mrazek and Carol Metzler masterfully facilitated the meeting. Others gave input, but did not attend: James Caccamo, Stephen Fawcett, David MacKinnon, David Olds, Dennis Prager, Heather Ringeisen, Mark Rosenberg, and Alex Wagenaar.

This book grew out of that project. Jaylan Turkkan, at the time at the National Institute on Drug Abuse (NIDA), conceived of the project. She believed that research on adolescent drug abuse and related problems had reached a point where a synthesis of existing knowledge and clarification of next steps for research and practice was in order. She secured partial funding for the project from NIDA and approached other funding agencies for support. The National Cancer Institute (NCI), the Offices of Behavioral and Social Science Research and of AIDS Research at National Institutes of Health (NIH), and the Robert Wood Johnson Foundation all agreed that the project had merit. After the effort began, the National Institute on Alcohol Abuse and Alcoholism (NIAAA) also provided funding. The funds were collected and routed to the Center via the National Science Foundation.

The planning and implementation of the project involved many. We thank Dr. Turkkan for her guidance in developing the team of people who worked on it. Robert Croyle and Cathy Backinger of NCI also provided guidance and support. Virginia Cain of the Office of Behavioral and Social Science Research at NIH provided input as well. Nancy Kaufman and Karen Gerlach at the Robert Wood Johnson Foundation all provided input at critical junctures. Judith Auerbach's guidance and encouragement was, at points, pivotal to our developing a viable plan for the project. We are also indebted to Jan Howard at NIAAA for her enthusiasm and straightforward feedback throughout the project. Although these individuals held the purse strings and went out of their way to be available to provide feedback and ideas, they gave us the flexibility to determine our own focus, directions, and projects.

Anna Katz was our assistant during our year at the Center. With patience, diligence, and enthusiasm, she researched topics, organized literature, created reference lists, corresponded with collaborators, arranged travel and meetings, and supported our team. We thank her profusely. We also thank Colette Lord, who helped with some of the literature searches and references. Kitty Moore at The Guilford Press provided valuable editorial suggestions to make the book more accessible.

CASBS provided a unique setting for our work. The Center staff provided considerable assistance throughout the year, and we thank them all. Lynn Gale helped in particular with the analysis of several data sets and provided important guidance about statistical procedures. She had a keen appreciation of what we were trying to accomplish and we greatly appreciated her moral support. Kathleen Much provided helpful input on editing and preparation of the manuscript.

The Director of the Center, Neil Smelser, and Associate Director Robert Scott exemplified the strongest traditions of academic institutions. At critical points, they made clear their support for what we were doing. We were touched by their solicitousness and appreciated their guidance. The Society for Prevention Research took over the project after the year at the Center ended, and we are particularly grateful to Jennifer Lewis, Denise Hallfors, and Ted Langevin for making this transition both possible and smooth.

The first author of this book left Palo Alto with a completed draft of the manuscript. The final version could not have been finished without the effort and enthusiasm of Christine Cody at the Oregon Research Institute. For months, she edited and refined the text; communicated with the coauthors; and clarified, supported, encouraged, and prompted all of us to do the things needed to bring this book to fruition. She did this with persistence, generosity of time and spirit, and good humor. Without her effort, this book might be languishing in a file drawer. We are deeply indebted to her.

Contents

1   Youth with Multiple Problems   1

Adolescent Problem Behaviors   2
A Public Health and Life Course Developmental
     Perspective   13

2   The Extent and Consequences of Multiple Problems   21

The Co-Occurrence of Problem Behaviors   22
Serious and Diverse Consequences of Multiple
     Problem Behavior   27
Implications for Prevention and Intervention   30

3   The Social Costs of Adolescent Problem Behavior   31
Ted R. Miller

Cost Concepts   33
Costing Methods by Problem Behaviors   38
Costs Imposed by Multiproblem Youth   44
Summary and Conclusions   55

4   Influences on the Development of Multiple Problems   57

A Life Course Developmental Perspective   60
Risk Factors throughout Development   63
Prenatal and Perinatal Development   63
Infancy and Early Childhood   69
Middle Childhood   74
Adolescence   80
Studies of Multiple Problems among Youth   89
Implications for Prevention and Intervention   92

5   Prevention of Adolescent Problems through Interventions   96
    in the Preteen Years
    Criteria for Identifying Effective Interventions   98
    Interventions for Prenatal, Perinatal, and Early
        Childhood Periods   104
    Interventions for School-Age Children   110
    Summary and Recommendations   121

6   Prevention Practices Targeting All Adolescents   127
    Family-Focused Interventions   128
    School Practices and Programs   132
    Media Campaigns   140
    Policies to Affect Adolescent Problem Behaviors   147
    The Value of Policy   168
    The Value of Federal Policies   169
    Summary and Recommendations   170

7   Interventions Targeting Adolescents   172
    with Behavior Problems
    Interventions for Delinquency and Antisocial Behavior   173
    Tobacco Use Cessation for Adolescents   201
    Summary and Recommendations   202

8   Comprehensive Community and Statewide Interventions   207
    Community Interventions   208
    Statewide Campaigns   215
    The Potential of Community Interventions   215

9   Integrating Science and Practice to Enhance   222
    the Well-Being of Children and Adolescents
    Developing Collaborative Partnerships
        with a Shared Vision   226
    Ongoing Assessment of Child and Adolescent Problems
        and Well-Being   231
    Empirically Supported Interventions across the Lifespan
        and across Multiple Levels of Influence   238
    The Innovating and Evaluating Society   247

    References   251

    Author Index   299

    Subject Index   309

HELPING ADOLESCENTS AT RISK

1

Youth with Multiple Problems

Sixteen-year-old Michael has just ended a stay in a juvenile detention center. Arrested twice—once for breaking and entering and once for an assault that followed a night of heavy drinking—Michael has problems other than his encounters with the legal system. He attends high school erratically and no doubt will soon drop out entirely. He smokes almost a pack of cigarettes a day and smokes marijuana frequently. Recently he has begun to experiment with harder drugs. Now, Michael has another surprise in store for him—his girlfriend is pregnant and she plans to tell him this as soon as she sees him after his release.

We have written this book for Michael and for the many other young people headed for deeply troubled lives. Research has helped us understand much about young people with multiple behavior problems and the cost of their actions to themselves and society. Research and clinical work have also helped us to identify numerous promising strategies to work with these multiproblem youth and to begin to reduce the number of teens who end up on a downward spiral. In this book, we lay out what we know about these young people. Our goal is to demonstrate actions that are more effective in order to alter the destructive path these children travel.

The existence of a small group of multiproblem youth has been clear, at least since Jessor and Jessor (1977) first described the phenomenon of deviance-prone youth. However, despite literally hundreds of studies showing that delinquency, substance use, and high-risk sexual behavior co-occur, the implications of this phenomenon for policy, practice, and research are not clear. They have been unclear because no one has brought all this information together and spelled out its significance

1

for research and practice. Prevention and treatment strategies typically focus only on a subset of problems. For example, we have programs to prevent academic failure, but we know little about whether these programs can prevent delinquency or drug abuse. In addition, we know that the family, schools, peers, and the community may (either positively or negatively) influence what happens to these teens. For example, with protective factors, such as a stable home life, involved parents, and teachers at school who never give up, even a teen beginning to get involved in problematic behavior can pull out of the downward spiral. Yet, when the child's father abandons the family, the mother works two jobs, and the child's acting out in school lands him or her in the principal's office more often than not, avenues narrow for the opportunity to resist the negative pull. We know that influences on the development of the multiproblem pattern begin while the child is still in the womb. Obviously, the time to intervene is when the potential for the developmental of problems is in its infancy. Despite our knowledge, we have not instituted widespread comprehensive, evidence-based approaches geared to deal with these problems before they lead to a cascade of increasingly destructive behavior patterns.

In Chapter 2, we document the extent to which multiproblem youth account for a large proportion of the occurrence of serious antisocial behavior, risky sexual behavior, drug and alcohol misuse, and tobacco use. In that chapter, we also show how multiple behavior problems lead to many problematic outcomes such as suicide and unwanted pregnancy. In Chapter 3, we show how to estimate the social costs attributable to the behavior of multiproblem youth. In Chapter 4, we identify the major factors that influence young people to develop these problems. Chapters 5–8 describe empirically evaluated interventions shown to reduce one or more of the problems that concern us. Chapter 5 focuses on interventions that target preadolescent influences on the development of multiple problem behaviors. It documents numerous strategies to follow for prevention of these problems and to promote successful adolescent development. Chapter 6 describes interventions designed to prevent problem behaviors among all adolescents. Chapters 7 and 8 describe interventions focused on helping adolescents who are already showing signs of problematic behavior. The final chapter examines issues involved in applying these scientific findings to help communities develop programs and policies to help not only youths in trouble but also those headed in that direction.

ADOLESCENT PROBLEM BEHAVIORS

We have chosen to focus on five adolescent problem behaviors: antisocial behavior (including aggressive social behavior and more serious acts such as stealing and assault), cigarette smoking, alcohol and drug misuse, and sexual behavior that risks pregnancy or disease. We chose these behaviors for several reasons. First, they represent the five most costly problems our society faces. Second, young people who engage in any one of these problem behaviors are highly likely to engage in the others. Third, many of the same biological and environmental factors influence the development of each these problems. Fourth, many of the prevention and treatment interventions previously developed have an impact on more than one of these problems. It is clear to us, therefore, that our society's efforts to lower the rates and costly consequences of each of these problems will benefit from comprehensive and coordinated strategies that simultaneously address the entire set of problems.

Most typical adolescents engage in some of these behaviors to some extent. For example, the majority of adolescents report committing some form of delinquent behavior at some point in their adolescence (Elliott, Huizinga, & Menard, 1989). Similarly, by the age of 17, 70–75% of adolescents drink alcohol, 25% have smoked marijuana, and 80% have engaged in sexual intercourse (Huizinga, Loeber, & Thornberry, 1993). Although we may argue about the desirability of these behaviors in any form, we would all have to concur that, at serious levels, these behaviors are deeply problematic for everyone concerned and can only lead to more difficulties. Therefore, we focus on types of behavior that most would agree are problematic because of the serious consequences they can and often do produce.

We call youth who engage in two or more of these behaviors "multiproblem youth." Because large numbers of youth begin to engage in these serious behavior problems only after they reach adolescence, our primary focus is on children between the ages of 11 and 18, although we look also at early precursors of these problems and the corresponding prevention strategies for use with younger children.

Serious Antisocial Behavior

Antisocial behavior consists of aggressive and criminal acts. The most serious forms of antisocial behavior are so-called index crimes, identified by the FBI as murder, aggravated assault, sexual assault, gang fights, car theft, theft of something worth more than $50, breaking and entering, or strong arming someone (Elliott et al., 1989). In addition, antisocial behavior is generally defined to include less severe delinquent offenses, such as buying stolen goods; carrying a hidden weapon; stealing something worth less than $5; prostitution; selling marijuana; hitting a teacher, parent, or student; disorderly conduct; selling hard drugs; joyriding; stealing something worth $5 to $50; and panhandling (Elliott et al., 1989). Some also distinguish violent from nonviolent crimes. Typically, they consider robbery, assault, rape/sexual assault, murder, and attempted murder as violent crimes. In this volume, we consider "serious antisocial behavior" to include index offenses as well as physical aggression perpetrated against other individuals.

Perhaps the most serious antisocial behavior is murder. Snyder and Sickmund (1999) estimate that juveniles committed 2,300 murders in 1997 in the United States, or 12% of all murders. The rate of murders committed by juveniles increased substantially between 1984 and 1993 but has declined since then to the same level as in 1986 (Snyder & Sickmund, 1999). Males account for most murders committed by adolescents and the recent decline in the murder rate resulted from changes in the rate among adolescent males. Juveniles are responsible for an even higher proportion of violent crimes besides homicide. Based on the National Crime Victimization Survey conducted by the Bureau of Justice, juveniles were involved in 14% of sexual assaults, 30% of robberies, and 27% of aggravated assaults in 1997. Similar to the pattern for murder, the rate of other serious violent crime increased from 1986 to 1993 but declined back to its 1986 level (Snyder & Sickmund, 1999). Nonetheless, juvenile involvement in violent crime is still an important and costly issue.

Cigarette Smoking

Cigarette smoking is the number one preventable cause of disease and death in the United States (U.S. Department of Health and Human Services [USDHHS], 2001). More than 400,000 Americans die each year of smoking-related illnesses (Centers for Disease Control and Prevention [CDC], 1989) and an additional 50,000 die from chronic exposure to secondhand smoke (CDC, 1989). This results in premature mortality that translates into 6 million years of life lost each year (Smoking-Related Deaths, 1993).

Adolescent smoking is a particularly important problem because most smokers begin smoking before the age of 18 (USDHHS, 1994). Estimates suggest that one-third of adolescents who begin smoking will eventually die of a smoking-related illness (Pierce, Gilpin, & Choi, 1999). Most of the problems associated with adolescent smoking appear later in life. However, some health consequences of smoking in adolescents are detectable, including increased respiratory infections and lessened lung capacity (USDHHS, 1994). Thus, preventing adolescent smoking is a high priority for public health (USDHHS, 2001).

Researchers have defined adolescent smoking in various ways, mostly in terms of self-reported smoking in the previous week or the previous month. Unlike occasional alcohol use, there appears to be no level of tobacco use that is advisable. Recent evidence, for example, shows that after even a couple of cigarettes, adolescents begin to exhibit some signs of addiction (DiFranza, 2000). However, most adolescents do not believe that tobacco is addictive until they are already addicted (Slovic, 2000). Figure 1.1 presents the monthly prevalence of smoking among 8th, 10th, and 12th graders from nationally representative samples of schools for the years 1991 to 2001. The data come from *Monitoring the Future,* a project that obtains data on adolescent problem behaviors from a nationally representative sample of high schools and middle schools (Johnston, O'Malley, & Bachman, 2000a, 2000b, 2000c; *Monitoring the Future,* 2003). The prevalence of youth smoking increased steadily from 1991 to 1996 in all grades and continued to increase for 12th-grade students in 1997. Further, despite much clamor about the problem, considerable activity designed to reduce youth smoking, and acknowledging that prevalence has shown a steady decline over the past 4 years, its prevalence was still higher in 2001 than it was in 1993 for 8th and 10th graders. On a positive note, there is a decrease shown in 12th graders in 2001 compared to the percentage shown for them in 1991 (Johnston, O'Malley, & Bachman, 2001).

Alcohol Misuse

Once considered a rite of passage, youthful high jinks, or "better than using drugs," underage drinking is now recognized as a serious public health problem. The National Household Survey on Drug Abuse, con-

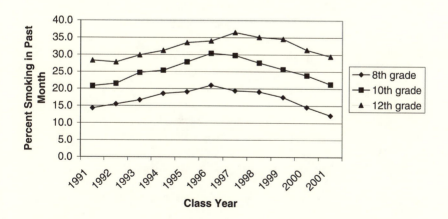

FIGURE 1.1. Trends in 30-day prevalence of tobacco use. Data from Johnston, O'Malley, and Bachman (2001) and *Monitoring the Future* (2003).

ducted by the USDHHS, is the only national household survey of drug
and alcohol use in the country and involves annual interviews of between 15,000 and 17,000 respondents (Substance Abuse and Mental
Health Services Administration [SAMHSA], 1998). Data from this survey indicate that 52% of 8th graders and 80% of 12th graders reported
having used alcohol at least once. By ninth grade, 25% of students reported having five or more drinks in a row in the previous month. Just
less than one-third of 8th graders and half of all 10th graders report being drunk at least once. Girls now consume alcohol at the same rate as
boys.

Binge drinkers are also responsible for a majority of the alcohol
consumed by young people. Recent analyses (Office of Juvenile Justice
and Delinquency Prevention [OJJDP], 2000) of data from the 1997 U.S.
National Household Survey on Drug Abuse (SAMHSA, 1998) show that
binge drinkers constituted 2.4% of 12- to 14-year-olds in that survey but
drank 82% of the alcohol consumed by that age group. They comprised
12.1% of 15- to 17-year-olds, but drank 88.5% of the alcohol consumed by this age group.

A large number of teenagers binge drink at least on occasion (see
Figure 1.2). In 2001, 29.7% of 12th graders, 24.9% of 10th graders,
and 13.2% of 8th graders reported consuming five or more drinks in a
row at least once in the 2 weeks before the survey. What is most alarm-
ing about these data is that the prevalence of binge drinking has varied
little within subsets over the past 10 years. The percentage of 10th grad-

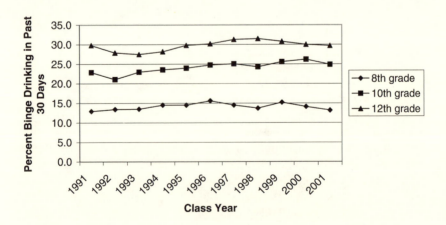

FIGURE 1.2. Trends in 30-day prevalence of binge drinking. Data from Johnston,
O'Malley, and Bachman (2001) and *Monitoring the Future* (2003).

ers having "been drunk" in the past month is the highest since 1991, when *Monitoring the Future* started including students in the 10th grade. The trends over the past 10 years demonstrate the frequent pattern of this high-risk drinking by grade level (Johnston, O'Malley, & Bachman, 2001; *http://monitoringthefuture.org/pubs/monographs/overview2000.pdf*).

Drug Dependence and Abuse

The terms "drug abuse" and "drug dependence" refer to patterns of drug use problematic for the user or for those around them (American Psychiatric Association, 1994). Abuse involves serious consequences of use, including one or more of the following: (1) failure to fulfill major role obligations; (2) absence, suspensions, or expulsions from school or work; (3) recurrent substance use in hazardous situations (e.g., while driving); (4) recurrent substance-related legal problems; (5) continued use despite persistent problems; or (6) conflict caused or exacerbated by use.

Dependence refers to an even more serious pattern in which a person uses a substance to the extent that it causes impairment or distress. At least three of the following can indicate dependence: (1) increased tolerance of the substance, requiring more to achieve the same effect; (2) withdrawal symptoms when not used; (3) greater or longer use than intended; (4) persistent desire for the substance; (5) much time spent seeking or using the substance; (6) reductions in social, recreational, or work activities; or (7) continuing substance use despite physical or psychological problems.

Not surprisingly, given these definitions, drug abuse is associated with crime and with numerous problems of physical health and psychological well-being (see Institute of Medicine [IOM], 1996, for a summary of the evidence). Among the health consequences associated with drug abuse are HIV/AIDS infections that result from injecting drug users sharing needles, unsafe sexual contacts with infected drug users, and mother-to-infant transmission of the virus. Experts now believe that injecting drugs is the number one risk factor for HIV infection (IOM, 1996). In addition, injection drug users have higher rates of viral and bacterial infections, including hepatitis, pneumonia, and endocarditis. Numerous psychiatric disorders co-occur with drug abuse. Drug abuse probably causes or heightens at least some of these disorders. Maternal drug use impairs fetal development. In addition, parents who abuse drugs are more likely to neglect or abuse their children.

We should distinguish drug dependence or abuse from drug use. Obviously one must begin use of a substance before dependence or abuse is established, but not all drug use leads to these problems. One of the problems with much of the research on adolescent drug taking is that the research simply examines the patterns of use without indicating the extent to which use is associated with dependence or abuse. As we shall see, young people who develop problematic use of drugs typically develop some of the other problems we are considering.

Given this caution, consider recent evidence on the prevalence of drug use among adolescents. Figure 1.3 presents data from *Monitoring the Future* on the percentage of students in 8th, 10th, and 12th grades reporting the use of marijuana in the past month. The data are for the years 1991–2001. Figure 1.4 presents data for the same years on the use of any other illicit drug during the prior month. Most school-based surveys do not provide in-depth information about the patterns of drug use; thus we do not know what proportion of the users of these drugs would meet the criteria for drug dependence or abuse.

Use of both marijuana and other illicit drugs increased from 1991 to 1996 across all three samples. However, in 1997, while prevalence of use leveled off or declined for 8th and 10th graders, the use of marijuana and hashish among 12th graders continued to climb until 1999. However, by 2001, prevalence rates for both marijuana and other illicit drugs had leveled off for all grade levels surveyed. Nonetheless, in 2001, more than 22% of 12th graders and nearly 20% of 10th graders reported marijuana use in the last month. Among 12th-grade students, 10.8% reported use of other illicit drugs. This was a 3.7% increase from 1991.

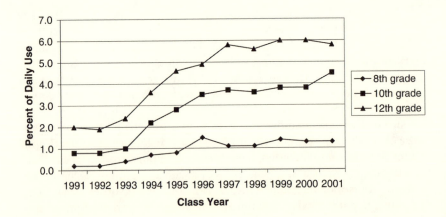

FIGURE 1.3. Trends in 30-day prevalence of marijuana/hashish use. Data from Johnston, O'Malley, and Bachman (2001) and *Monitoring the Future* (2003).

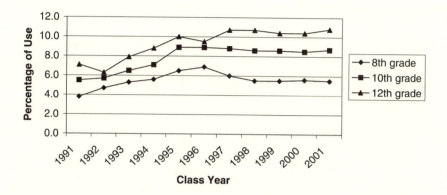

FIGURE 1.4. Trends in 30-day prevalence of illicit drug use (other than marijuana/hashish). Data from Johnston, O'Malley, and Bachman (2001) and *Monitoring the Future* (2003).

Risky Sexual Behavior

Sexual activity is a normal part of adolescent development, but it also carries risk. Sexual intercourse obviously can lead to unwanted pregnancy and the possibility of contracting a sexually transmitted disease, including AIDS. By "risky sexual behavior," we mean engaging in sexual intercourse without using birth control or condoms and having sex with multiple partners—practices that have been associated with increased risk of contracting AIDS or other sexually transmitted diseases, or unwanted pregnancy.

According to the Alan Guttmacher Institute (1999; *http://www.agi-usa.org/pubs/fb_teen_sex.html#tp*), each year in the United States about 10% of 15- to 19-year-old women become pregnant and 78% of those pregnancies are unplanned. During the 1990s, the teen pregnancy rate declined in the United States. However, it is still much higher than in any other developed country, twice as high as the pregnancy rate in England, and nine times higher than in Japan or the Netherlands.

Sexually transmitted diseases have long been a problem among adolescents. Each year, one in every four sexually experienced teens acquires a sexually transmitted disease (Alan Guttmacher Institute, 1999). Chlamydia and gonorrhea rates among adolescents are often higher than among adults. In some studies, researchers have found as many as 15% of sexually active adolescent women to have the human papillomavirus, some strains of which have a link to cervical cancer. The Guttmacher Institute also reports a higher hospitalization rate for acute pelvic inflammatory disease among adolescents than among older women. Typically caused by untreated gonorrhea or chlamydia, pelvic inflammatory disease can lead to infertility and ectopic pregnancy.

The risk of contracting AIDS has increased the dangers associated with sexual behavior. The CDC (1998) reports that, through 1997, there were 2,953 cases of AIDS reported among adolescents. Although that number is relatively small, HIV infection typically occurs long before the diagnosis of AIDS. Thus, the fact that there were 22,000 AIDS cases reported among 20- to 24-year-olds through 1997 is probably due in large measure to HIV infections occurring during adolescence. The rate of AIDS is disproportionately higher among Hispanic and African American adolescents than among Caucasian youth. HIV infections are particularly high among homeless youth, juvenile offenders, and high school dropouts (CDC, 2000a).

According to the most recent Youth Risk Behavior Survey (CDC, 2000b), about half of high school students have had intercourse. About 16% of them reported having had four or more sexual partners in their lifetime, a behavior that is associated with a higher risk of sexually transmitted disease. Fifty-eight percent of sexually active adolescents surveyed in 1999 indicated that they had used a condom at their last intercourse. Yet, 42% of young people were still engaging in unprotected sex. The use of birth control pills declined from 20.8% in 1991 to 16.2% in 1999. This may be due, in part, to the increased use of condoms. Nonetheless, these numbers imply that a substantial proportion of adolescents are at risk for pregnancy.

Racial, Ethnic, and Gender Differences in These Behaviors

Racial and ethnic groups and genders differ in their reported rates of most of these behaviors. For example, boys are more likely to commit violent crimes (Blum et al., 2000; OJJDP, 2000) and property crimes (OJJDP, 2000). Arrest rates for white male youth are lower than for black or Hispanic youth, but girls' arrest rates do not differ by ethnicity (Snyder & Sickmund, 1999). Despite this, black, Hispanic, and white males ages 12–16 reported similar rates of destroying property and carrying a handgun over the last 12 months, based on 1997 data from the National Longitudinal Survey of Youth (Center for Human Resource Research, 2001). That study also found that black males were slightly more likely to report committing assault (21%) than the Hispanic (13%) and white (15%) males (Snyder & Sickmund, 1999). However, Blum et al. (2000) found that both black and Hispanic youth were significantly more likely than white youth were to report weapon-related violence.

Differences exist also in substance use. White adolescents are significantly more likely to become cigarette smokers than are black,

Hispanic, or Asian adolescents (Blum et al., 2000; Pierce, Giovino, Hat-ziandreu, & Shopland, 1989). According to the latest *Monitoring the Future* data, white and Hispanic adolescents have higher levels of illicit drug use than do black youth (*http://monitoringthefuture.org/pubs/mono-graphs/overview2002.pdf;* Johnston, O'Malley, & Bachman, 2003).

Finally, youth risky sexual behaviors differ for males and females and for different ethnic groups. According to data from the Youth Risk Behavior Survey (CDC, 2000b), a higher proportion of males than females reported having had multiple partners in the last 3 months. More African American males reported multiple partners than did white or Hispanic males. Condom use was also highest among African Americans males and females. Table 1.1 provides a breakdown of these data.

What should we make of ethnic differences in the rates of these problems? Our answer is, "Not much." As Blum et al. (2000) have pointed out, the amount of variance accounted for by gender, race, and ethnicity is relatively small and a focus on these variables often tends to "negatively portray minorities . . . while only marginally advancing our understanding of the factors that contribute to the behaviors under study" (p. 1883). Differences due to these variables are small relative to other factors that distinguish young people engaging in problem behaviors from those who do not. It is easier to manipulate those other variables, including family, school, peer, and neighborhood factors. Thus, whether one is concerned with preventing crime among African American or white youth, one will need to be concerned about altering family, peer, school, and neighborhood influences.

Certainly, these data provide some guidance about where society might concentrate its resources in trying to prevent problems. For example, the higher rate of HIV/AIDS among African American youth (CDC,

TABLE 1.1. Adolescent High-Risk Sexual Behavior by Ethnicity and Gender

	White (%)		African American (%)		Hispanic (%)	
	Male	Female	Male	Female	Male	Female
Two or more partners last 3 months						
9th grade	10.0	5.8	25.3	13.2	11.2	2.3
12th grade	8.0	6.2	34.2	10.7	12.5	6.1
Used a condom at last intercourse						
9th grade	67.4	51.1	75.7	79.9	73.5	61.3
12th grade	54.8	45.1	70.7	60.9	60.8	34.9

Note. Data from Centers for Disease Control and Prevention (2000b).

2000a) points to the need for preventive programs targeting this population. However, it still seems a mistake to make too much of the differences. Even if white youth are more likely than black youth to take up smoking, we should target all youth with antismoking campaigns.

Finally, there is a legitimate fear that emphasis on racial or ethnic differences in the rates of these problems could contribute to stigmatizing particular minority groups.

With respect to gender differences, the differences in antisocial behavior are most noteworthy. Even at an early age, boys are more likely than girls are to exhibit aggressive behavior that may eventually develop into the various forms of antisocial behavior. Moreover, although no one has adequately studied it, we suspect that older antisocial boys influence much of the problem behavior of adolescent girls by encouraging them to get involved in drug use and risky sexual activity. This certainly justifies efforts to prevent the aggressive and antisocial behavior among boys. Yet, even if fewer girls manifest antisocial behavior, its consequences are no less serious. Thus, it seems important to ensure that these behaviors be prevented among all young people, but we need to be alert to differences in the factors that lead to problem behavior development.

What Are the Costs to Society?

Undoubtedly, the costs to society are enormous (see Chapter 3). Cost estimates of youthful violence and related property crime in the United States were at $165 billion in 1998. The estimate for binge drinking is $29 billion, for cocaine and heroin abuse $21.7 billion. High-risk sexual behavior cost $48 billion, mostly for quality of life lost. The cost of youth smoking during 1998 was a relatively low $79 million. However, the lifetime cost of smoking for those ages 12 to 20 in 1998 is approximately $1.8 trillion. We offer a detailed analysis of how to measure costs to society in Chapter 3.

Clearly, even modest improvements in our ability to prevent young people from engaging in these behaviors could have substantial benefits in reducing health care costs, property damage, lost productivity, and harm to the quality of life of these young people (and others whom they harm).

Why Focus on These Problems?

We do not focus on depression, suicide, or anxiety disorders—the so-called internalizing disorders—in this volume except if they occur with two or more of the problems we discuss. These problems are not as highly clustered with antisocial behavior, substance use, and sexual behavior as the latter behaviors are with each other. For example, Loeber, Stouthamer-Loeber, and White (1999) found in their study of Pittsburgh boys that persistent internalizing problems were unrelated to persistent substance use, except when persistent delinquency was also present. Moreover, risk factors for depression, suicide, and anxiety often differ from those for the focal problems of this book. Adequately dealing with them would require a much larger volume.

Nonetheless, these internalizing problems overlap to some extent with the ones on which we focus here. For example, Fergusson, Horwood, and Lynskey (1994b) reported that adolescents with conduct problems, early sexual activity, and marijuana use were significantly more likely than young people without these problems to report problems with mood, suicide ideation, and low self-esteem. White (1992) concluded that, although psychological problems such as depression do not consistently cluster with other problem behaviors, they do predict future drug use. This implies that some adolescents may use drugs to cope with psychological problems. At the same time, Aseltine, Gore, and Colten (1998) reported that depression and substance use did not co-occur significantly in a representative sample of 900 9th-, 10th-, and 11th-grade students from three high schools in Boston.

These findings suggest that, although one is unlikely to address the bulk of anxiety, depression, and suicide problems by targeting youth who engage in serious antisocial behavior, substance misuse, and risky sexual activity, interventions targeting such multiproblem youth will sometimes need to address depression and related problems. In addition, strategies designed to prevent the development of the problems we do focus on may very well contribute to lowering the incidence of depression, suicide, and anxiety problems.

A PUBLIC HEALTH AND LIFE COURSE DEVELOPMENTAL PERSPECTIVE

A public health perspective recognizes the importance of preventing problems along the life course in order to influence the actual number of teens who develop and display multiple behavior problems. The essence of the public health perspective is its focus on affecting the incidence or prevalence of a problem in an entire population rather than affecting only individuals. The perspective differs from the one found in many systems dealing with youth development, where the focus is typically on whether an individual young person has been affected. Prevention scientists and public health-oriented practitioners emphasize the idea that helping individual young people has limited social impact if the total number with a particular problem remains the same. Our ultimate goal should be to reduce the total number of young people who engage in one or more problem behaviors. To do this, we must consider the entire populations of youth.

Focusing on multiproblem youth may not seem to be in keeping with this view, because it singles out a subgroup of young people. However, we advocate greater attention to multiproblem youth precisely because they contribute such a large proportion to our social problems. In fact, it may be that interventions that do not deal with this subgroup will have limited impact because they fail to affect the young people most likely to engage in multiple and more serious levels of problem behaviors.

Life Course Development

We organize information about multiproblem youth according to a life course developmental perspective (Baltes, Reese, & Lipsitt, 1980). According to this model, normative age-related changes, historical and cultural circumstances, and unique life events influence a child's development. Important genetic and biological conditions interact with these environmental and social experiences to influence the way a child develops. Thus, the child's biological systems mature as the child simultaneously develops skills and behavioral propensities over time, and these processes are interdependent. For example, in adolescence, many changes conspire to affect the adolescent's choices about educational goals or potential careers. Hormones, personality traits, peer pressure, school success, parental expectations, and social demands all influence their decision making. We can think of the life course of this development as a "trajectory" or path. As young people develop, they may or may not move toward an increasing number of problem behaviors, depending on the unfolding interplay between the characteristics they bring to current situations and the nature of those situations.

These developmental changes occur in the context of economic and cultural conditions that also proscribe or constrain behavior: Teens experience adolescence during a recession in a different manner from teens that reach adolescence during an economic boom. A child whose father dies during adolescence will likely have a different high school experience than one whose father suddenly makes it big. What can seem like a small shift in the adolescent's world can substantially alter that child's developmental course.

Michael, the teen we introduced at the beginning of this chapter, was only 8 when he began to be engaged in high rates of aggressive and disruptive behavior. Shunned by his peer group, he started spending more time with kids like himself, prone to deviant behavior. When his parents were unable to provide consistent consequences to help control his aggressive behavior, and teachers threw up their hands, he ended up seeking out acceptance from kids like himself. As a result, he became involved in delinquent acts, smoking, alcohol, and other drug use.

To start even younger, evidence suggests that delivery complications during birth are associated with the development of violent behaviors when those infants reach adolescence, but only in cases in which mothers express rejection of the infant (Raine, Brennan, & Mednick, 1994). Presumably, birth complications in some way affect the functioning of infants, and when they are born into a family in which they are not wanted, their family may not be able to cope with their behavior. This interaction between the characteristics of children and their environment sets them on a path toward delinquency. Although we do not yet know the precise mechanism that leads to these developments, the implications of this research are clear: Helping families of babies with birth complications to provide effective environments for their children may help to prevent delinquency. Interventions to prevent birth complications from occurring in the first place could potentially accomplish the same end.

These examples suggest that if we want to understand the development of multiproblem behavior—or of nonproblematic behavior—we need to consider how the characteristics of the child or adolescent at any point in time interact with the ways that the environment influences subsequent development. Furthermore, understanding these influences leads to possible strategies for preventing serious problems from occurring.

If our concern is with preventing multiproblem behavior among teens, do we need to consider their entire lifespan from the prenatal period through adolescence? The answer is emphatically, "Yes." We can identify—at every point in the lifespan—both individual characteristics and aspects of the environment that predict the later development of one or more problems. Each points to an opportunity to promote successful development and prevent the development of problems.

Table 1.2 presents a schematic of this framework, organized by phases of development and factors that influence those phases. Biopsychosocial characteristics involve attributes a child brings to the environment based on biological and behavioral predispositions established genetically and in earlier development. The environment consists of "social fields" (Kellam, Ling, Merisca, Brown, & Ialongo, 1998; Kellam & Van Horn, 1997), which are the primary social environments with which the developing child interacts. The obvious and most frequently studied environmental influences on child and adolescent development involve the family, peers, and school. As we show in Chapter 4, the individual characteristics of the child, as well as multiple facets of the envi-

TABLE 1.2. Sources of Influence and Life Course Development

				Phases of development			
Influences	Prenatal	Perinatal	Infancy	Early childhood	Middle childhood	Early adolescence	Adolescence
Child[a]	×	×	×	×	×	×	×
Family	×	×	×	×	×	×	×
Peer				×	×	×	×
School				×	×	×	×
Media				×	×	×	×
Neighborhood				×	×	×	×
Community				×	×	×	×

[a]The biopsychosocial characteristics of the child.

ronment, influence development throughout childhood and adolescence. Certain well-established individual characteristics, family conditions, peer processes, and school practices make problem behavior particularly likely to develop. Others promote the development of skills, orientations, and social involvements that make problems less likely. Communities that ensure nurturing families and schools and that promote positive peer group formation will prevent many adolescent problems.

Other aspects of the environment, such as neighborhood and community characteristics, are also important for youth development. These directly influence youth and play a role in family, schools, and peer groups. A range of policies influence tobacco use and the use of alcohol and the problems associated with their use. For example, laws making alcohol and tobacco less accessible to youth can prevent their use (Forster, Wolfson, Murray, Wagenaar, & Claxton, 1997; Holder, 1998; Holder & Blose, 1987).

The ×'s in the table depict our estimates of the phases in which each influence comes into play to affect the developing young person directly. However, the table does not depict the influences of these fields on each other. Throughout development, the child's individual characteristics both react to and influence interactions with family members, teachers, and peers. Neighborhood and community conditions influence the family. Schools and families influence peer groups. Neighborhood and community conditions influence the practices of schools.

In addition to what their social sphere produces, children bring their own array of genetic predispositions; biological characteristics; and cognitive, behavioral, and affective capacities. Children with low impulse control and an auditory learning disability will have a tougher time sitting in their seat in school and are less likely to learn to read at a developmentally appropriate time. These individual characteristics influence how the child reacts to the environment. These environmental influences in turn shape the continuing development of the child's biological and behavioral responses.

How does a social field or environment affect a child's behavior? There are a few fundamental principles. Chief among them is the principle that *consequences* influence behavior (Biglan, 2003a). An obvious example is, when children receive positive reinforcement for good behavior, they will more likely do the expected next time around. In the economic arena, the cost of goods obviously influences buying patterns (e.g., Landsburg, 1993). At every stage of development, in every social field, the consequences of both prosocial and problematic behavior influence children's development. Michael, for example, learned early in life that hitting and swearing got his parents to give in to his requests. Others learn to get their own way by asking in a more appropriate and respectful manner. Indeed, the relative costs and benefits of problematic and nonproblematic behavior are pivotal in making it more or less frequent, although individual characteristics may make some children more responsive than others to particular types or patterns of consequences.

A second obvious influence involves *stressful life events*. These can be one stressful event—such as a death in the family—or ongoing stressors—such as crowded neighborhoods with high crime rates and ineffective police and school systems. Teachers or parents who scream at children in frustration, parents who quarrel openly and without resolution in front of their children, and peers who taunt others create stressors in a child's life. Stressors have direct and negative effects on physiological and psychological functioning as well as on behavior. Environmental stressors influence the level of hormones released in the body, which in turn influences both the structure and function of particular brain areas (Anisman & Merali, 1999). Communities that wish to ensure young people's successful development must minimize stressful events for young people and those around them.

The environment also creates opportunities for and places limits on young people's behavior. For example, ready availability of substances creates opportunities for their use. Settings in which early adolescents are unsupervised present opportunities for them to experiment with a full range of behaviors such as vandalism, precocious sexual behavior, and substance use (Richardson, Radziszewska, Dent, & Flay, 1993). Settings that limit opportunities, such as supervised recreation programs, make such experimentation less likely.

Behavior can be neither discouraged nor promoted if others are not aware of it. How adolescents are monitored and watched by parents, schools, and communities will affect how often problem behaviors are noted. Parents who know where their kids are, are aware of what they are doing, and interact with them regularly are in a much better position to reinforce desirable behavior and to prevent or penalize risky behavior. Schools must set up systems to detect problem behavior, but they must also have systems for recognizing desirable behavior. Communities that have systems for detecting such problems as drunken driving can significantly reduce fatal car crashes (Holder et al., 2000).

The process of *persuasion* is also important, especially the way in which media influence behavior. In general terms, young people come to view objects and activities more or less favorably, depending on the contexts in which they view those activities. For example, when cigarette smoking appears in a context of exciting and desirable activities, it will appear more favorably (USDHHS, 1994). We can examine the extent to which young people's environments persuade them to view problem behavior favorably. Examining the media to which they are exposed is especially important.

Group norms influence behavior. Norms refer to the extent to which a behavior occurs in a group and the extent to which others are likely to approve it. Young people are more likely to engage in a behavior to the extent that they perceive that others engage in the behavior or would approve of their engaging in it. Peer-group norms are especially influential for problem behavior, but families, schools, neighborhoods, and communities have normative influences.

Finally, young people's social environments can cultivate social, verbal, cognitive, artistic, and athletic skills through *skill training*. In many educational situations (e.g., when a child is learning to read, do simple arithmetic, or play a new sport), the skill training is obvious. Skill training can occur with social behavior as well. For example, a child learns new skills when his parent teaches him how to handle a problem with his older brother. A parent can learn from a therapist who teaches her how to how to discipline without hitting. Skill training is a complex process that usually includes modeling behavior, instruction, opportunities for the child to practice the new skill, and reinforcement of gradual improvements in skills and performance. In building communities in which most children develop successfully, it is essential to examine whether their everyday environments are organized to teach them desirable skills and minimize opportunities for them to learn problematic behaviors.

To understand how children develop and how to intervene to prevent problems, we must look at all these mechanisms and how they operate within families, schools, peer groups, neighborhoods, and communities to shape the biological and social characteristics that children carry forward into adolescence. As Chapter 4 describes in detail, consequences, stressors, opportunities and limits for behavior, monitoring, skill building, persuasion, and group norms all contribute to the development of problem behavior. This information defines points of intervention helpful for changing the life course of children such as Michael.

A Focus on Communities

The community is a natural focus for efforts to reduce the prevalence of youth problem behaviors. Local communities generally organize schools, family services, police practices, juvenile justice, media, and business (Biglan, 1995). These communities could also effectively implement efforts to change any of the proximal influences on problem behaviors and can most effectively mount comprehensive interventions at that level. Interventions that include media and community organizing or that combine school, family, and peer-group interventions are difficult or impossible to evaluate in smaller units. Communities are also the natural unit for assessing population-based outcomes. By focusing on community-level measures of the prevalence of drug use and abuse, we have the opportunity to move to the ultimate goal of public health research, namely, to affect entire populations.

Experimental Evaluation

In this book, we rely heavily on experimental evidence of the effects of programs and policies. We have reached a point in the development of the behavioral sciences when it is reasonable to demand experimental evidence of the efficacy of practices that claim to be of value. Practitioners have experimentally evaluated numerous policies and programs, and the resources and technical knowledge to conduct experimental evaluations are increasingly available. For the most part, we restrict our attention to programs and policies previously experimentally evaluated. As will be seen, there is still plenty to discuss.

Critics will argue that requiring experimental evidence of the effects of a preventive or treatment intervention may cause us to overlook valuable programs. There are undoubtedly valuable programs not yet evaluated but which are making a difference in the lives of young people. The problem, however, is that we do not know which ones they are.

We are not suggesting that a community interested in improving outcomes for its young people could not make progress by adopting some practices not experimentally evaluated. We simply suggest that a community would be on firmer ground by starting with the implementation of programs and policies already shown by experimental evaluation to be of value in some other setting. There is no guarantee that they will work, but they are a better bet than unevaluated practices.

Prevention and Treatment

Societies expend the bulk of their resources for dealing with common problems of human behavior on treatment of the problems rather than on their prevention (Mrazek & Hagerty, 1994). In most cases, it would probably be more cost-effective and humane to organize societies so that problems never occur, rather than to wait until they do and attempt to ameliorate them. However, given the current state of our knowledge, we take the view that both treatment and prevention practices should be included in any organized effort to address the problem of multiproblem youth. Research in recent years has identified both treatment and prevention practices that can affect these problems. It is unlikely that even the best prevention program will prevent every instance of a problem. Why would we want to forego the opportunity to ameliorate the problems that do develop, if efficacious interventions are available?

Moreover, the prevention–treatment distinction is, to an extent, a false dichotomy. Many of the most effective preventive practices are themselves "treatment" procedures. For example, nurse home visitation helps poor, young mothers to improve their health habits and parenting practices and thereby prevents adolescent problems such as delinquency (Olds, Henderson, Cole, et al., 1998). It both treats and prevents. Virtually any treatment program targeting children has the potential to prevent the development of problems in adolescence because problems in childhood make so many adolescent problems more likely.

As will be shown in Chapters 5–8, the few available cost-effectiveness analyses suggest that preventive interventions can save considerable public and private money. At the same time, even our best approaches cannot reach and affect every child. Some children will develop serious problems despite our best efforts, and approaches must be in place to reduce these problems after they develop. Thus, we must adopt the best preventive and intervention approaches if we wish to have an impact on not only the prevalence of problems currently but also the emergence of problems in the future.

2

The Extent and Consequences
of Multiple Problems

When Michael is 19, the authorities arrest him for driving while intoxicated. This is his third arrest in 6 months and the judge finally sends him to jail. In jail, he goes through an involuntary detoxification and develops seizures that require medical attention. His doctor notices the tracks on his arms and gives him a warning about HIV risk. Although the jail staff offers counseling to Michael for his drug abuse, he refuses. When he gets out of jail, he gets drunk, goes to his girlfriend's house (the mother of his child), gets into an argument with her, and beats her up.

Michael is heading toward a multitude of troubles in life. Each of his problem behaviors makes it harder to move away from the other problem behaviors. His aggressive tendencies get him into conflict with people who could nurture and guide him—if he did not get angry with them so often. His use of alcohol and other drugs increases his aggressive tendencies and undermines his occasional attempts to get his life in order. In addition, his aggressiveness, drug abuse, and sexual risk taking lead to numerous other difficulties.

In this chapter, we show how common and pernicious patterns of multiple problem behaviors are among young people. The tendency for problem behaviors to co-occur is one of the most common findings in studies of adolescent development, but the extent to which it occurs is still not appreciated sufficiently and the deleterious consequences of patterns of multiple problem behaviors have not been adequately documented.

THE CO-OCCURRENCE OF PROBLEM BEHAVIORS

Documentation of the co-occurrence of problem behaviors is volumi-
nous and growing. Numerous studies show that delinquent or antisocial
behavior correlates with drug use, cigarette smoking, and risky sexual
behavior. For example, antisocial individuals are more likely to use illicit
drugs other than marijuana (Elliot et al., 1989), to develop drug abuse
problems (Robins & McEvoy, 1990), and to sell drugs (Elliott et al.
1989). In addition, young people who display delinquent behavior are
more likely to have intercourse, less likely to use condoms (Metzler,
Noell, Biglan, Ary, & Smolkowski, 1994), and more likely to be involved in coercive sexual encounters (Biglan et al., 1990).

It has been repeatedly documented that young people who smoke
cigarettes are more likely to engage in antisocial behavior, use alcohol
and other drugs, and engage in risky sexual behavior. Willard and
Schoenborn (1995) provide a good example of the evidence in a study of
a large and nationally representative sample of individuals ages 12–21
years. They found that current cigarette smokers were substantially
more likely than nonsmokers to use alcohol heavily, use marijuana, carry
a weapon, be involved in a fight, or be sexually active.

National youth self-report surveys such as *Monitoring the Future*
reveal a strong relationship between binge drinking and illicit drug use
(Johnston et al., 2001). However, it is not only binge drinking that can
lead to serious problems for adolescents. The National Highway Traffic
Safety Administration (2001) reports that in 2000, 20% of those under
15 killed in automobiles were in alcohol-related crashes. The percentage
of behavioral problems, suicide, homicide, depression, and health-
related problems was much higher among adolescents who drink alcohol
than among those who do not (Hanna, Hsiao-ye, & Dufour, 2000; National Center for Health Statistics, 1997; National Institute on Alcohol
Abuse and Alcoholism, 1996; SAMHSA, 1999; White, Hansell, & Brick,
1993, all cited in Leadership to Keep Children Alcohol Free, 2001).

Much research has linked crime and violence to drug abuse. Some
crime results from drug abusers stealing to support drug habits and some
stems from the violent nature of the drug distribution system. The Institute of Medicine report on drug abuse (1996) reviews evidence that
when drug abuse co-occurs with certain psychiatric disorders, the likelihood of violence rises substantially, especially for lower-socioeconomic-
status males. There is also substantial evidence that drug abuse and dependence co-occur with other diagnosable disorders, including conduct
and oppositional/defiant disorders, anxiety disorders, and depression
(Glantz, Weinberg, Miner, & Colliver, 1999; IOM, 1996).

We have previously documented the general finding that risky sexual behavior may lead to our other problems. An analysis completed with data from the National Longitudinal Study of Adolescent Health (Lindberg, Boggess, & Williams, 1999), a nationally representative sample of 12,105 adolescents in grades 7–12, also demonstrates the relationship between risky sexual behavior and multiple behavior problem status. In that analysis, the researchers defined risky sexual behavior as unprotected sex; 12% of the youth reported engaging in the behavior. Of these youth, 76% reported that they engaged in at least one other problem behavior.

Multiproblem Youth and the Seriousness and Duration of Problems

Youth who engage in multiple problems have more serious levels of each problem and are less likely to improve. Brown, Gleghorn, Schuckit, Myers, and Mott (1996) found that among young people admitted for treatment of drug abuse, those with conduct disorders had greater posttreatment use of alcohol. White and Labouvie (1994) found that adolescents who engage in higher levels of delinquent behavior have psychological problems that are more serious and that young people who are delinquent and using drugs have the highest levels of psychological problems. Stice, Myers, and Brown (1998) found that within a sample of adolescents who had been treated for substance abuse problems and had relatively low rates of substance use at treatment entry, those who also had delinquency problems were significantly more likely to have problem substance use 2 years later. Elliott et al. (1989) reported that the most serious offenders also have the highest rates of offense. Zhang, Wieczorek, and Welte (1997) found that the prevalence of violent behavior was especially high when adolescent males were both heavy drinkers and high in aggression and hostility. White, Loeber, Stouthamer-Loeber, and Farrington (1999) found the severity of drug use related to the frequency of violence.

The Robustness of These Relationships

Studies of nationally representative samples of youth have shown the interrelationships among our focal problem behaviors (e.g., Elliott et al., 1989; Osgood, Johnston, O'Malley, & Bachman, 1988). These interrelationships also occur in community samples (e.g., Fergusson, Horwood, & Lynskey, 1994b; Huizinga et al., 1993; Loeber, Farrington, Stouthamer-Loeber, & Van Kammen, 1998a; McGee & Newcomb, 1992) and in numerous samples of youthful offenders (Chaiken & Chaiken, 1990; Dembo et al., 1992). They have been shown using correlational and factor-analytic techniques (e.g., Ary et al., 1999; Donovan & Jessor, 1985; Donovan, Jessor, & Costa, 1988; Osgood et al., 1988) as well as with analyses of categorical data (e.g., Bergman & Magnusson, 1991).

Both longitudinal and cross-sectional studies have studied these relationships. For example, Duncan, Duncan, Biglan, and Ary (1998) examined relationships among the growth parameters for tobacco, alcohol, and marijuana use. Using latent growth modeling, they found that change in the use of these three substances over an 18-month period formed a higher-order substance use growth construct. Those who increased use of one substance were likely to increase use of the others and those who decreased use of one were likely to decrease use of the other two.

White et al. (1999) looked at longitudinal relationships between substance use and violence in a sample of 506 boys in Pittsburgh, Pennsylvania. In general, alcohol and marijuana use predicted later violence. In addition, earlier violence predicted later substance use. For boys who had used marijuana by age 13, the odds of violence between the ages of 14.5 and 18.5 were 5.4 times greater than they were for boys who had not used marijuana by age 13. This was true even when earlier aggressive behavior and other risk factors were controlled. Similarly, for boys who had used alcohol by age 13, the odds were 2.2 times greater than for those who had not drunk that they would engage in later violence—even when earlier violence and other risk factors were controlled. Among boys who were violent by 13, the odds were 2.4 times greater that they would use alcohol between the ages of 14.5 and 18.5 than they were for boys who were not violent.

Researchers have replicated these relationships across diverse ethnic groups, including the following:

- Mexican Americans and American Indians in Oregon communities (Barrera, Biglan, Ary, & Li, 2001).
- Urban American Indians (Howard, Walker, Walker, Cottler, & Compton, 1999).
- African Americans in urban areas (Barone et al., 1995; Ensminger, 1990; Fagan, Weis, & Cheng, 1990; Farrell, Danish, & Howard, 1992; Zimmerman & Maton, 1992).
- Urban black and Hispanic adolescents (Barone et al., 1995).

Problem interrelationships have occurred in countries other than the United States, including New Zealand (Fergusson, Horwood, & Lynskey, 1994b) and Holland (Ferdinand & Verhulst, 1994; Garnefski & Diekstra, 1997).

Although many studies have not included females, many have. These studies show that problem behaviors are interrelated among adolescent girls (Ary, Duncan, Biglan, et al., 1999; Ary, Duncan, Duncan, & Hops, 1999; Barone et al., 1995; Biglan et al., 1990; Donovan & Jessor, 1985; Donovan et al., 1988; Ellickson, Saner, & McGuigan, 1997; Ensminger, 1990; Farrell et al., 1992; Fergusson, Horwood, & Lynskey, 1994b; Lindberg et al., 1999; Tildsley, Hops, Ary, & Andrews, 1995). Yet, there are some differences in the relationships according to gender. Fergusson, Horwood, & Lynskey (1994b) found that more girls fell into a cluster involving sexual activity and marijuana use and more boys fell into a cluster involving conduct disorder, police contacts, and marijuana use. Lindberg et al. (1999) found that 31% of boys were involved in two or more risk behaviors, but only 26% of girls were. White (1992) found that for girls, delinquency and violence loaded less strongly on a problem behavior factor than they did for boys. White, Brick, and Hansell (1993) found that although prevalence rates for alcohol use were similar for male and female adolescents, rates of aggression and alcohol-related aggression were lower for females.

There is some evidence that these relationships may not be as robust among early adolescents as among older adolescents (Gillmore et al., 1991). However, the general pattern of co-occurrence of antisocial behavior with other problem behaviors is evident in samples from 1st grade (e.g., Loeber et al., 1998b) to 12th grade (Osgood et al., 1988). McGee and Newcomb (1992) found problem behaviors intercorrelated for both early and later adolescents. The factor was composed of substance use, social conformity, and academic orientation factors for early adolescents; it also included factors for sexual involvement and criminal behavior for later adolescents. Willard and Schoenborn (1995) reported that the relationships between smoking and other problem behaviors were "stronger at younger ages, but remained consistent, though somewhat attenuated, among youth 18–21 years of age" (Willard & Schoenborn, 1995, p. 2).

White has argued that the relationship between drug use and delinquency is "spurious," in the sense that one behavior does not automatically lead to another. Rather, the interrelationships stem from the fact that they share some common influences (White & Hansell, 1998; White & Labouvie, 1994). Indeed, as we see in Chapter 3, many etiological factors influence the development of two or more of these youth problem behaviors. However, whatever the underlying reasons for these relationships, the fact remains that young people who engage in one of these problems are also more likely to engage in the others. From a public health perspective, the important question is whether there is a subgroup of young people who manifest multiple high-risk behaviors and whether targeting this group could bring about substantial reductions in a variety of social and health problems.

Comparison and Analysis of National Survey Studies

We completed our own analysis of data from four national surveys of youth to assess what proportion of children who display one problem behavior also display one or more other types of problem behavior. The four surveys that we used in this analysis included the 1999 National Household Survey on Drug Abuse (USDHHS, 2000a), the 1999 Youth Risk Behavior Survey (YRBS; CDC, 2000b), the 1999 *Monitoring the Future* survey (Johnston et al., 2001), and the 1996 Health Behaviors of School Children Survey (World Health Organization, 2001). The percentages presented in Table 2.1 were weighted averages from these surveys.

It is noteworthy that our definitions of problem behavior differed somewhat across surveys as not all the surveys contained the same items. Violence reflected involvement in frequent or serious fights and/or weapon carrying. Smoking reflected self-reports of smoking three or more cigarettes in the past month. We define binge drinking as drinking five or more alcoholic beverages on one occasion in the last month. Illicit drug use includes use of marijuana, cocaine, or inhalants during the last 30 days and/or methamphetamine or heroin use during the lifetime. We define high-risk sex as youth having sexual intercourse without protection (YRBS data served as the source of information on this particular problem behavior).

Table 2.1 shows the proportion of young people who have any given problem who have at least one other problem. For example, the first column and first row show that nearly 99% of 12-year-olds who report smoking also report at least one other problem. In general, Table

TABLE 2.1. Percentage of Youth with a Given Problem Who Have at Least One Other Problem

Age (years)	Smoking	Binge drinking	Illicit drug use	Violence	High-risk sex
12	98.9	95.3	93.2	25.1	
13	87.1	91.8	84.8	31.6	
14	86.0	88.9	88.7	50.8	75.7
15	89.5	89.1	87.7	62.0	74.7
16	86.2	84.9	90.0	71.1	78.6
17	87.9	88.3	90.9	77.9	69.3
18	85.3	88.3	88.9	87.3	77.5
19	89.1	86.0	94.5	86.8	77.5
Average	87.6	87.5	90.3	62.7	74.9

Note. Data from 1999 National Household Survey on Drug Abuse (USDHHS, 2000a), 1999 Youth Risk Behavior survey (CDC, 2000b), 1999 *Monitoring the Future* survey (Johnston et al., 2001), and 1996 Health Behaviors of School Children Survey (World Health Organization, 2001). The percentages presented were weighted averages from these surveys.

2.1 shows that a young person engaging in one problem behavior is highly likely to engage in at least one other. This suggests that at least some of our strategies for reducing the prevalence of adolescent problems will need to recognize the high likelihood that one or more other problems will accompany any given problem.

Our data are also consistent with previous research examining the co-occurrence of behavior problems by age. Specifically, the overall finding of high co-occurrence is robust across ages, with a higher overlap between antisocial behavior and other problem behaviors at older ages, and a higher overlap between smoking and other problem behaviors at younger ages.

SERIOUS AND DIVERSE CONSEQUENCES OF MULTIPLE PROBLEM BEHAVIOR

Although the relationships among our focal behavior problems (antisocial behavior, alcohol and drug misuse, cigarette smoking, and risky sexual behavior) are well established, less attention has been paid to how much the behavior of multiproblem youth accounts for a host of other negative social and health outcomes. The policy question is what portion or percentage of a variety of negative outcomes can we attribute to multiproblem youth.

We explored this policy question in detail with data from the 1998 National Household Survey of Drug Abuse (NHSDA; USDHHS, 2000a, 2000b).[1] The primary purpose of this self-report survey is to obtain prevalence rates of drug and alcohol use in households across the United States. The NHSDA employs a stratified sampling method. The 1998 survey was the 18th such survey completed since 1971. For the purposes of our analyses on multiple problems of youth, we used weighted estimates (corrected for sampling and missing data) for individuals ages 12–20 years. We defined multiple problem youth as those youth who evidenced two or more of our focal behavior problems, operationalized as follows:

- *Serious antisocial behavior:* Involved in a serious/gang fight in the past year, physically attacked someone in the past year, carried a handgun in the past year, arrested for one or more violent offenses in the past year.

---

[1]For further methodological details concerning this survey, see the report by the Office of Applied Studies, SAMHSA (USDHHS, 1994).

- *Smoking:* Three or more cigarettes smoked in past 30 days.
- *Alcohol misuse:* Binge drinking in past 30 days.
- *Drug misuse:* Any use of any illicit drug in past 30 days and/or illicit drug dependence in the past year.
- *Risky sexual behavior:* Currently pregnant and/or arrested and booked for prostitution in the past year (this definition was limited by available NHSDA data).

Figure 2.1 presents the relationship between multiple problem status and harmful outcomes for youth in the NHSDA data set. We present data for youth (ages 12–20) who reported no problem behaviors, only one problem behavior, or more than one. The top, black bar in each set shows the proportion of the subgroup in the population. The lower bars represent the percent of all the harmful outcomes in each category (e.g., drunk driving) attributed to each "problem group." These harmful outcomes included:

- *Drunk driving:* Driving under the influence of alcohol in the past 12 months.
- *Violent arrest:* Times arrested and booked for assault, robbery, or murder in past 12 months.

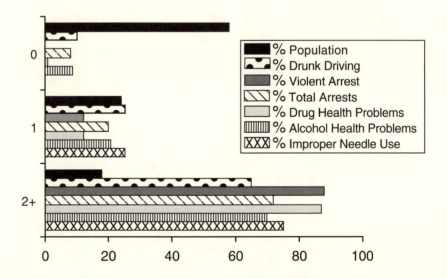

FIGURE 2.1. Proportion of youth with zero, one, or two problems and the proportion of other problems they account for. Data from 1994 National Household Survey on Drug Abuse (Office of Applied Studies, 1995).

- *Total arrest:* Total number of arrests in the past 12 months.
- *Drug health problems:* Health-related problems due to illicit drug use.
- *Alcohol health problems:* Health-related problems due to alcohol use.
- *Improper needle use:* Sharing or not properly cleaning needles used to inject drugs.

As can be seen in Figure 2.1, multiple problem youth are responsible for a much greater proportion of harmful outcomes than the other youth in the sample, especially relative to the small percentage of the total population that they represent. Although they are less than 20% of the population, they account for 75% of all improper needle use, 70% of health problems associated with alcohol, 87% of health problems associated with drug abuse, 72% of total arrests, and 88% of arrests associated with violence.

We examined the relationship between multiple problem status and negative health and social outcomes separately for males and females in the NHSDA sample. The results are highly consistent across genders. We also examined the data separately for black, white, and Hispanic respondents and found highly similar results across ethnicity. Finally, we examined the results for children ages 12–17 only, as many youth interventions target this age. The importance of the multiple problem youth group in terms of contribution to negative social and health outcomes is particularly apparent for these ages of youth.

Given that we tie our risky sexual behavior definition heavily to pregnancy, we also examined the relationship between multiple problem status and pregnancies in the NHSDA sample. This seemed particularly relevant to the children ages 12–17 years in the sample. Pregnancy at or after age 18 is not necessarily a negative social outcome; however, teenage pregnancy is widely considered problematic in our society. The analysis of percentage of pregnancies accounted for by the multiple problem group reveals that this group (12% of the youth population) accounts for 58% of the teenage pregnancies in this sample.

Our analysis of multiple problem youth suggests that incremental increases in problem behaviors produce disproportionate increases in negative social and health outcomes. These results support the argument that multiple problem youth may be a particularly important group to target in prevention and treatment programs. In Chapter 3, we present data on specifically how costly these youth are to our society. In Chapter 4, we examine the factors that influence the development of multiple problems of youth.

IMPLICATIONS FOR PREVENTION AND INTERVENTION

Despite the wealth of evidence, no one has fully delineated the implications of the multiproblem behavior phenomenon for the development of effective prevention strategies. We believe that the empirical evidence warrants the following conclusions.

- A subgroup of multiproblem youth exists who engage in multiple problem behaviors including antisocial behavior, cigarette smoking, binge drinking, marijuana use, hard drug use, and risky sexual behavior. Although few young people engage in all the problems, engaging in any one of them makes it quite likely that they will engage in others.
- Higher rates and serious levels of problem behavior characterize these multiproblem youth.
- Successful targeting of these young people has the potential to prevent a substantial proportion of a wide range of problems, including antisocial behavior, tobacco, alcohol, and other drug use, improper needle use, health problems associated with alcohol and drug use, and drunk driving.
- Conversely, prevention strategies that target one or a few problems may be ineffective with this multiproblem subgroup. For example, drug prevention strategies that focus on changing perceived norms for use (e.g., Hansen & Graham, 1991; Johnston, O'Malley, & Bachman, 1999) may be sufficient to deter substance use among members of peer groups whose norms support use of cigarettes or marijuana but are otherwise not deviance prone. However, they may have little impact on young people who are heavily involved in a variety of problem behaviors.

3

The Social Costs of Adolescent Problem Behavior

TED R. MILLER

This chapter examines the costs to society of having young people with multiple problem behaviors. Most people recognize intuitively that young people who break into homes, drink and drive, or abuse drugs are doing harm to themselves and others, but public discussions about these problems seldom take into account empirical analysis of the cost of those harms.

Why consider costs? One reason is that costs provide a single compact measure that summarizes such diverse outcomes as dropouts from high school, rapes, broken legs, and drug overdoses. Legislators, media, and the public can readily grasp costs. Costs communicate problem size clearly and illuminate policy relevance. For example, a minor's consumption of one can of beer results in an average of $1.15 in medical and work loss costs (Levy, Miller, & Cox, 1999). Yet, that beer costs only $.75, including $.35 of gross profit (Miller Brewing Company, 2000). Can $1.15 of social harm for a $.35 profit possibly be worth it?

Another reason for assessing annual costs is to compare the importance of different problems in a fair way. For example, the interpersonal violence attributable to underage drinking costs almost 20 times what associated suicides cost (Levy et al., 1999). As Weimer and Vining (1989) point out, however, cost differentials alone do not tell us what in-

tervention investments make the most sense. Because resources are always scarce, the priorities for investment may be the interventions that
will yield the greatest problem reduction for the funds available, even if
they address only narrow parts of the overall problem.

Consistent with the youth problems examined in the previous chapter, this chapter considers the costs of a series of problems or harms
related to high-risk behavior by youth. We were able to find or derive
costs for the following problems:

1. Violent crime—events where a youth deliberately killed or injured someone or attempted to injure someone, including all
   child abuse and neglect by youth.
2. Property crime related to violence or substance abuse—burglary,
   larceny/theft, and motor vehicle theft committed by violent
   youth or substance-abusing youth.
3. Binge drinking—drinking five or more drinks of alcohol on one
   occasion. Binge drinking substantially impairs motor skills and
   judgment. It increases the risk of injury and death while driving
   and injury from non-motor vehicle trauma, such as drowning
   and fires.
4. Heroin and/or cocaine abuse—youth using these addictive drugs
   at least three times in the past year, which puts a youth at great
   risk of developing a need to maintain their regular administration well into adulthood.
5. High-risk sex—youth having heterosexual or male homosexual
   intercourse without protection. High-risk sex poses risks of infection, including HIV and sexually transmitted diseases, and unwanted pregnancy.
6. Smoking—smoking tobacco products, which are highly addictive, at least three times in the past month. This level of tobacco
   use poses a severe risk of dependency, resulting in premature
   death.
7. High school dropout—youth leaving high school before graduation and thus not completing the requirements of a high school
   diploma. Dropout often results from high-risk sex, substance
   abuse, or delinquency. As such, it may be an additional outcome
   of these problems. Because it is not specific to any one problem,
   however, we chose to cost this problem separately rather than
   trying to allocate its incidence among those problem behaviors.
8. Suicide acts—often link to other high-risk youth behavior or
   stem from victimization of other youth by risk takers. Although
   we explore the link to substance abuse, we largely cost suicide

acts separately. Many, but not all, probably result from high-risk youth behavior.

COST CONCEPTS

It is possible to evaluate the cost of an event from a number of different perspectives. As recommended by the U.S. Panel on Cost-Effectiveness in Health and Medicine (Gold, Siegel, Russell, & Weinstein, 1996), we estimated costs from society's perspective, also called social costs. That perspective enumerates all costs associated with social problems: costs to victims, families, government, insurers, and taxpayers.

This contrasts with methods in which costs to government, to insurers, or to employers are computed separately. When evaluating minimum-drinking-age laws, driver blood alcohol limits, and other laws that interfere with personal freedom, economists often focus only on external costs—the costs to people other than the person whose behavior is constrained. The rationale is that high external costs justify public intervention. However, this chapter does not differentiate external or government costs from internal costs. Thus, in our data, government would not recoup all the cost savings that resulted from reducing youth behavioral problems; others would reap much of the savings.

The societal cost perspective poses conundrums when applied to problem behaviors. Some economists argue that money stolen is not a societal cost. Rather, it is a transfer of income from the rightful owner to the thief. Applying this same logic, a smaller group of economists would claim a date rape gave sexual pleasure to the rapist, a benefit that is lost if the rape is prevented. This obviously goes against most people's understanding of the basic social contract. Our method of costing adopts William Trumbull's (1990) approach. We do not count gains criminals and sinners get illegally as societal benefits, nor do we view prevention of those gains as a loss. In proscribing these actions, legislatures implicitly state that the gains are ill gotten and do not benefit society.

Costs can be prevalence or incidence based. Prevalence-based costs measure all problem-related expenses during one year, regardless of when the problem occurred. For example, the prevalence-based cost of lung cancer in 1996 measures the total health care spending on lung cancer and its sequelae during 1996, including spending on patients diagnosed years earlier. Prevalence-based costs are computed by summing all costs incurred during the year. They are used to understand health care spending, evaluate cost controls, and describe the cumulative burden that society currently bears because of past problem behaviors. We estimate the prevalence-based costs that youth problem behaviors caused during 1998.

Incidence-based costs sum the lifetime costs expected to result from problems that began during a single year. For example, the incidence-based cost of lung cancer in 1996 estimates present and future medical spending associated with all lung cancers diagnosed in 1996. Incidence-based costs are computed by multiplying the number of new victims times lifetime cost per victim. They measure the savings that prevention can yield. We provide incidence-based estimates of costs per youth involved by problem behavior (e.g., the cost of a teen's criminal career).

Investments earn interest. In incidence-based costing, therefore, it is necessary to discount future costs to present value. This demonstrates the amount needed to invest today to pay future costs as they arise. The Panel on Cost-Effectiveness in Health and Medicine (Gold et al., 1996) recommends that all cost-savings analyses include an estimate at a 3% discount rate to accommodate cross-study comparisons. We used that recommendation.

Cost Categories and Measurement Methods

Our costing efforts largely update or extend existing estimates. We separated societal burden of youth problem behavior into four cost categories.

Medical costs include emergency transport, medical, hospital, rehabilitation, mental health, pharmaceutical, ancillary, and related treatment costs, as well as funeral/coroner expenses for fatalities and administrative costs of processing medical payments to providers.

Other resource costs include police, fire, legal/court, prison/probation, foster care, and child protective services, plus the costs of property damage or loss. A difficult question here is whether to include intervention costs (e.g., the spending on security guards and alarm systems, police patrol and ambulance stations, or the National Highway Traffic Safety Administration) in problem costs. A reasonable guideline is to include these costs only when evaluating a problem or intervention impact that is so large that eliminating it would substantially reduce the need for these prevention services. For example, eliminating alcohol-attributable violence would reduce total violence by perhaps 15%, with an even smaller effect on violence by strangers (Harwood, Fountain, & Fountain, 1999; Harwood, Fountain, & Livermore, 1999; Miller, Fisher, & Cohen, 2001). That might marginally reduce security spending but it would not greatly reduce it. Therefore, this chapter excludes intervention costs.

Because they are paid out of pocket, travel-delay costs for uninjured travelers delayed by road crashes and the injuries they cause and employer productivity losses caused by temporary or permanent worker absence (e.g., the cost of hiring and training replacement workers) are included as resource costs. One could argue for counting these costs as work losses instead.

Work loss costs include victims' wage losses, the replacement cost of lost household work, fringe benefits, and the administrative costs of processing compensation for lost earnings through litigation, insurance, or public welfare programs such as food stamps and Supplemental Security Income. Victim work loss has two components: short-term losses during acute recovery and lifetime losses due to death or permanent work-related disability. Children under age 15 will not lose work in the short term. When injured children are impaired sufficiently that they would not have been able to work if they had been employed, someone else generally will lose work while serving as a caregiver. We assume work loss by family and friends equals the loss that normally occurs when an adult suffers a comparable injury. For other age groups, the value of lost work depends on the work that someone of the victim's age and sex normally would do and the amount such an individual would earn. We can estimate household workdays lost from the days of paid work lost (Miller, 1993). These days are valued at the wages paid for comparable tasks (e.g., cooking, cleaning, and childcare).

Quality of life includes the value of pain, suffering, and quality-of-life loss to victims and their families. While measuring medical and other resource costs and work losses in monetary terms is obviously possible to do, placing a monetary value on pain, suffering, and lost quality of life is challenging and controversial. For this reason, we first quantify this portion of burden with a nonmonetary measure, quality-adjusted life years (QALYs). A QALY is a health outcome measure that assigns a value of 1 to a year of perfect health and 0 to death (Gold et al., 1996). The duration and severity of the health problem determine the QALY loss. The fraction of perfect health lost for each year that a victim is recovering from a health problem or living with a residual disability is estimated and then summed over years. When people die, economists assume a loss of a full QALY per life-year, a conventional assumption that ignores preexisting conditions and the general decline in health as people age. As Gold et al. (1996) recommend, like costs, we discount future QALY losses to present value at a 3% discount rate.

The most practical way to assess health-related quality of life losses from a community viewpoint involves a two-step process. In the first step, one creates a set of scales for rating health states (i.e., physical and emotional health status). The public then answers polls to determine how society values the different health states relative to optimal health and to death. A good measure allows people to rate some fates as worse than death.

In the second step, either patient survey/observation or expert physician judgment is used to estimate the temporal pattern of health status changes over time that result from a medical problem. The rating scale then is used to estimate lost utility (an economist's measure of the relative value people place on different goods). The result is an estimate of the QALYs lost to the medical problem.

How do we put a monetary figure on QALYs? For death, pain, suffering, and lost quality of life are best valued in dollars using an approach economists call willingness to pay. This approach derives the value of pain and suffering by asking people what they are willing to pay for or by studying what people actually pay for small changes in their chance of death or injury. The value of reducing the risk of death, aggregated over many people, yields the value of a statistical life. For example, suppose a study estimated that the average person spends $300 on optional auto safety features that reduce the chance of dying prematurely by 1 in 10,000. Dividing $300 by the 1 in 10,000 probability yields a $3 million value per statistical life. That value has two components: (1) the value of the foregone future work and (2) the value of the pain, suffering, grief, lost companionship, and lost quality of life. The value of lost future work is known. Subtracting it leaves the value of the intangibles (Arthur, 1981; Miller, Calhoun, & Arthur, 1989). Importantly, when this subtraction-based method is used to value lost quality of life, the total cost of an injury or illness becomes insensitive to the work-loss estimate and is determined by the risk reduction value.

The values for lost quality of life in this book use the estimated mean value of statistical life across 67 studies that Miller (1990, 2000) rated as technically sound. The estimated mean value of statistical life in the United States is $3.25 million in 1999 after-tax dollars. This value is conservative. Individual value estimates vary widely around it, with a standard deviation of $.7 million if only studies that Miller (1990) considered sound are included. Miller (1990) modified many published values to remove inappropriate biases. Without these somewhat arbitrary adjustments, Viscusi (1993) recommends a value of $3–5 million. Fisher, Chestnut, and Violette (1989) recommend a $1–8 million range, and a meta-analysis (Miller, 2000) suggests a $3.3–4.5 million range, with a best estimate of $3.7 million. Although these uncertainties seem quite large, they are no larger on a percentage basis than the uncertainty ranges around many intervention effectiveness estimates.

Depending on the nonfatal outcome considered, in order of preference, we used one of three methods to place a dollar value on pain, suffering, and lost quality of life:

1. Monetization of estimated QALY loss.
2. Analysis of jury awards for noneconomic damages.
3. Multiplication of work losses by the average ratio of QALYs to work loss across all nonfatal injuries to get a low-cost order-of-magnitude estimate.

Working from a general equilibrium model of the economy, Miller et al. (1989) show that the value of a statistical life times the percentage utility loss associated with a nonfatal outcome equals the willingness to pay to avoid that outcome. QALY systems measure the desired utility loss if calibrated so that optimal health has a value of 1, death has a value of 0, and fates worse than death are allowed.

We can estimate the value of reducing risk by one QALY readily from the value of statistical life by:

1. Assuming the value per QALY does not vary with age or sex.
2. Subtracting lifetime work loss from the value of statistical life to avoid double-counting.
3. Dividing the remainder by the expected years of healthy lifespan saved per life saved (discounted to present value). Multiplying the discounted years of expected healthy life lost for someone in a specific age group times the QALY value and dividing by the mean discounted all-victim lifespan yields a value of a statistical life tailored by age and sex.

With a $3.25 million value of statistical life, a QALY of healthy life expectancy is worth $135,000 (at a 3% discount rate in 1999 U.S. dollars). Although validation of this QALY value has been limited, some investigations support QALY use as a reasonable estimate. Miller et al. (1989) used it to accurately predict values of asthma risk reduction obtained in a subsequent survey. For assaults (Miller, Cohen, & Wiersema, 1996), consumer product injuries (Lawrence, Miller, Jensen, Fisher, & Zamula, 2000), and drunk driving (Smith, 1998), the pain and suffering component of jury verdicts can be predicted well from QALY losses (r^2 0.5 in log-linear regressions), with juries valuing QALYs consistent with a value of statistical life of $1.9–4.4 million. Thus, QALY costs measure real and tangible losses. The theoretical framework for the jury verdict method comes from Cohen (1988), Viscusi (1988), and Rodgers (1993). The basic notion is that pain and suffering to a survivor can be approximated by the difference between the amount of compensatory damages awarded by a jury minus the actual out-of-pocket charges associated with the injury. Miller et al. (1996) estimated pain and suffering for physical assaults from log-linear jury verdict regressions, then compared the results with QALY estimates by diagnosis group (from Miller, Pindus, Douglass, & Rossman, 1995). Some individual estimates varied significantly, but the incidence weighted mean estimates from the two methods varied by only 5%. Thus, it is reasonable to mix medically based QALY estimates and ones estimated from U.S. jury verdicts.

In the hopes of avoiding controversy, we present both QALYs expressed as years lost and monetized QALYs. The strongest argument for monetizing QALYs is to permit comparisons between health sector investments and investments in other sectors. Valuing quality of life may be unfamiliar or disquieting. Given the wide range for the value of a statistical life and the slim validation of the implied QALY value, it also is difficult and controversial. Nevertheless, the ease of dealing with a single measure of costs, plus the ability to compare between health and other sectors make it a valuable supplement to economic cost and QALY loss estimates.

COSTING METHODS BY PROBLEM BEHAVIORS

We relied on prior studies whenever possible in estimating the costs of youth problem behavior. We found studies of the costs of heroin and cocaine abuse (Cohen, 1998), criminal careers (Cohen, 1998; Miller et al., 1996; Miller et al., 2001), high school dropout (Cohen, 1998), and underage drinking (Levy et al., 1999). We also found fragmentary studies of high-risk sexual behavior (notably Trussell, Koenig, Stewart, & Darroch, 1997; Wang et al., 2000) and smoking (Adams & Melvin, 1998; Cromwell, Bartosch, Fiore, Hasselblad, & Baker, 1997; Manning, Keeler, Newhouse, Sloss, & Wasserman, 1991). Every study probed only one of the annual costs of high-risk behavior or lifetime costs resulting from youthful risk taking. Considerable reanalysis was required to arrive at comparable, contemporaneous cost estimates for the various behaviors.

This section details the methods used. All costs are in 1999 dollars. It describes how we estimated the costs of a high-risk youth and the annual costs of youth problem behavior. We costed seven behaviors: high-risk sex, binge/heavy drinking, regular drug use, violence, smoking, high school dropout, and medically treated or fatal suicide acts. Dropping out and suicide acts, although not behavioral problems focused on in this book, tie closely with the focus behaviors and youth who practice them or are victims of them. We chose to cost them separately rather than trying to apportion dropout and suicide costs among the target behaviors.

For each behavior costed, we estimated the number of adolescents with this behavioral problem in a recent year, the lifetime of costs resulting from their misbehavior during that year (essentially a prevalence-based estimate of the costs of problem behavior), and the likely temporal course and incidence-based cost of a career of misbehavior. Where possible, we used published cost estimates. Typically, we adjusted these estimates to make them comparable to the costs for other behaviors. The most frequent adjustments were to change the discount rate (used to convert future costs to present value) to 3% and to estimate work-related and QALY costs.

Underage Drinking

Levy, Miller, Cox, and Spicer (2001) estimate costs attributable to underage drinking (meaning that they involved alcohol and would not have arisen if the adolescents involved were not drinking). We replaced their alcohol-related crime and suicide costs with the crime and suicide costs used in this book.

From 1998 National Household Survey on Drug Abuse (NHSDA) data, we calculated that 91% of all alcohol consumed by adolescents ages 12–20 was consumed by the 4,817,000 adolescents who reported binge drinking (five or more drinks in one day) during the past 30 days. We consider those adolescents high-risk drinkers and assume they are responsible for all costs attributable to underage drinking. From NHSDA, we estimated the average temporal course of binge drinking before the 21st birthday, which allowed us to compute the cost per high-risk adolescent drinker. Unlike the career costs for youth smokers or heroin/cocaine abusers, our career costs for underage drinkers stop at the 21st birthday. If these youth would experience more drinking problems as adults than those who did not start drinking underage, our career costs are underestimates. Several studies suggest that delayed initiation could have averted some adult drinking problems (e.g., Hingson, Heeren, Jamanka, & Howland, 2000).

Heroin/Cocaine Abuse

We started from Cohen's (1998) estimated lifetime costs for a heavy adolescent user of cocaine (including crack) or heroin, but excluded the money spent on the drugs consumed. Cohen shared his costing spreadsheets with us, which facilitated converting his cost model to a 3% discount rate. We recomputed the crime costs.

The number of youth using heroin or cocaine at least three times in the past year (roughly Cohen's definition of a heavy user) came from the 1998 NHSDA. We used Cohen's cost model and the NHSDA incidence estimate to compute the costs of adolescent heroin/cocaine abuse in

1998, exclusive of crime costs. With data from the 1997–1998 waves of the NHSDA, we updated Cohen's estimate of the career heroin/cocaine usage of people who started using heroin or cocaine before age 21, then used this information to compute the costs per career of heroin/cocaine use initiated before age 21.

The rate of hospital-admitted youth suicide acts involving heroin/cocaine and the cost per act came from pooled 1997 hospital discharge data from 19 states that coded injury causes. The pooled data cover 52% of U.S. youth. Miller, Romano, and Spicer (2000) describe the costing methods. The incidence estimate is conservative because some injury discharges lacked required cause codes or their intent was coded as unknown.

We did not cost drug abuse by youth who did not abuse heroin/cocaine. A portion of the abuse costs for those youth is included in the costs of criminal careers, high school dropouts, and suicide acts, as well as in the alcohol abuse costs, which largely capture the costs of youth who abuse both alcohol and other drugs except heroin/cocaine.

High-Risk Sex

For the cost analysis, the limited information available for costing forced us to define high-risk sexual behavior as unprotected sex. Costs of female heterosexual, male heterosexual, and male homosexual sex were estimated separately and then summed. Little is known about the incidence of sexually transmitted diseases with lesbian sex, although it appears to be modest (Roberts, Sorensen, Patsdaughter, & Grindel, 2000). Therefore, we omitted the associated costs.

Female Heterosexual

Trussell et al. (1997) provided the annual risk of sexually transmitted diseases (STDs), including HIV/AIDS, herpes simplex, human papillomavirus, syphilis, gonorrhea, chlamydia, trichomoniasis, and pelvic inflammatory disease, and of pregnancy from unprotected sex by female adolescents. The percentage of live births to mothers ages 10–19 that were unintended and unwanted or mistimed (unintended hereafter) came from a 1995 national survey (summarized in Wang et al., 2000), and the number of births and abortions from U.S. Vital Statistics (U.S. Census Bureau, 1998). We assumed that the percentage of pregnancies that were unintended was equal for births and miscarriages to 10- to 19-year-old females and that all abortions in this age range resulted from unintended pregnancy. Further, we assumed that all 833,000 unintended pregnancies of adolescent mothers in 1996 (85.55% of the total) resulted from unprotected or other high-risk sex. Dividing the total by the annual 29.7% pregnancy risk associated with unprotected adolescent sex (Trussell et al., 1997) yields an estimate that 2,805,000 female adolescents had unsafe sex in 1996. Trussell's risk data let us compute the resulting STD cases.

Trussell et al. (1997) gives the medical costs per adolescent STD case and live birth. We used its cost estimates from 1993 Medstat data. Medstat pools health care claims data on more than 3 million people who get health insurance through their own or a family member's employer. Wang et al. (2000) gives 1993 Medstat costs for pregnancies that are not carried to term and for prenatal care. These costs were multiplied times the 1996 outcome distribution for pregnancies to women under 21 (U.S. Census Bureau, 1998), yielding medical costs per unintended pregnancy.

Work loss equals the sum of wages and fringe benefits lost. When illness causes work loss, household work losses also are included. We restricted work loss due to live birth an average of 2 years earlier than desired to wage-related losses of $10,535 per live birth (from Maynard, 1996, inflated to 1999 dollars and roughly adjusted to a 3% discount rate). For HIV, we found data on QALY loss to age 65 (essentially healthy years equivalent [HYE] loss) from Holtgrave and Pinkerton (1997), but not lifetime work loss under recent treatment regimens. We assumed the same percentage of lifetime wage and household work and QALYs were lost (both computed at a 3% discount rate). We conservatively assumed other STDs of adolescents resulted in just 2 days of lost wage work (often by a parent, not the teen) and no lost household work. Finally, we assumed that the ratio of QALY losses to work losses for HIV applied to the other conditions, which allowed us to estimate QALY losses for those conditions.

The unit costs were multiplied by the incidence of STDs and unintended pregnancies to obtain annual costs. Dividing by the number of adolescent females practicing unsafe sex yielded an annual cost per high-risk adolescent female. To compute lifetime cost per high-risk adolescent female (or male), we assumed that unsafe sex practices started at age 16 and lasted until adolescence ended at age 20 (and possibly beyond, but practices after age 20 are not relevant in costing this adolescent risk).

Male Heterosexual

Faulkner and Cranston (1998) report that 1.18 times as many adolescent males as females in high school are heterosexually active in Massachusetts. We assume that ratio applies to all adolescents. We assume unprotected sex and STD rates and costs do not vary by sex (except that males do not suffer pelvic inflammatory disease). Our assumption implies that 3,306,000 male adolescents practice high-risk sex and allows us to compute male heterosexual STD costs from female costs.

Male Homosexual

From Faulkner and Cranston (1998), we estimate that the ratio of homosexually active males to heterosexually active females is 0.0805. From Pinkerton, Holtgrave, DiFranceisco, Stevenson, and Kelly (1998) and Trussell et al. (1997), we estimate that HIV risk is 5.84 times higher for male homosexual than heterosexual adolescents. We assume that ratio applies to other male STDs and that the cost per STD case does not vary by type of partner. That allows us to compute male homosexual STD costs from female STD costs.

Youth Violence

The costs per youth crime came from Miller et al. (1996) and Miller, Fisher, and Cohen (2001). Adjudication and sanctioning costs came from Cohen (1998). We converted the costs to a 3% discount rate. We used 1998 crime incidence by perpetrator age from the Bureau of Justice Statistics (U.S. Government Printing Office, 2000). We adjusted for underreporting of sexual assault and added violence against victims under age 12 with factors from Miller et al. (1996). Child abuse and neglect data came from Miller et al. (1996) and Miller, Levy, Cohen, and Cox (2001). The percentage of motor vehicle thefts by youth came from the 1996–1998 waves of the NHSDA, with three waves required to get an adequate sample size. We used Cohen's (1998) ratios of robberies to property crimes by substance abuse involvement, but adjusted the motor vehicle theft count downward to match the youth-involved total. Our cost estimate omits the many burglaries and larcenies/thefts committed by nonviolent youth who were not using drugs or alcohol. For comparison purposes, we also computed the total cost of violence in the United States in 1998.

For violent crime analyzed by type, we used data from the *1997 Survey of Inmates in Federal and State Prisons* (U.S. Department of Justice, 1999) and the *1986 Survey of Youth in Detention* (the only national survey of this population; U.S. Department of Justice, 1994). Using these data, we estimated the percentage of youth using heroin/cocaine, other drugs only, alcohol only, or both alcohol and other drugs at the time of their crime and the percentage of crimes committed to get money to buy drugs while not drugged or drinking. Cohen (1998) provided factors used to estimate property crime involving substance abuse from similar data about robberies. The estimates apportion crimes between violent perpetration and substance abuse without double counting.

We used Cohen's estimate of duration and intensity to cost a violent crime career that started in adolescence. We computed the number of violent crime careers by dividing the annual number of violent youth crimes not involving heroin/cocaine or alcohol (excluding child abuse and neglect) by the annual number of violent crimes per youth predator from Cohen (1998).

Youth Smoking

We computed four components of youth smoking cost:

1. Costs of adolescent girls smoking during pregnancy and until their children reach age 6.
2. The excess medical costs over a smoker's lifetime less the cost savings resulting from early death.
3. The work loss and QALY loss over a lifetime of smoking.
4. The costs of secondhand smoke exposure.

Because the addictiveness of smoking causes this behavior to persist for many years, we believe it is fair to attribute lifetime smoking costs to youth smoking.

NHSDA data suggested how to define a smoker. They showed that binge drinking rates of adolescent daily smokers matched binge drinking rates of adolescents who smoked on at least three occasions in the past 30 days but were much higher than rates for adolescents who had smoked only once or twice in the past 30 days. Given this clear break, we defined a smoker as someone who smoked on at least 3 days in the past 30; 6,234,000 adolescents ages 12–20 smoked in 1998 by this definition.

Adams and Melvin (1998) provided differential risk and medical cost data for delivery complications stemming from smoking during pregnancy. Smoking increases the risk of ectopic pregnancy, placenta previa, abrupto previa, and preterm premature rupture of membrane but reduces preeclampsia risk. The medical cost data were obtained from 1993 Medstat. For pregnancies that miscarried due to smoking, we used data from Wang et al. (2000) to estimate the number and cost savings from pregnancies that otherwise would have been aborted. The remaining miscarriages resulted in loss of a lifetime of work and QALY losses (computed with a standard age-earnings model and a 3% discount rate). The number of adolescent females who smoked during pregnancy came from 1998 Vital Statistics (CDC, 2002).

Stoddard and Gray (1997) indicated that children under age 6 living with smokers experience $140 more in medical costs of respiratory illnesses annually (in 1999 dollars). We estimated parental work loss and quality of life loss to these respiratory problems from the medical costs using Tolley, Kenkel, and Fabian's (1994) estimates of respiratory illness costs per case by cost category. We applied the respiratory illness costs only to children whose mothers smoked during pregnancy.

Added lifetime medical cost for a smoker came from Manning et al. (1991). QALY loss per smoker came from Cromwell et al. (1997), with wage losses assumed proportional. We computed the costs of second-hand smoking from smoking's lifetime costs for all smokers and the ratio of 0.37 annual smoking-related cardiovascular deaths of secondhand smokers per cardiovascular death due to primary smoking from Glantz and Parmley (2001) and He et al. (1999).

High School Dropout

The cost per high school dropout came from Cohen (1998), adjusted to a 3% discount rate. Cohen's estimate ignores the health behavior impact that results from being poorly educated. The number of high school dropouts in 1999 came from the National Center for Education Statistics (U.S. Department of Education, 1999).

Youth Suicide Acts

Costs per medically treated or fatal youth suicide act and the number of nonfatal acts that were medically treated but not hospitalized were computed with the methods described in Miller et al. (2000). The number of suicide deaths came from 1998 Vital Statistics (CDC, 2002). Hospitalized incidents, their substance abuse involvement, and their costs were computed from pooled, cause-coded 1997 hospital discharge censuses from 19 states. These 19 states house 52% of U.S. youth. We assumed their youth suicide act rate matched the U.S. rate. If instead we estimated incidence with the methods in Miller, Romano, and Spicer, the estimate would be within 5% of the estimate we used. We adjusted estimates of nonfatal incidence in 1997 to 1998 in proportion to the relative numbers of youth suicide deaths by year. From the 1999 Youth Risk Behavior Survey (YRBS; Kahn et al., 2000) we estimated that a youth who attempts suicide averages two suicidal acts, with 0.7% fatal and 28% of nonfatal acts requiring medical treatment.

COSTS IMPOSED BY MULTIPROBLEM YOUTH

To estimate the extent of the costs of these problems that could be attributed to multiproblem youth, we multiplied the total cost for each problem by the percentage of youth who we estimate have multiple problems.

As the previous chapter explained, those percentages were averages from four surveys (with some surveys not covering all ages). We used the 1999 NHSDA (USDHHS, 2000a), the 1999 YRBS (Kahn et al., 2000), the 1999 *Monitoring the Future* survey (Johnston, O'Malley, & Bachman, 2000c), and the 1996 Health Behaviors of School Children survey (World Health Organization, 2001). There was one exception: we used only YRBS data to assess high-risk sex behavior, because the other surveys collected minimal data about sexual risk taking. Because NHSDA personal interviews, some of them not conducted in private, detected lower rates of substance abuse than written surveys, we view the four-survey averages as conservative. We also computed costs using multiproblem rates with averages from just the other three surveys, obtaining a range.

Cost of All Youth Problem Behavior in 1998

Table 3.1 presents the prevalence-based costs of all youth problem behaviors in 1998—not just the costs attributable to multiproblem youth. As noted previously, these costs include continuing effects of conditions that started in 1998, such as a lifetime disability caused by an assault in 1998. They do not include the lifetime health consequences or criminal careers that result from someone establishing an addiction in 1998.

Problem behaviors cost $435.4 billion in 1998. This total included $16.6 billion in medical spending, $35.9 billion in other resource costs, $121.1 billion in work losses, and suffering and quality-of-life losses val-

TABLE 3.1. Social Costs by Cost Category and QALY Losses from High-Risk Youthful Behavior, Total and per Youth Ages 12–20, United States, 1998

Cost category	Total cost	Cost per American youth[a]
Medical	16,637,000,000	470
Other resources	35,899,000,000	1,020
Work	121,052,000,000	3,430
Quality of life	261,799,000,000	7,430
Total	$435,387,000,000	$12,350
QALYs lost	1,939,000	0.05

Note. Costs are prevalence-based (in 1999 dollars, with future consequences discounted to present value at a 3% discount rate). Averages computed from 1999 NHSDA Youth Risk Behavior Survey, 1999 *Monitoring the Future* survey, and 1996 *Health Behaviors of School Children* survey.

[a]Averaged across youth with problems and youth with no problems.

ued at $261.8 billion (all computed at a 3% discount rate). Some of these prevalence-based losses—although resulting from deaths, injuries, and illnesses in 1998—were deferred to later years, but they all resulted from problems active in 1998. For example, the person paralyzed by a gunshot wound fired by a drugged youth in 1998 faces a lifetime of suffering and work loss.

The cost per U.S. youth may be more understandable. In 1998, these youth problems cost an average of $12,300 per youth ages 12–20 (and much more per problem youth, as explored later). This is averaged across all U.S. youth in this age range, not just across youth with problems. These problems consumed $1,500 in resources per youth, led to $3,400 in future work losses, and imposed $7,400 in quality of life losses. In just 1 year, the average youth lost 20 days of HYE due to these problems.

These losses included 1.94 million years of healthy life. To put that loss in perspective, consider that when a youth reaches age 21, with our 3% discount rate, in present value terms, a healthy lifespan of 23.1 years awaits. The health losses were thus the equivalent of 84,000 young lives.

Estimating total costs to society for all youth across the number of cost categories that must be considered *and* across all these individual problems is complex. Apportioning these costs among problem behaviors is difficult because they are interlocked. For example, youth committed 70% of their crimes while drinking or under the influence of drugs. Similarly, most high school dropouts and suicide acts involved risk-taking teens or the consequences of their risk taking. Table 3.2 classifies the costs by problem behavior but lumps all crime costs and all suicide costs. During 1998, violent youth committed crimes that cost $165.8 billion. Crime was the largest cost of youth risk taking. Next came high school dropout at $142 billion and high-risk sexual behavior at $48 billion. Not counting associated crime and suicide costs, substance abuse cost $64 billion. Counting them raises substance abuse costs to $168 billion. This figure largely excludes costs of abusing illicit drugs other than heroin and cocaine.

Tables 3.3–3.7 provide alternate, more detailed views of the prevalence-based costs of intertwined youth crime and substance abuse problems and details of the costs of high-risk adolescent sexual behavior. We did not apportion the costs of high school dropout among the other risks and segmented only the suicide risks linked to alcohol and drugs. Remember that our figures involving antisocial behavior include only a portion of crime by youth: violent crimes plus property crimes committed by violent or substance-abusing youth. Thus, our figures underestimate the total cost of all youth crimes.

In the short term, youth smoking causes minimal costs, almost all

TABLE 3.2. Total Social Costs and QALY Losses from High-Risk Youthful Behavior by Risk Category, United States, 1998, Excluding Costs of Adult Behavior Initiated before Age 21

Risk category	Medical	Other resource	Work loss	Quality of life	Total cost	QALYs lost
Violence and related property crime	5.7 B	30.8 B	12.7 B	116.7 B	165.8 B	864,000
Binge drinking[a]	3.2 B	5.0 B	5.1 B	28.7 B	42 B	213,000
Cocaine and/or heroin abuse[a]	644 M	148 M	5.4 B	15.5 B	21.7 B	115,000
High-risk sex	6.8 B		8.1 B	33.3 B	48.1 B	246,000
Smoking	99 M		81 M	239 M	419 M	2,000
High school dropout			87.1 B	54.5 B	141.6 B	404,000
Suicide acts	221 M	11 M	2.6 B	12.9 B	15.7 B	95,000
Total	$16.6 B	$35.9 B	$121.1 B	$261.8 B	$435.4 B	1,939,000

Note. Costs are prevalence-based (in 1999 dollars). B, billion; M, million.
[a]Excludes costs of crime and suicide acts related to substance abuse.

TABLE 3.3. Social Costs of Youth Violent Crimes and Property Crimes Committed by Violent Offenders, by Drug and Alcohol Involvement and Cost Category, United States, 1998

Substances involved	Medical	Other resource	Work loss	Quality of life	Total cost	QALYs lost
Heroin or cocaine	1.3 B	8.7 B	3 B	26.6 B	39.6 B	197,000
Alcohol and other drugs	1.3 B	2.4 B	972 M	8.3 B	13 B	62,000
Alcohol only	933 M	4.7 B	2.2 B	19.1 B	26.9 B	141,000
Other drugs only	352 M	5.6 B	2.9 B	28.4 B	37.2 B	210,000
None	1.8 B	9.4 B	3.6 B	34.3 B	49.1 B	254,000
Total	$5.7 B	$30.8 B	$12.7 B	$116.7 B	$165.8 B	864,000

Note. Costs are prevalence-based (in 1999 dollars). B, billion; M, million.

TABLE 3.4. **Social Costs of Youth Violent Offenses and Property Crimes Committed by Violent Offenders, by Type of Crime and Cost Category, United States, 1998**

Crime	Number of cases	Medical	Other resource	Work loss	Quality of life	Total cost	QALYs lost
Rape	587,000	2 B	1.9 B	1.5 B	57.6 B	$63 B	427,000
Murder	6,114	137 M	1.0 B	6.9 B	14.8 B	$22.8 B	109,000
Assault	3,463,000	2.3 B	17 B	3.7 B	30.5 B	$53.5 B	226,000
Robbery	336,000	185 M	2.8 B	335 M	2.3 B	$5.6 B	17,000
Child abuse and neglect	422,000	968 M	552 M	365 M	11.2 B	$13.1 B	83,000
Burglary	375,000	2 M	1.4 B	6 M	130 M	$1.5 B	1,000
Larceny	1,643,000	12 M	3.1 B	15 M	0	$3.1 B	0
Motor vehicle theft	432,000	3 M	3.1 B	23 M	136 M	$3.2 B	1,000
Total	7,264,114	$5.6 B	$30.9 B	$12.8 B	$116.7 B	$166 B	864,000

Note. Costs are prevalence-based (in 1999 dollars). B, billion; M, million.

TABLE 3.5. Social Costs of Binge Drinking by Problem and Cost Category, Ages 12–20, United States, 1998

Problem	Medical	Other resource	Work loss	Quality of life	Total cost	QALYs lost
Impaired driving	1.2 B	2.1 B	3.3 B	13.5 B	$20.1 B	100,000
Violence	2.2 B	8.5 B	5 B	47.4 B	$63.1 B	351,000
Property crimes	4 M	1.8 B	11 M	65 M	$1.9 B	500
Burns	2 M	0	63 M	130 M	$195 M	1,000
Drowning	3 M	0	159 M	278 M	$440 M	2,000
Suicide	20 M	1 M	233 M	1.2 B	$1.4 B	9,000
Fetal alcohol syndrome	373 M	0	140 M	244 M	$757 M	2,000
Alcohol poisoning	10 M	0	17 M	325 M	$352 M	2,000
Abuse treatment	1.1 B	0	0	0	$1.1 B	0
Total	$4.9B	$12.4 B	$8.9 B	$63.1 B	$89.3 B	467,500

Note. Costs are prevalence-based (in 1999 dollars). B, billion; M, million.

TABLE 3.6. Costs of Cocaine and Heroin Abuse by Problem and Cost Category, Ages 12–20, United States, 1998

Problem	Medical	Other resource	Work loss	Quality of life	Total cost	QALYs lost
Drug treatment	378 M	0	0	0	$378 M	0
Medical care	350 M	0	679 M	1.3 B	$2.3 B	10,000
Risk of death[a]	23 M	22 M	4.8 B	15.4 B	$20.2 B	114,000
Violence	1.2 B	5.6 B	2.9 B	25.2 B	$35 B	187,000
Property crimes	7 M	3 B	17 M	106 M	$3.1 B	1,000
Drug possession	21 M	54 M	34 M	257 M	$366 M	2,000
Nonfatal suicide acts	11 M	0	9 M	293 M	$314 M	2,000
Total	$1.99 B	$8.7 B	$8.4 B	$42.6 B	$61.7 B	316,000

Note. Costs are prevalence-based (in 1999 dollars). B, billion; M, million.
[a]Includes suicide deaths.

51

TABLE 3.7. Social Costs of High-Risk Sex by Problem and Cost Category, Ages 12–20, United States, 1998

Problem	Medical	Work loss	Quality of life	Total cost	QALYs lost
HIV/AIDS	680 M	2.2 B	8.9 B	$11.7 B	65,000
Pelvic inflammatory disease	219 M	20 M	85 M	$324 M	1,000
Other sexually transmitted diseases	478 M	835 M	3.4 B	$4.7 B	25,000
Unintended pregnancy	5.4 B	5.1 B	20.9 B	31.4 B	155,000
Total	$6.8 B	$8.2 B	$33.3 B	$48.2 B	246,000

Note. Costs are prevalence-based (in 1999 dollars). B, billion; M, million.

related to pregnancy or children's respiratory illness. Tobacco, however, is highly addictive. The youth who smoked in 1998 will cause $2.6 trillion in associated incidence-based costs over their lifetimes (Table 3.8), with 27% of that cost due to secondhand smoke. The $37 billion in anticipated medical costs of smoking far exceeds the combined medical costs of all other youthful risk taking in 1998. This estimate of the medical cost includes the offsetting Medicare cost savings from lifespan truncation. The 14.1 million healthy life years that these 6.3 million young smokers and their victims will lose equates to more than 610,000 lives.

Cost of a Single Lifetime Career of Each Problem

As noted earlier, the costs of many youth problems are not limited to the time of adolescence but continue into adulthood. Therefore, we are interested in the costs of the career of a youth who engages in a particular

TABLE 3.8. Lifetime Cost of Smoking for All Smokers Ages 12–20, United States, 1998

Cost category	Total cost
Medical	$37 B
Work	$658 B
Quality of life	$1,900 B
Total	$2,595 B
QALYs lost	$14,078,000

Note. Costs are incidence-based (in 1999 dollars discounted to present value at a 3% discount rate). B, billion.

problem behavior. Violence, cocaine or heroin abuse, and smoking are problem behaviors that typically continue and thus incur costs into adulthood. As shown in Table 3.9, the incidence-based costs are highest for youth criminals who are violent when not drinking or using drugs and for those addicted to cocaine or heroin. The costs of binge drinking shown here include all costs of alcohol-involved crime. In reality, some of those crimes would occur even if the perpetrators were sober. They are costs of a high-risk behavior complex that involves drinking and committing violent acts. Because of pregnancy and its complications, girls face higher costs than boys do when practicing risky sex or smoking. The costs per smoker would be much higher if they were not so far in the future.

Of course, as documented previously, most youth who engage in one of these problems engage in other problems. The last row of table 3.9 gives the cost for each youth who engages in *all* of the problems under consideration, including dropping out of high school and attempting suicide.

Total Costs of Multiproblem Youth

Table 3.10 shows the total prevalence-based costs of youth who had *two or more* of the focal problems in 1998, including costs due to two related nonfocal problems: dropping out of high school or attempting suicide. The costs are broken down by cost category. We estimate that multiproblem youth accounted for 77–80% of the total cost of youth behavior problems. Thus, they cost society $335–350 billion in 1998. The costs include $12–13 billion in medical costs, $24–26 billion in other resource costs, $102–103 billion in work loss costs, and $196–207 billion in quality of life costs. About 1.5 million years of healthy life—the equivalent of 63,000–66,500 young lives—were lost.

The social costs imposed by multiproblem youth are so large that one needs a yardstick to comprehend them. In 1999 dollars, the $340 billion cost of high-risk youth behavior during 1998 is:

- Slightly less than the $394 billion cost of all violence in the United States in 1998.
- Slightly less than the annual cost of U.S. highway crashes ($418 billion; Miller, Lestina, & Spicer, 1998).
- About three times the total alcohol sales in 1999 ($113 billion; Miller Brewing Company, 2000).
- More than one-third of total spending on medical care for adults and children combined in 1999 ($943 billion; U.S. Office of Management & Budget, 2000).

TABLE 3.9. Number of Problem Youth Ages 12–20 and Cost of One Youth's High-Risk Career by Type of Risk, United States, 1998

Risk category	Number of youth	Medical	Other resource	Work loss	Quality of life	Total cost	QALYs lost
Violent criminal	300,000	20,900	511,000	141,100	424,600	$1,097,600	3.14
Binge drinker[a]	4,817,000	3,700	9,600	6,900	48,600	$68,800	0.36
Cocaine/heroin abuser[a]	674,000	28,300	128,100	122,900	614,500	$893,800	4.55
High-risk sex partner	6,337,000	4,900	0	5,600	23,500	$34,000	0.17
Female	2,805,000	9,800	0	9,600	40,700	$60,100	0.30
Male	3,532,000	1,000	0	2,500	9,800	$13,300	0.07
Smoker	6,286,000	5,800	0	104,700	302,400	$412,900	2.24
High school dropout	519,000	0	0	167,800	105,100	$272,900	0.78
Suicide attempter[b]	99,000	2,800	100	26,800	143,300	$173,000	0.96
Youth with all problems	Unknown	55,000	632,200	486,500	1,333,400	$2,507,100	9.88

Note. Costs are incidence-based (in 1999 dollars).
[a]Includes costs of crime and suicide acts related to substance abuse of $51,100 per binge drinker and $221,700 per drug abuser.
[b]Excludes those whose suicide acts were not medically treated and recognized as suicide acts by the medical provider or not coded as suicide in Vital Statistics mortality data.

TABLE 3.10. Ranged Estimates of Costs of Multiproblem Youth by Cost Category, United States, 1998

Cost category	% Multiple from four data sets	% Multiple from three data sets
Medical	12,319,000,000	12,884,000,000
Other resource	23,782,000,000	26,480,000,000
Work loss	101,999,000,000	103,287,000,000
Quality of life	196,446,000,000	207,200,000,000
Total cost	$334,546,000,000	$349,851,000,000
QALYs lost	1,455,000	1,535,000
Life-equivalents	63,000	66,500

Note. Multiproblem youth are defined as having two or more of the following problems: violent criminal, smoker, risky sexual behavior, cocaine/heroin abuser. Costs include costs of those behaviors plus costs of related suicide attempts and school dropout. The first column averages data from YRBS, *Monitoring the Future*, Healthy Behavior of Children, and NHSDA databases. The second column excludes NHSDA data. See text for details. Costs are prevalence-based (in 1999 dollars).

Added to these costs are those associated with extending the consequences of youth behaviors into adulthood, including violent criminal careers, binge drinking, cocaine/heroin abuse, high-risk sexual behavior, smoking, and high school dropout (see Table 3.9). In total, these represent social costs of $2.5 million over the career of each youth who had all of the problems.

SUMMARY AND CONCLUSIONS

In this chapter, we estimated cost to society of young people with multiple problem behaviors. As in any effort to estimate total societal costs and adjust for a wide variety of economic considerations, there are caveats. For example, we lack perfect estimates for any of the problems and lack any cost estimate for some problems associated with this youth subpopulation (e.g., vandalism, eating disorders, and fires started by cigarettes or by young children of adolescent parents). However, we believe that our analysis provides reasonable and somewhat conservative dollar estimates of the damage wrought by these multiproblem youth.

This chapter first estimates the costs to society for the series of problems most likely to involve youth. Looking across all U.S. youth, the average cost of problems per youth during 1998 was about $12,300. This estimate includes costs for underage drinking, heroin/cocaine abuse, high-risk sex, violence, smoking, school dropout, and suicide. Using these estimates, the health losses for 1998 were equivalent to 84,000 young lives.

These costs were specific to adolescence, but social costs for problems that begin in adolescence extend throughout adulthood. This means that these estimates will increase over time as careers of high-risk behavior continue. Table 3.9 gives estimates for a career of high-risk behavior. Violence yields the highest total to society of over $1 million per youthful career. As we will see in the next three chapters, many effective prevention and treatment programs cost only a fraction of this per youth to provide. Even if we look only at dollars, not at wasted or harmed lives, the potential for savings is enormous.

Applying the costs for individual problems to the population of youth who are involved in multiple problem behaviors gives a total cost to society of $335–350 billion for misbehavior in 1998. This represents 77–80% of the costs of the youth behavioral problems analyzed individually. This means that interrupting the life course of multiple problem youth is likely to have tremendous payoff for society. This payoff also translates into improved lives for these youth and the victims and family members they harm by their problems.

While this chapter provides reliable estimates of costs associated with youth problems and the costs associated with combinations of these problems, we make no claims that these are the final or only estimates possible. The implication of these estimates is that 1.5 million years of healthy life were lost, the equivalent of 63,000–66,500 young lives. In sum, the total cost to society for youth problems, the substantial amount of this cost accounted for by youth who engage in multiproblem behavior, and the great burden these problems represent show the import of multiproblem youth.

From a public policy perspective, these cost estimates provide strong support for the importance of investing in reducing these problems. Investing can lower both the costs associated with problem behaviors during adolescence and the longer-term costs when these behaviors persist into adulthood.

4

Influences on the Development of Multiple Problems

When we last left Michael, he was 19 and just out of jail. We also know that by age 8, he was already showing some real problems with aggressive behavior. However, his problems started long before that. Michael's mother worked throughout her pregnancy to help her husband support their other three children. Her job in a local deli was fast-paced and stressful. She and her coworkers enjoyed their cigarette breaks, although she tried to cut down to only one pack a day during her pregnancy.

Michael was born prematurely. When he was a toddler, his mother found it hard to cope with his frenetic activity level, inability to obey, and aggression. Maybe if she had been able to stay home, hadn't fought with Michael's father over his drinking and job loss, and didn't have four children to raise, she would have been better able to deal consistently with Michael. In fact, she was often worried and for a time took medication for depression. Michael's father was home more often when he was out of work, and he and Michael's mom argued more about how to handle Michael. They found fault with almost everything that he did and frequently yelled at him. Michael discovered very early that if he cried or threw a fit, his parents might back down. Causing trouble with his siblings also succeeded in getting his parents' attention. When yelling did not work, hitting did the trick.

In kindergarten, Michael found it hard to stay in his seat, which irritated his teacher. He tried his usual strategy of yelling and even hit her once. Not surprisingly, he was sent into the hallway more days than not. Soon he noticed that he could not read as well as the other kids. They laughed when he tried to read aloud and he reacted to their teasing by getting back at them. Eventually, other kids began to leave Michael alone. His only friend was another boy who also got into trouble a lot.

As he got older, Michael did badly in school, although he did advance from elementary to middle school. At home, things changed after his dad left. His mother occasionally yelled at him, but her interest in disciplining him began to slip away. Because his mother worked two jobs, Michael was alone after school and tended to wander around the neighborhood. This was not a close neighborhood with people watching out for each other; most people were in transit, in search of a better place to live. On the street, Michael watched the older kids, who hung out together and smoked. He kept his distance though, because one kid threatened him with a knife when Michael asked for a cigarette. He still bought cigarettes occasionally from a local convenience store, where the clerk believed that they were for his mother.

When Michael entered middle school, it did not take long before he was spending time in detention. As he connected with the other kids, he encountered new temptations. One day on the way home from school, these other kids offered him alcohol in exchange for some cigarettes. It was easy for these kids to get beer from the older kids, who bought it at a local shop where the employees never checked to see if they were of legal age. He began to hang around with these kids, although he sometimes fought with them and found them hard to deal with. When drinking, he felt better and worried less about his trouble in school.

One afternoon, Michael and his friends skipped class to drink in the parking lot of the liquor store. Two police officers drove up, threatened to arrest them, and took them to their homes. Michael's mother was at work, but one of the officers called her and told her about the incident. She assured the officer that she would handle the situation. When she came home, she yelled at Michael for embarrassing her, he responded by swearing, and she threw a hairbrush at him. He retaliated by slapping her face. She ran into the bedroom to get away from him, but the next day, she seemed to have forgotten the whole thing. Michael met his friends as usual in a neighborhood parking lot; he joked about what had happened with his mother and they all laughed. They had the whole weekend ahead of them and it looked like it would be a fun one.

Our biography of Michael shows some of the risk factors that influence the life trajectory of children who end up in trouble. In this chapter, we present a systematic framework for understanding these influences. They occur at many levels, from the individual to the community, and often build on one another over time. All along the way, there are crucial turning points that can accelerate or diminish a young person's development of problems. Understanding these influences is vital for understanding how we might prevent problem development.

In our review, we attempt to capture the complex, interactive nature of risk for multiple problem outcomes in youth. As Wachs (2000) stated, "Whether one is involved in research, intervention, or public policy, we need behavioral models of theoretical causal sequences and intervention strategies that honor existing complexities that underlie individual human behavioral developmental variability. Through an understanding of these complexities, we will be better able to promote both competence and resilience for a greater number of individuals" (p. 334).

Few studies have systematically examined how risk and protective factors contribute to youth having *multiple* problems. Rather, they have typically focused on studying influences on a single problem. This strategy is not consistent with the fact that most youth with one problem have a number of others. It likely stems from the fact that most research on youth problems has been funded by agencies that are focused on only one or a few of the problems. Yet, as we showed in Chapter 2, many teens that develop one behavior problem also develop others. Therefore, studies of "delinquent" teens also include large numbers of participants who smoke, use alcohol or drugs, and engage in risky sexual behavior. Not surprisingly, therefore, many of the same risk factors emerge in studies of these supposedly different populations.

As a result, we have attempted to identify factors shown to influence the development of more than one of the problems we are discussing. In most cases, all we can say is that the factor appears to contribute to a number of different problems, but we cannot be sure that it necessarily makes all problems more likely in a given individual. We need further research to determine which factors contribute to problems in isolation and which contribute to the development of multiple behavior problems.

At the same time, consistent findings that similar risk factors underlie various youth behaviors suggest that preventive and treatment intervention programs focusing on these particular risks will be more useful and cost-effective than those focusing on risk factors unique to one problem or another. One potential benefit is that ameliorating these risks may prevent different problem behaviors in different children. Alternatively, these preventive and treatment intervention efforts may be particularly useful in preventing multiple problems in the same individual. Given that multiple-problem adolescents (and boys in particular) are responsible for a large share of criminal outcomes and mental health services needs in the United States (Loeber, Farrington, Stouthamer-Loeber, & Van Kammen, 1998a), prevention and intervention efforts aimed at this group should provide us with substantial payoff over time.

A LIFE COURSE DEVELOPMENTAL PERSPECTIVE

As indicated in Chapter 1, we examine risks using a life course developmental perspective (Baltes et al., 1980). This perspective examines the child's biological, cognitive, social, and emotional development in interaction with the environment. It also emphasizes the changing societal expectations for the child's behavior as he or she develops. Kellam and his colleagues linked these social task expectations to proximal social fields (i.e., immediate social situations or experiences; Kellam, 1990; Kellam & Rebok, 1992). Cultural and historical norms also have a large influence on how we expect children to behave at any phase in development.

A central issue in the study of development is how a child's characteristics at any given point contribute to later development. Elder and Caspi (1988) describe two mechanisms by which problem behavior at one point may contribute to growing difficulties. First, "interactional continuity" involves the child's negative behavior contributing to others withdrawing their demands, thereby rewarding and perpetuating the child's negative behavior. Second, "cumulative continuity" involves current behavior problems contributing to the development of further problems. For example, a child's negative behavior leads to rejection by well-adjusted peers, thus decreasing the child's exposure to positive peer influences while increasing his exposure to deviant peer influences.

This life course developmental perspective is not rigidly deterministic. Any given influence affects the probability of a behavior developing, but the existence of a given risk factor in the life of a child by no means guarantees that a problem will develop. We can think of risk factors as fluid characteristics altered by a person's behavior and by other factors in the environment (Zucker, Fitzgerald, & Moses, 1995).

We are concerned with protective factors as well as risk factors. Protective factors are assets that can offset or reduce the impact of risk factors. In particular, developmental transitions such as puberty or entry into the working world often provide turning points when a child enters or leaves a high- or low-risk trajectory. However, other unique events that occur outside the context of developmental transitions can also provide such turning points. For example, an antisocial boy might become attracted to a girl who is more socially conforming than he is. By socializing with her and her friends, he might be motivated to conform to societal rules and to control his antisocial behavior. Attention to potential protective factors (e.g., association with prosocial peers) will also guide us in our attempts to reduce the incidence and prevalence of youth problem behaviors.

Protective factors for youth problem behaviors that have been noted consistently include high intelligence, a resilient temperament, a close bond with a prosocial adult, and exposure to clear and consistent standards that prohibit aggression and substance use (Catalano & Hawkins, 1995). Recent work on the study of developmental assets points to other potential, less well-examined protective factors (Scales & Leffert, 1999). These include exposure to a caring and supportive school climate, a community that values its youth, parents who have high expectations for the youth, and the youth's own feeling of control over his or her future. Although our focus is predominantly on risk factors, we acknowledge that attention to potential protective factors also has great relevance for the prevention of youth problem behaviors.

Intuitively, factors that promote positive development could also reduce the development of problems, and factors that impede problems may also promote positive development—but these possibilities have not been widely explored in the context of the development of the problems that concern us here. Until researchers in the "assets" and "problems" camps come together to examine problems and assets conjointly, they will continue to base these speculations on intuition rather than on evidence.

A Note on Gender and Ethnicity

Researchers have devoted less attention to girls than to boys in studying the emergence of the behavior problems addressed in this book. Researchers commonly examine etiological factors in samples containing both boys and girls. They then report, "There were no gender differences." We treat this conclusion with some skepticism, especially in cases in which the study samples were small. Simply finding that boys and girls do not differ "on average" in some risk factor does not mean that the risk factor operates the same way for boys and girls. Physical aggression and alcohol abuse are far less frequent in girls than in boys. Thus, researchers need larger samples in order to obtain the statistical power necessary to accurately assess whether the relationships between risk factors and negative outcomes differ for girls versus boys.

As pointed out in Chapter 1, researchers have noted differences in the rates across ethnic groups for youth problem behaviors such as cigarette smoking, alcohol use, weapon-related violence, and sexual intercourse (e.g., Blum et al., 2000). However, as Blum et al. (2000) point out, ethnic group differences tell us little about the social or environmental forces that determine behavioral outcomes in youth from different ethnic groups. We agree with their argument that there is little utility in focusing exclusively on variables such as race and gender. We cannot modify these variables and, in fact, they are only "markers" for possible forces that operate on child development. More complex, process-oriented analyses that look at how risk factors operate within and across ethnic and gender groups will ultimately give us more information that is useful in our attempts to reduce adolescent risk behaviors.

Attention to ethnic differences in the context of more complex developmental processes is likely to be beneficial in terms of prevention and intervention. For example, ethnic differences in youth problem behaviors suggest that factors that differentially affect ethnic groups might be important risk factors for particular youth problem behaviors. Members of an ethnic minority group may be at higher biological and psychological risk (e.g., poor prenatal and medical care and lack of psychological and social services), as well as increased stress exposure resulting from prejudice and discrimination. Ethnicity is also associated with proximal factors such as teacher expectations for achievement. We may make a correlation (through segregation and discrimination in the work force) with disorganized neighborhoods and less shared responsibility for monitoring neighborhood children (Wachs, 2000). Moreover, ethnic differences are not fully separable from cultural differences, which in turn may influence the relationship between proximal risk factors and youth behavior problems. Lack of attention to these cultural influences will hamper the implementation and ultimate success of prevention efforts.

Given this perspective, a caveat is in order. As with gender, relatively little information is available about ethnicity as it relates to risk-outcome relationships (especially in the context of the development of multiple behavior problems), although we present information whenever it is available. Perhaps researchers feel that considering these issues can lead only to harmful outcomes for ethnic minority groups. We believe the opposite; that is, careful consideration of these issues can lead to more culturally appropriate interventions that produce better outcomes for ethnic minority groups. How risk and protective factors play out and which ones predominate in the development of multiple behavior problems in girls and in diverse samples warrants further study (Foster & Martinez, 1995).

Risks Often Travel in Packs

Risk factors tend to cluster. For example, antisocial alcoholic men are more likely to become partners with antisocial and alcoholic women (Jacob & Leonard, 1986; Zucker, Ellis, Bingham, Fitzgerald, & Sanford, 1996), increasing the chances that they will have difficulty socializing their children. Antisocial alcoholism is also associated with downward social mobility (Zucker, Ellis, Bingham, & Fitzgerald, 1996), and offspring in these families, even early in life, are developmentally more disadvantaged; they have more learning disabilities and intellectual deficits than do offspring from alcoholic but not antisocial families (Poon, Ellis, Fitzgerald, & Zucker, 2000). Whether some of these factors cause others is not well understood. Nonetheless, as these factors continue to accumulate, they can interact and propel the child toward the development of later problems.

The fact that risks "travel in packs" complicates efforts to understand and deal with risk factors. For example, when family conflict, association with deviant peers, and poor academic performance occur together, teens are particularly likely to begin using drugs early and to use a greater quantity of illegal substances (Duncan et al., 1998). It is difficult to be sure how these factors interact to produce problems, and it is a greater challenge to address each factor when it occurs in the context of the other factors. Other findings indicate a linear association between the number of risk factors to which a child is exposed and negative behavioral outcomes (Rutter, 1979; Sameroff, 1998, 2001). This implies that youth with multiple problems are likely to encounter numerous, intertwined risk factors, all of which probably need to be addressed.

Risk factors may also nest within each other. For example, poor parental monitoring appears more likely in socially disorganized neighborhoods (Sampson & Raudenbush, 1999). This nesting has important implications for intervention. Several levels of environmental factors may need altering in order to reduce the risk for multiple-problem outcomes. We should expect that if one risk factor for youth problem behavior exists, it is more likely that other risk factors will be present. Treatment or prevention efforts will be particularly challenging in these circumstances.

RISK FACTORS THROUGHOUT DEVELOPMENT

The remainder of this chapter describes the influences that shape behavior problems throughout the lifespan of children and adolescents. Although we introduce and discuss a risk factor in the first developmental phase during which it becomes relevant, most factors occur and are potent across several phases of development. Different factors, however, may have different effects on behavior, depending on the developmental phase in which they occur. We attempt to capture this point in Table 4.1, in which we present the important risk factors for each developmental phase and list risk factors across all relevant phases.

PRENATAL AND PERINATAL DEVELOPMENT

The earliest phase of human development occurs within the mother's womb. The growth of the body and the central nervous system are its

TABLE 4.1. Major Risk Factors for the Development of Multiple Problem Behaviors

	Prenatal and perinatal	Infancy and early childhood	Middle childhood	Puberty and adolescence
Individual	Genetic predisposition	Genetic expression of risk traits Negative affect, impulsivity, and over/underarousability	Genetic expression of risk traits Negative affect, impulsivity, and over/underarousability Executive cognitive deficits	Genetic expression of risk traits Negative affect, impulsivity, and over/underarousability Early (girls) or late (boys) puberty
Family	Prenatal and perinatal complications, including maternal smoking, alcohol and drug use	Poor quality of mother–child interaction Parenting: Poor monitoring; parent–child conflict; harsh and inconsistent discipline	Parenting; poor monitoring; parent–child conflict; harsh and inconsistent discipline	Parenting; poor monitoring; parent–child conflict; harsh and inconsistent discipline
Peers			Poor peer relations/ rejection	Association with deviant peers
School			Academic difficulties	Transition to middle and high school

Neighborhood and community	Environmental stress	Environmental and psychosocial stress (e.g., violent events and discrimination)	Environmental and psychosocial stress (e.g., violent events and discrimination)	Environmental and psychosocial stress (e.g., violent events and discrimination)
		Presence/absence of public drinking and tobacco alcohol outlets	Physical availability of weapons/substances/ tobacco and alcohol outlets (e.g., density of outlets)	Availability of weapons/ substances/tobacco and alcohol outlets (e.g., density of outlets)
Economic	Poverty (inadequate nutrition)	Poverty (stimulus deprivation)	Poverty (neighborhood disorganization)	Poverty (neighborhood disorganization)
		Concentration of tobacco and alcohol outlets	Economic availability of tobacco and alcohol (low prices and low cost to acquire)	Economic availability of tobacco and alcohol (low prices and low cost to acquire)
			Cost of weapons	Cost of weapons
				Poor job opportunities

most salient characteristics. Growth, migration, and differentiation of cells are the core features of development in the brain. From the first trimester of pregnancy through infancy, the body overproduces neurons and the connections between them. Then a pruning process occurs that lasts at least through adolescence. Each of these aspects of brain growth is crucial to optimal, overall brain functioning.

It is important to note that the mother's womb (and hence the fetus) exists in—and is highly affected by—familial, community, and economic circumstances (Brown, 1999). For example, animal studies have demonstrated that malnutrition during prenatal development relates to reductions in cortical volume and number of cortical synapses in the fetal brain (Levitsky & Strupp, 1995).

Genetic Influences

Current knowledge concerning gene expression of complex behavior patterns (traits)—such as the ones that concern us here—indicates that genes, the network of intermediate traits that they influence, and the environmental contexts that dampen or enhance their expression interact in complicated ways during the entire lifespan (Sing, Haviland, Templeton, Zerba, & Reilly, 1992). The expression of genes and the development of the cells of the brain and nervous system depend on the actions of hormones, neurotransmitters, and growth factors, which, in turn, are influenced by the environment in which we develop (Gottlieb, 2000; Sing, Haviland, & Reilly, 1996).

Michael—whose mother is poor, is in a stressful marriage, and has few friends—may develop differently in the womb than a genetically identical Michael whose mother had a comfortable income, a happy marriage, and adequate social support. These differences are due evidently to different patterns of hormonal secretions and other chemical responses to social stressors. In addition, it is important to recognize that genetic risk does not always operate in the same manner across different stages of life; genes may express themselves in a measurable way at one age but may not play any role at another.

Some genetic aberrations, regardless of environment, appear to predict a different course and outcome for a developing fetus. For example, chromosome defects can lead to disorders such as fragile X and Down syndrome. These direct gene-to-outcome relationships are typically quite rare and are attributable to single gene effects. However, genetic research on youth problem behaviors such as serious antisocial behavior, smoking, risky sexual behavior, and alcohol and drug misuse has not revealed any one-to-one correspondence between a particular genetic defect and the occurrence of one or more of these behaviors. In fact, these behavioral syndromes are virtually certain to be the product of multiple genes, operating in interaction with environments that affect the manner and timing of their expression. Such disorders are referred to as complex genetic disorders or, alternatively, in the language of medical genetics, as "multifactorial diseases."

Evidence for genetic contributions in the development of problem behaviors comes from studies of twins and of adoption (e.g., Cadoret, Cain, & Grove, 1980; Kendler, Karkowski, Neale, & Prescott, 2000). These findings are not surprising in light of what we now know about genetic influences on the development of physiology and about physiological influences on behavior. Because our genetic makeup shapes our brain and physiology, at some level it must also shape our behavior. Yet, equally important, the awareness that these disorders have complex genetic influences as well as complex environmental and learned components is essential to our understanding of their causal structure (cf. Cloninger & Gottesman, 1987). If we divide the "pie" of risk factors for youth problem behaviors, genes are one portion of that pie and social environmental effects comprise other portions. However, the interactions between these involved genes and the environment contribute to individuality and to the development of the multiproblem youth.

What does it mean, then, that genetic influences exist for youth problem behaviors? Is this knowledge of any use to us in planning interventions for these youth problems? We think that information about genetic influences makes several contributions. First, it may help to refine our understanding of how problems develop. For example, it can clarify the precise way in which children become vulnerable to environmental influences. This may help us to pinpoint precisely when and why environmental factors have their effects, which may refine our ability to ameliorate the effects of environmental risk factors. Second, we may be better able to define subgroups of young people who are vulnerable to environmental risk factors based on genetic screening. Finally, we may be able to identify pharmacological interventions that can prevent or ameliorate the effects of environmental risk factors.

Exposure to Teratogens and Stress

Aspects of the mother's behaviors and her social environment are also risk factors for youth problem behaviors during the prenatal phase. One maternal behavior that affects youth outcomes is cigarette smoking during pregnancy. Smoking during pregnancy predicts the development of conduct disorder in boys (Wakschlag et al., 1997), early onset of arrests in African American males (Gibson, Piquero, & Tibbetts, 2000), and persistent criminal behavior in males (Brennan, Grekin, & Mednick,

1999). Weissman and colleagues linked it to substance abuse in adolescent girls (Weissman, Warner, Wickramaratne, & Kandel, 1999) and Brennan and colleagues to hospitalization for substance abuse in men and women later in life (Brennan, Grekin, Mortensen, & Mednick, 2002). Not surprisingly, researchers have also linked maternal tobacco smoking during pregnancy to offspring tobacco smoking (Griesler, Kandel, & Davies, 1998; Isohanni, Moilanen, & Rantakallio, 1991). Researchers have attempted to control for a variety of potential confounds that could explain these associations (e.g., fathers' criminal behavior, mothers' alcohol use during pregnancy, socioeconomic status, inadequate parenting processes, and low birthweight; Brennan et al., 1999; Fergusson, Woodward, & Horwood, 1998; Wakschlag et al., 1997; Weissman et al., 1999). Despite these statistical controls, the maternal smoking–offspring antisocial behavior relationship remains significant.

There are probably both biological and social reasons for the relationship between maternal smoking during pregnancy and youth problem behaviors. Genetics may play a role (Fergusson, 1999) and maternal neglect or maltreatment may increase risk for negative behaviors in some of these children (Chessare, Pascoe, & Baugh, 1986). Moreover, nicotine may have a direct effect on the developing brain. In animal studies, King (1996) found prenatal nicotine exposure related to changes in serotonin receptor sites and alterations in the vasopressin system. King and colleagues found these physiological changes, in turn, linked to aggressive behavior and substance abuse outcomes in both animals and humans. Thus, maternal cigarette smoking may set off a chain of biological and environmental factors that act together to increase risk for youth problem behaviors (King, 1996).

Researchers studied maternal stress during pregnancy in association with outcomes of serious mental health problems, such as schizophrenia (Huttunen & Niskanen, 1978). Recent animal studies on stress and early brain development suggest that maternal stress might also play a role in increasing risk for youth behavior problems such as aggression and substance abuse (Dawson, Ashman, & Carver, 2000; DeKloet, Korte, Rots, & Kruk, 1996). In rat populations, prenatal stress increases the response of the hypothalamus–pituitary–adrenal (HPA) axis, and specifically increases glucocorticoids, which can have harmful effects on the developing brain (Gunnar, 1998). Interestingly, these detrimental effects on the brain do not occur if the mother provides additional postbirth stimulation by stroking, grooming, or licking her newborn (Francis, Champagne, Liu, & Meaney, 1999). Thus, optimal or at least improved parenting skills may compensate for or undo the negative impact of prenatal stress in humans as well as in animals (Gunnar & Chisholm, 1999).

This interaction highlights the fact that physiological and neurological deficits or weaknesses do not translate directly into behavior problem development. Rather, the biological profiles of children provide different levels of challenge to parents and community caretakers. In cases in which parenting and caretaking adjust to these differing levels of physiological capabilities, we can prevent many of the potential deleterious behavioral outcomes. Unfortunately, genetic and physiological deficits are more likely to occur in social environments that are less than optimal (Moffitt, 1993; Zucker et al., 1995). The interplay of biological and social problems—more than either in isolation—likely increases the risk that vulnerable youth will display behavior problems such as delinquency and substance abuse.

INFANCY AND EARLY CHILDHOOD

Temperament

Research consistently shows that children largely inherit temperament (Goldsmith, Lemery, Buss, & Campos, 1999; Phillips & Matheny, Jr., 1997; Schmitz, Saudino, Plomin, Fulker, & DeFries, 1996). Thus, children show tendencies to be shy, aggressive, difficult to soothe, fearful, anxious, extroverted, introverted, and so forth in their elemental forms early in life (Houck, 1999). As the baby becomes a toddler, the manifestation of temperament becomes more complex and subjected to environmental influences, eventually forming a basis for what we typically think of as the individual's personality.

Temperamental traits that have been specifically associated with risk for delinquency and drug abuse include impulsivity, negative affect, extroversion, aggressiveness, high activity levels, risk taking, proneness to anger, and depression (Friedman, Granick, Bransfield, Kreisher, & Khalsa, 1995; Tarter et al., 1999). Biological and environmental factors contribute to the course and longevity of these characteristics. However, they remain somewhat stable throughout the lifespan in the absence of severe psychosocial or physical trauma. Interestingly, each of these traits has been associated with specific biological and physiological responses to environmental stimuli that appear to provide the foundation for their development. There is some evidence, nevertheless, that even these biological bases of behavior may be alterable given appropriate and targeted interventions (Raine et al., 2001).

From the earliest stages of development, the child's temperament influences his or her long-term behavioral outcomes. The infant does not develop in isolation, however, and the surrounding social environment in which he or she grows is highly influential in determining eventual youth behavioral functioning outcomes.

Mother–Infant Interactions

The family is the dominant social field that influences development during infancy and early childhood. Historical and cultural characteristics and economic conditions, in particular, influence family practices and behaviors, which in turn affect the developing child. One critical influence in this phase of development is the type of interaction that develops between the infant and his or her primary caregiver (Shonkoff & Phillips, 2000). A pattern of synchronous interactions in which the mother responds sensitively to the infant's needs results in what developmental psychologists call "secure attachment" (Ainsworth, Blehar, Waters, & Wall, 1978). This interaction pattern allows the mother, and later fathers and other adults, to help the infant develop cognitive and behavioral capacities that are essential to further development (DeWolff & van IJzendoorn, 1997). On the other hand, a pattern in which the mother is unresponsive to the child's emotional needs or is impatient and uncomforting can lead to insecure or disorganized attachment (Shonkoff & Phillips, 2000). Researchers link disorganized attachment in infancy to aggression in childhood (Lyons-Ruth, Easterbrook, & Cibelli, 1997), as well as to conduct disorders and substance abuse disorders in adolescence (Rosenstein & Horowitz, 1996). Walsh related adult retrospective reports of poor parental attachment to drug abuse and promiscuity (Walsh, 1995).

Stress, poverty, maternal smoking, maternal or paternal alcohol and illicit drug use and abuse, and maternal depression all reduce the likelihood that parents will provide effective care giving and that the child will develop secure attachment relationships. This probably occurs because each of these factors contributes to the mother being irritable or insensitive, to a child with a difficult temperament, or to both of these conditions (e.g., Eiden & Leonard, 1996; Eiden, Peterson, & Coleman, 1999). Expression of genetic factors may also play a role here by increasing the likelihood that some children will be difficult to soothe and that some mothers will be more easily irritated than others.

The quality of the mother–child interactions influences the role the child's temperament plays in the development of later problems. Having a difficult temperament as a youngster predicts diverse problems in childhood and adolescence. Specifically, Henry and his colleagues linked negative emotionality and poor behavioral control at age three to receiving convictions for violent crime during adolescence (Henry, Caspi, Moffitt, & Silva, 1996). Undercontrol at age 3 also predicts personality characteristics at age 18, which in turn predict an increased likelihood of alcohol dependence, risky sexual behavior, and violent crime at age 21 (Caspi et al., 1997). We cannot completely disentangle this from parenting, however. Infants whose temperaments are characterized as highly active, easily distressed, and difficult to comfort have an increased likelihood of eliciting insensitive care giving and developing disorganized patterns of attachment (Seifer, 2000).

Children with difficult temperaments clearly are more difficult to parent than children who are easy to soothe and can regulate negative affect more readily. Not surprisingly, then, the mother's skill at handling a difficult child influences how much a difficult temperament in infancy affects later development. Problematic development is more likely to occur when both the mother and infant display difficult patterns of behavior, as with Michael's case outlined at the beginning of this chapter. Bates, Pettit, Dodge, and Ridge (1998) found that a resistant temperament predicts later behavior problems only in families with poor parental control and not in families with high parental control. Similarly, temperament difficulties in children are significantly more likely to be associated with later delinquency and aggression when parents suffer from alcoholism and antisocial behavior themselves (Wong, Zucker, Puttler, & Fitzgerald, 1999).

Parenting behaviors appear to be the crucial moderating factor here. In high-risk families, temperament problems in children lead to negative parent–child interactions and these parent–child interactions then contribute to an increased risk for delinquency and aggression. These findings imply that we might prevent the development of difficult mother–infant interactions and insecure attachment by intervening to help parents learn effective patterns of care giving and ways of coping with factors that contribute to insensitive care giving. Parents of children with difficult temperaments may be most in need of this assistance.

Coercive Family Processes

Coercive interactions involve patterns in which one family member engages in behavior that is aversive to another family member, the other responds in an aversive way, and the aversive behavior of the second person prompts the first person to desist from being aversive. For example, Michael learned very early that yelling or hitting was quite effective at getting his mother to withdraw her demands. We call this process negative reinforcement (Patterson, Reid, & Dishion, 1992). Careful and extensive studies in which observers coded family interactions in the homes of families with aggressive youngsters indicate that family members achieve frequent, albeit brief, respites from the aversive behavior of other family members by behaving aversively themselves (Patterson & Dishion, 1985, 1988; Patterson, Reid, & Dishion, 1998). Aversive behaviors on the part of parents include requests to do chores, commands, criticism, and scolding. Aversive behaviors of the child include whining, crying, refusing to follow requests, ignoring, pouting, hitting, yelling, and criticizing the parent.

Human beings are sensitive to environmental contingencies. Both rewarding and aversive events that follow behavior influence the future probability of that behavior for both children and adults. Thus, an irritable, whiny 3-year-old quickly learns that whining has the reinforcing effect of decreasing her mother's request for compliance (e.g., "Pick up your dirty clothes"). Similarly, when the parent withdraws the request, the child's whining ceases. This in turn reinforces the parent's withdrawal of the demand because it allows the parent to escape the whining (which to most adults is aversive). Over time, children learn that such behavior can—and does—influence the behavior of their parents and others who interact with them.

Parenting practices play a major role in sustaining and increasing aggressive behavior throughout childhood. The child's and the parent's biological predispositions may influence the likelihood of negative parent–child interactions as well. For example, a child might have an irritable temperament resulting from genetic factors or prenatal trauma that shapes parents' harsh and inconsistent style (Shonkoff & Phillips, 2000). In these instances, a synergy is likely to make the problems both more severe and more intractable.

It may be that harsh and inconsistent parenting contributes to children's aggressive behavior only for children with problematic temperaments. We note this caveat because substantial evidence suggests that a cluster of child temperament characteristics relating to impulsivity (quickness of response), negative affectivity (i.e., irritability), and impertinence are early precursors of aggressive behavior as well as long-term adolescent and adult outcomes involving violence, alcohol dependence, dangerous driving, and risky sexual behavior (Caspi et al., 1997). The earlier the appearance of these manifestations of behavioral undercontrol, the more reasonable it is to posit a biologically driven link. At the same time, the literature we have just reviewed, as well as the work we describe later, suggests that environments that either facilitate or dampen these biologically based characteristics play a major role in whether these early vulnerabilities sustain themselves into adolescence and adulthood.

Childcare

In 1995, according to the U.S. Census Data Report, there were about 9.5 million children under age 5 in a childcare setting before entering elementary school. This number represents 48.5% of children under 5. It includes center-based childcare, Head Start, and family childcare. The U.S. Census Bureau estimates that children under 5 spend an average of 19.5 hours per week in childcare. Preschoolers (3–5 years old) spend an average of 28 hours per week in childcare (U.S. Census Bureau, 1995).

The characteristics of these settings have an influence on the development of problem behavior. Children who receive poor-quality childcare with high levels of problem behavior and poor caregiver–child relationships have been found to be higher on aggressiveness and disruptive behavior as late as second grade (Howes, 1988; Peisner-Feinberg et al., 1999; Peisner-Feinberg et al., 2001). However, a close relationship between a childcare provider and the child is associated with fewer behavior problems in preschool through second grade, especially among children whose mothers have fewer years of education (Peisner-Feinberg et al., 1999, 2001). Phillips, McCartney, & Scarr (1987) found that the quality of childcare accounted for a significant amount of the variance in child sociability, even when family background and time in childcare were controlled for. The experience of the center director predicted child aggression and hyperactivity, as well as sociability.

In a study that generated some controversy (National Institute of Child Health and Human Development Early Child Care Research Network, 2001), it was found that the number of hours in childcare was positively related to caregiver reports of children's aggressive behavior at 24 and 36 months. However, positive care giving in childcare related negatively to both caregiver reports and observations of children's aggression. Given the huge proportion of children in childcare, the most important implication of this study would seem to be that it is important to ensure high-quality care.

Investigators have detected the deleterious effects of poor childcare in adolescence. Two studies have shown that quality childcare in early childhood can reduce the likelihood of pregnancy during adolescence (Campbell, Ramey, Pungello, Sparling, & Miller-Johnson, 2002; Schweinhart, Berrueta-Clement, Barnett, Epstein, & Weikart, 1985). Researchers found effects for delinquency (Schweinhart et al., 1985) and substance use (Campbell et al., 2002).

Economics and Parenting

Throughout childhood, parents invest in their children by spending time with them and by purchasing goods and services such as books, schooling, and medical care to promote their optimal development. In formal economic models, this investment process is described by a household production function, where an output called "child quality" is produced by combining inputs of parental time and purchased market goods. One general insight based on economic models is that teen mothers and parents in disadvantaged economic conditions face economic environments that discourage or impede investments in positive child outcomes. This general insight is supported by Weinberg's work (Weinberg, 2001) demonstrating that lower socioeconomic status results in direct limits on monetary incentives that can be used to influence children's behavior, as well as increased reliance on other incentives such as corporal punishment.

It is easy to see the connection between economic hardships and other, more proximal, risk factors for youth behavior problems. Economic hardship can create stress and malnutrition in the prenatal and postnatal environments. We have already discussed the potential negative consequences of inadequate nutrition on prenatal brain development. Inadequate nutrition after birth can also reduce the infant's exploratory behavior and response to the environment, which in turn might lead to fewer enriched person–environment interactions and further detriments to brain development (Wachs, 2000). Stress can also have detrimental effects on the development of the brain during infancy, and on behavioral outcomes later in childhood. For example, children exposed to early environmental stress are more likely to respond to later stresses with conduct problems (Werner & Smith, 1982) than those not exposed to earlier stress.

Attachment to parents moderates the relationship between early stressors (e.g., institutional rearing in orphanages) and later physiological stress sensitivity (Gunnar & Chisholm, 1999). Just as the behavior of mothers of rat pups could ameliorate the stresses that their infants had experienced, positive parent–child interactions can overcome the effects of early environmental stressors. Unfortunately, some evidence suggests that difficult work conditions and economic hardship can have detrimental effects on parenting as well (McLoyd, 1995; Whitbeck et al., 1997), making it less likely that positive parenting will compensate for or protect against the effects of stressors.

MIDDLE CHILDHOOD

The beginning of elementary school marks the beginning of middle childhood. It is the point at which instruction in reading and math begins in earnest (though a good preschool will already have started children on these skills). It is also a point at which peer interactions become increasingly important (Kellam, 1990). At the same time, the family remains an important social field, and school, family, and peer group act in conjunction to shape the child development.

Many of the youth problem behaviors that concern us begin to appear during the last part of this phase of development. Although a small percentage of children engage in serious delinquent behavior, substance use, or sexual intercourse prior to age 10, those who do have much greater risk for a variety of long-term negative outcomes than youth who begin these behaviors during the teenage years. Early onset of tobacco and alcohol use increases the risk for substance abuse in later childhood and in adulthood (Grant & Dawson, 1997; Lewinsohn, Rohde, & Brown, 1999).

The Significance of Early Aggressive Behavior

Aggressive behavior is a particularly important risk factor for later problem development. It increases the risk for later youth problem behaviors, including early sexual behavior, persistent delinquency, tobacco use, alcohol abuse, and drug abuse in males (Brook, Cohen, Whiteman, & Gordon, 1992; Kellam, Brown, Rubin, & Ensminger, 1983; Lipsey & Derzon, 1998; Robins & McEvoy, 1990; Tremblay & Schaal, 1996), and cigarette smoking, marijuana use, and early pregnancy in females (Woodward & Fergusson, 1999).

Table 4.2 illustrates this point. It shows when aggression, drug and alcohol use, tobacco smoking, and sexual activity commonly begin to occur among children and adolescents. Aggressive behavior begins in early childhood, whereas smoking and alcohol use usually do not occur until middle childhood, and marijuana and other drug use and sexual behavior typically do not occur until early adolescence or later. In addition, as noted earlier, early-onset aggression tends to persist over time and to be associated with other, later behavior problems of multiple types. These characteristics make early aggressive behavior a potentially important focal point for early intervention programs.

In work done especially for this volume, Derzon did a meta-analysis of studies of the relationships between aggressive behavior and later behavior problems. He found that in studies of aggressive children between the ages of 0 and 9, aggressive behavior predicted (1) later aggressive and disruptive behavior before 9 (mean correlation = .54) and at 10–14 (.42); (2) criminal offenses before 9 (.40) and at 10–14 (.24); (3) serious offenses, violence, or selling drugs at ages 15–18 (.15); (4) recidivism at 15–18 (.19); (5) cigarette use at 15–18 (1.4); (6) alcohol use at 15–18 (.14); (7) binge drinking at 15–18 (.18); and (8) marijuana use at 10–14 (.29) and 15–18 (.14).

Patterson, Forgatch, Yoerger, and Stoolmiller (1998) reported the rate of arrest among boys who were above the median on a multimethod measure of aggressive social behavior in grade 4. They had a .46 probability of arrest before age 14, while the rate among those below the

TABLE 4.2. Developmental Emergence of Multiple Problem Behaviors

Prenatal and perinatal	Infancy and early childhood	Middle childhood	Puberty and early adolescence	Adolescence
	Aggression	Aggression	Aggression	Aggression
		Tobacco use	Tobacco use	Tobacco use
		Alcohol use	Alcohol use	Alcohol use
			Other drug use	Other drug use
			Sexual behavior	Sexual behavior

median was .056 and the overall rates was .257. Thus, 80% of arrests were attributable to those above the median in fourth-grade aggression (.257 − .056)/ .257 = .80)

Patterson, Debaryshe, and Ramsey (1989) provide an explanation of why aggressive behavior contributes so powerfully to the development of diverse problems. Children who enter school with aggressive behavior problems have a significant chance of academic failure and peer rejection (Walker, Colvin, & Ramsey, 1995). Children exposed to numerous coercive encounters in the family arrive at school with highly practiced sets of aggressive behavior for interacting with teachers and peers. They are less likely to follow teachers' instructions and more likely to challenge them, making it more difficult to establish good relationships with their teachers. This makes it less likely that they will learn basic academic skills such as reading (Kellam & Anthony, 1998). As they fall behind academically, their disruptive classroom behavior escalates, leading to more negative interactions with teachers that may have the indirect effect of undermining parental involvement in school due to their negative interactions with school personnel (e.g., receiving multiple calls that their child is disruptive). At the same time, their aggressive behavior toward peers makes it more likely that peers will reject them. This can mean that they have few friends—at least among young people who would support the development of social skills and prosocial behavior. As a result, they are likely to become friends with other rejected children and thereby form deviant peer groups. Such peer groups appear to be the final training ground (Patterson et al., 1989) for a wide variety of problematic behaviors.

Of course, as the correlations presented previously show, aggressive behavior in childhood is by no means a guarantee of future trouble. Many aggressive children will not go on to develop other problems and early onset aggression will not characterize all multiple problem youth. Therefore, early aggression cannot be the sole target of early intervention, but it would appear to be exceedingly unwise to ignore it.

Academic Problems

Intellectual deficits also contribute to academic difficulties in some of these youths. Individuals with an IQ at the 33rd or lower percentile in early childhood have a threefold increase in risk for later conduct problems (Moffitt, 1990; Schonfeld, Shaffer, O'Connor, & Portnoy, 1988). Lynam and colleagues found a negative relationship between IQ and delinquency across different ethnic groups, apparent when race, class, and test motivation are statistically controlled (Lynam, Moffitt, & Stouthamer-Loeber, 1993).

Low IQ scores may reflect general or specific cognitive difficulties. Neuropsychological evidence suggests that specific deficits in executive cognitive function are especially potent risk factors for later conduct problems, overt aggression, and substance abuse (Moffitt, 1990; Moffitt, Lynam, & Silva, 1994; Pihl & Peterson, 1991; Schonfeld et al., 1988). Executive function deficits include poor ability to plan, difficulty in inhibiting behaviors, difficulty in sustaining attention, and deficits in verbal processing. Deckel and Hesselbrock (1996) linked executive cognitive dysfunction prospectively to alcohol consumption in high-risk youth and Glantz and Leshner (2000) linked it to drug abuse. The significant relationship between executive functioning deficits and aggressive behavior may also explain the high comorbidity rates noted for conduct disorder and attention-deficit/hyperactivity disorder (ADHD). Low arousability of the nervous system characterizes hyperactivity and ADHD, in particular, in the area of the brain that is responsible for higher-order cognitive skills and behavioral inhibitions. When ADHD exists with patterns of serious aggression and disruptive behavior, the likelihood for later conduct problems and substance abuse increases substantially (Chilcoat & Breslau, 1999; Disney, Elkins, McGue, & Iacono, 1999).

Executive functioning deficits noted in elementary school children may initially result from, or might reflect, physiological causes. These deficits can also reflect early parenting that involved less use of language, less provision of learning experiences (e.g., fewer books, age-appropriate games, or work spaces for the children), or some combination of genetic/biological predispositions and environmental stimulation. Regardless of the causes, however, children with poor academic skills will be more challenging to teach effectively, just as children with poor behavioral skills are particularly difficult to manage at home and at school. Unfortunately, these problems interact: Children who are hard to manage may fail to learn the essential academic skills on which future lessons build, and children who fall behind may be increasingly frustrated by academic demands they cannot meet. When teachers and school systems lack the resources to break this cycle in mainstream classrooms, children may experience repeated failure or may be tracked into special education classes or classes for the behaviorally disordered. As noted later, classroom clustering of children in this manner is likely to perpetuate the same problem behaviors that it is attempting to control (Kellam, Ling, et al., 1998).

Peer Relations

Peer relationships assume increasing importance as the child matures in middle childhood. As noted previously, children who enter elementary school with poorly developed skills for coping with social situations may find it difficult to make friends. Children are particularly likely to reject their aggressive and disruptive classmates (Newcomb, Bukowski, & Pattee, 1993). These children also have impoverished cognitive skills for thinking through problem situations (Crick & Dodge, 1994). Aggressive children, particularly boys, justify their aggressive behavior and see ambiguous situations as motivated by hostile intent of others (Crick & Dodge, 1994). When rejected children make friends, their companions are likely to be younger children or similarly rejected peers (George & Hartmann, 1996; Ladd, 1983). This aggregation of rejected children not only exposes children to others with similar negative interaction styles but also restricts their opportunities to learn better social and problem-solving skills by observing and interacting with their more skilled peers.

Exposure to peers who display deviant behavior has important negative effects, as we will see in discussions of adolescence. These negative effects begin early. One large school-based study has found that boys who were rated by their teachers as highly aggressive in first grade and who were in first-grade classrooms with high general levels of overt aggression were significantly more likely than controls to be rated as highly aggressive in sixth grade (Kellam, Ling, et al., 1998). Interestingly, for girls, if they were aggressive in the first grade they were likely to be aggressive in the sixth grade, regardless of the general level of aggressiveness in the classroom.

Exposure to Trauma

Traumatic experiences can and do occur with unfortunate frequency during childhood. Correlational data suggest that experiences of one form of trauma—sexual abuse—during childhood often lead to risky sexual behavior (Pierre, Shrier, Emans, & DuRant, 1998), conduct disorder (Lynskey & Fergusson, 1997), cigarette smoking (Acierno et al., 2000), and alcohol and other substance abuse (Kilpatrick et al., 2000) during adolescence. There is some disagreement, however, over whether associated risk factors such as inadequate parenting or low socioeconomic status might better explain these relationships (Rind & Tromovitch, 1997). Given the potentially complex effects of a variety of stressors on physiological and psychological functioning, further attention and study seem warranted concerning the process by which child sexual abuse victimization may increase the risk for multiple problem behaviors in adolescence.

Media Influences

Huesmann, Moise, and Podolski (1997) reviewed the evidence that children are exposed to a heavy diet of media, including television, movies, videos, video games, radio, music CDs and videos, and the Internet. They found estimates that children between the ages of 10 and 11 watch about 28 hours of television a week and that teens watch about 23.5 hours (Comstock & Paik, 1991, as cited by Huesmann et al., 1997). Less evidence is available on exposure to other forms of media, but one study showed that 67% of girls and 90% of boys played video games and, for the boys, half of the games were violent (Funk, 1993, as cited by Huesmann et al., 1997).

Numerous experimental studies that manipulate young people's exposure to violent media have shown that exposure increases aggressive behavior (Huesmann et al., 1997). Correlational studies have shown repeatedly that young people who are more aggressive also view television that is more violent. Of course, this could be because the more aggressive youths prefer such media. However, other studies show that levels of exposure to violent media predict later aggressive and criminal behavior, even after controlling for initial levels of aggressive behavior. Researchers replicated the relationship between viewing habits and later aggression in elementary school children in the United States, Israel, Finland, and Poland (Huesmann et al., 1997). Nevertheless, cross-cultural comparisons with Japan reveal that the relationship between media violence and aggressive behavior is not a simple one-to-one correspondence. Japan has some of the highest levels of violence portrayed in its media and the lowest levels of violence in its society.

Of course, the media do not deliberately attempt to increase the rate of aggressive behavior in children. However, in the case of tobacco smoking, the media actually attempts to increase youth problem behavior in a direct and deliberate manner—through specific advertisements and promotions (Wakefield, Flay, Nichter, & Giovino, 2001). Advertising campaigns for particular cigarette brands increase adolescent use of the advertised brand more than they do for adults. Longitudinal studies have shown that a predilection for cigarette ads among 10- to 12-year-olds predicted initiation of smoking and choice of brand smoked, and that ownership of promotional items such as T-shirts, caps, and jackets predicted the initiation of smoking (Biener & Siegel, 2000; Pierce, Choi, Gilpin, Farkas, & Berry, 1998; Sargent et al., 2000).

ADOLESCENCE

Although G. Stanley Hall's characterization of adolescence as a period of storm and stress does not apply to everyone, it does characterize the lives of some children as they go through puberty (Arnett, 1999). The developmental phase of puberty includes hormonal changes, development of adult sex characteristics, onset of menstruation in girls, and physical growth spurts. These physical changes are accompanied by increased interest in dating and sexual relationships, greater parent–child conflict, and— among girls—increased depression (Paikoff & Brooks-Gunn, 1991; Wachs, 2000). Youths' cognitive capacities increase during the teenage years. Nevertheless, adolescents often fail to think in terms of their longer-term futures, and this makes them vulnerable to engaging in risky behaviors that may have serious consequences for their health and safety.

Indeed, during this phase of development, the majority of youth begin to engage in at least low levels of one of the risky behavior problems that concern us here (Huizinga et al., 1993). Why is it reasonably normative in the United States for adolescents to experiment with socially prohibited behaviors that—if taken to an extreme—cause great difficulties? One hypothesis involves a primary task of adolescence, which involves answering the question, "Who am I?" In struggling to establish an identity as separate from their parents, adolescents often want to be adults in their own right. According to the "development as action in context" model, adolescents attempt to gain control over their own development through their choice of peer groups, their dating relationships, and their entry into the work force (Silbereisen & Noack, 1988). What we have termed "youth problem behaviors" may have functional significance in this regard. Drinking, smoking, and early sexual activity might be seen as pseudo-adult behaviors; they permit adolescents to achieve their goal of adult identity formation (Siegel & Scovill, 2000) as well as to increase their perceived control over at least some aspects of their lives, which they feel are dominated by parents, teachers, and other adults. Furthermore, some teens report that substance use is a component of some of their preferred leisure activities, selected based on primary motivations for contact with peers and potential dating partners (Silbereisen & Noack, 1988).

Beginning in early adolescence, children's expectancies about the effects of alcohol also change. Whereas earlier in childhood they often associated negative outcomes with drinking, they now begin to appreciate positive expectancies as well—for example, they begin to see the social benefits of drinking (Miller, Smith, & Goldman, 1990). Indeed, several studies by Siegel and his colleagues (e.g., Siegel & Scovill, 2000) have shown that adolescents participate in risky behaviors not in proportion to the risks involved but, rather, in proportion to the perceived benefits.

Puberty and Hormones

Most people who read the phrase "puberty and hormones" instinctively think about the gonadal hormones—testosterone and estrogen. Indeed, some hypothesize that gonadal hormones increase youth problem behaviors in puberty. In particular, many consider testosterone a risk factor for overt aggression in males. This connection has intuitive appeal, especially as it would help to explain large gender differences noted in physically aggressive behavior. Research on testosterone in puberty, however, does not suggest a direct causal connection to physical aggression. That is, early-maturing, high-testosterone boys are not the most aggressive boys. Instead, research on hormonal changes of adolescence suggests that the timing of maturation relates to youth behavior problems in a more complex manner. Specifically, both early and late maturation have links to increased risk for problems, and these effects appear to be gender specific.

Contrary to what one might think, late pubertal maturation is associated with aggression in boys. Susman and her colleagues (Susman, Nottelmann, Dorn, Inoff-Germain, & Chrousos, 1988) elucidate this process by suggesting that, as adrenal hormones rise in response to stress in the environment, they may suppress the increase in gonadal hormones associated with the start of puberty. This suppression of gonadal hormones, in turn, results in delayed physical maturation. Delays in physical maturation can produce additional stressors (e.g., increased peer harassment due to being different from other boys his age), and the cycle continues. In this scenario, high levels of stress may be the relevant risk factor for increased aggression and acting out in late-maturing boys. Here, as described earlier, the interplay between the environment and biology—rather than either acting in isolation—appears crucial.

The picture is different for girls. Here, early maturation is a risk factor for delinquency, substance use, risky sexual behavior, and school dropout (Tarter et al., 1999), which likely result, in part, from environmental influences such as increased contact with peers involved in risky behavior (Silbereisen, Petersen, Albrecht, & Kracke, 1989), particularly males (Caspi, Lynam, Moffitt, & Silva, 1993). Later maturation appears to be a protective factor for girls in this regard. Interestingly, a recent prospective longitudinal study found that positive relationships in the family, and particularly positive father–daughter interactions, predicted later pubertal maturation in girls (Ellis, McFadyen-Ketchum, Dodge, Pettit, & Bates, 1999).

As they transition into adolescence, children often report that they get less pleasure from their standard daily activities than they did before (Larson & Richards, 1994). This might increase their desire to look for more stimulation and reward in the environment through high-risk activities and experimentation with drugs and alcohol (a functional basis of youth problem behavior). Once having received this positive stimulation from drugs and alcohol, teens exposed to high levels of stress may be particularly likely to continue to engage in risky behaviors. In a series of studies in rats, Goeders (2002) demonstrated that exposure to environmental stressors increased the reinforcing saliency of cocaine. If these results generalize to humans, they suggest that the immediate positive effects of risky behaviors may be particularly strong for those exposed to high levels of stress.

Continuing Genetic Influences

Many mistakenly believe that genetic factors affect the child early in the lifespan and that environmental effects replace those factors as the child gets older. In fact, the opposite has been found for intelligence and, perhaps, for antisocial behavior. That is, genetic influences may be stronger in adolescence than they are in childhood. Interestingly, a qualitative as well as a quantitative change in genetic factors occurs during adolescence: the genetic influences that affect antisocial behavior in early adolescence overlap with, but are not the same as, the genetic influences that affect antisocial behavior in later adolescence (Reiss & Neiderhiser, 2000).

Genetic factors may also play a role in relationships between environmental variables and adolescent outcomes (Harris, 1998; Reiss, Neiderhiser, Hetherington, & Plomin, 2000). For example, the correlations found between parenting behavior and child outcome could be due to genetic influences as well. Investigators assess the genetic effect on the relationship between two variables (e.g., mother's negativity and child antisocial behavior) by looking to see if the correlation between the variables gets larger among families with higher genetic similarity than in families that share little genetic similarity (e.g., families with an adopted child). If it does, then genetic influences may—at least in part—account for the increased association.

A recent study that employed this method concluded that genetic influences could almost entirely explain the relationship between harsh parenting and antisocial outcome in adolescence (Reiss et al., 2000). Yet, consider what "genetic influences" might mean in this context. It is possible that the genes for antisocial behavior increase antisocial acts in both the mother (in the form of harsh discipline) and the adolescent (in the form of aggression). It is also possible that the child's genetic makeup will evoke parental behaviors, which in turn influence the child's behavior (e.g., heritable temperament [irritability] provoking particular negative reactions [hostility] by mothers, which in turn makes the child more antisocial). Still another possibility is that genes may influence the child to seek out certain situations or activities in the environment (e.g., risky situations), which in turn influence both the child's level of aggression and the parent's disciplinary reactions. This is an example of gene activation. Each of these possibilities implies that the expression of genetic potential is alterable but suggests a somewhat different tack for prevention and intervention efforts. For example, a gene–environment correlation might indicate that some (and likely many) parents of antisocial adolescents will have difficulty in applying new parenting strategies—their own temperament being to their detriment.

Thus, we should not interpret any of these potential genetic influences to mean that the youth's behavior is unchangeable. In addition, most of these genetic influences involve substantial interaction with some environmental component. Relevant to this point is evidence that genetic and environmental factors appear to interact with one another in the prediction of early adolescent substance use (Legrand, McGue, & Iacono, 1999) and drug abuse (Cadoret, Troughton, O'Gorman, & Heywood, 1986). Previous adoption studies have noted that genetic influences are not deterministic. In other words, a nurturing and positive environment can overcome genetic risk.

Parenting Practices and Parent–Adolescent Interaction

Parents continue to serve an important role in youth behavior problems as children mature into adolescence, with parent monitoring and parent–adolescent communication becoming particularly important during this period. Teens increasingly engage in activities outside the home as they mature and spend many more hours with their peers. As we will see later, ample evidence suggests that association with aggressive, disruptive, or drug-using peers promotes more of the same during adolescence. Indeed, the high-risk behaviors that concern us here (drug, alcohol, and tobacco use; risky sex; and serious antisocial behavior) commonly occur in situations in which no adults are present.

It is not surprising, therefore, that parents who take an "out of sight, out of mind" approach to the teenage years set themselves up for trouble. While defined in several ways, parental monitoring has generally included the supervision of the child's activities. The parents ask where the child is, what the child is doing, and who is with the child. With this definition goes the assumption that parents who regularly monitor the child's whereabouts and activities will also limit the child's opportunities to participate in risky situations.

Research strongly supports the association between the absence of parental monitoring and diverse adolescent problem behaviors (Ary, Duncan, Duncan, & Hops, 1999; Duncan et al., 1998). Low rates of parental monitoring correlate with adolescent delinquent and disruptive behavior (Barber, 1996; Patterson & Dishion, 1985) as well as smoking and alcohol use (Dishion, French, & Patterson, 1995), both concurrently and longitudinally. Poor monitoring by parents also can lead to spending time with antisocial peers (Patterson & Dishion, 1985), which in turn increases the likelihood that a teenager will engage in antisocial or drug use activity. Parental monitoring is clearly an important influence on the behavior of teenagers.

Another aspect of family life that comes into play during early and mid-adolescence involves how families communicate about conflict. As children age, they increasingly seek autonomy and independence and wish to spend more time away from the home and in new situations. This creates new challenges for parents, who must balance the teen's wishes for autonomy with appropriate supervision and monitoring.

Families can avoid acrimonious conflict over these situations as teens mature, but how they manage conflict is quite important. Investigators who observe and code how families interact when discussing issues about which they disagree show that negative interaction and poor skills at talking through problems characterize families with a son or daughter diagnosed with conduct disorder or arrested for delinquency (Hanson, Henggeler, Haefele, & Rodnick, 1984; Sanders, Dadds, Johnson, & Cash, 1992). Negative interaction styles also predict self-reports of alcohol use (Brody & Forehand, 1993). Poor problem solving during family discussions also predicts harsh and/or inconsistent parenting 2 years later (Rueter & Conger, 1995).

Negative parenting continues to be important when children become adolescents. A study by Ary, Duncan, Duncan, and Hops (1999) illustrates how family interactions, parenting, and monitoring evolve and interact over time in the development of diverse problem behaviors. The researchers first assessed 608 adolescents when they were between the ages of 14 and 17. The adolescents were then assessed 1 year later and again at 18 months post baseline. Families with high levels of coercive exchanges at the outset also had low levels of positive family interactions. A year later, these families showed lessened levels of parental monitoring. Poor monitoring predicted greater association with deviant peers. Both poor monitoring and deviant peer associations predicted engagement in diverse problem behaviors 6 months later.

Peer Influences

As noted previously, Patterson et al. (1989) argue that deviant peer groups are the final training ground for diverse problem behaviors, including substance use and delinquency. In fact, association with drug-using peers is perhaps the most replicated correlate of adolescent alcohol, tobacco, and drug use (Biglan & Smolkowski, 2002). Evidence also suggests that whereas peer, parent, and individual risk factors directly influence the type of drug use (e.g., marijuana vs. alcohol vs. tobacco), only peer factors directly influence the frequency of drug use (Brook, Whiteman, & Gordon, 1982). Not surprisingly then, peer substance use has been found to be related to alcohol problems in adolescence, not just to alcohol use (Windle, 2000). Association with substance-using peers also correlates with increased risky sexual behavior in adolescence (Kowaleski-Jones & Mott, 1998; Metzler et al., 1994).

In theory, peers could promote problem behavior in various ways: by instigating it directly, by modeling it, by encouraging or pressuring others into joining them in deviant activities in the interest of friendship, or by teaching less sophisticated teens to be more expert at it. Investigators based one well-documented mechanism on observations of how boys interact with their friends. High-risk adolescents and their peers reinforce each other's talk about deviant behavior by laughter and attention. In contrast, boys who are not aggressive respond to talk about nondeviant topics with laughter. Patterns of talking positively with a friend about deviant activities predict later substance use and delinquency, even when researchers statistically control for earlier levels of delinquency (Dishion, Capaldi, Spracklen, & Li, 1995; Patterson, Dishion, & Yoerger, 2000).

The deviant peer context helps to explain why both conduct disorder and antisocial personality disorder are associated with drug abuse. Conduct-disordered children may engage in both delinquent behavior and drug use in the context of their deviant peer group. They are more likely to transition to abuse and dependence because they have few alternative sources of reinforcement (Patterson et al., 1989) and perhaps because the stressful environments in which they live make them more susceptible to the reinforcing effects provided by drugs (Goeders, 1998).

School Influences on Development

Adolescence typically involves one or two changes in schools—the transition from elementary into middle school or junior high and the transition to high school. Eccles and Midgley (1990) note that the organization of most junior high and middle schools runs contrary to the developmental needs of children at this age. Compared to elementary schools, middle and junior high schools are more likely to emphasize competition and social comparison, offer fewer decision-making choices, disrupt social networks, and provide less supportive contacts with teachers. These changes in the school environment no doubt contribute to the stress encountered in adolescence.

Harassment and bullying in which one student teases or physically attacks another is unfortunately common in middle schools. Such victimization contributes to the development of problem behavior. In a recent study of over 15,000 students in 6th–10th grade across the United States, 10% reported that they were victims of repeated bullying by their peers (Nansel et al., 2001). Rusby, Forrester, and Biglan (2002) reported on victimization at a middle and high school in a small Oregon community. They found victimization significantly related to deviant peer association, aggressive behavior, and delinquency in both middle school and high school. Victimization in middle school predicted the further development of aggressive behavior in high school, and deviant peer associations in middle school predicted further increases in victimization in high school. Victimization appears to be particularly important for girls; victimized girls engage in greater substance use in middle school and escalate deviant peer involvement and alcohol use in high school.

Neighborhood and Community Influences

Relevant risk factors at the neighborhood and community level include social disorganization, exposure to violence, low neighborhood attachment, and high rates of mobility. The availability of weapons, cigarettes, alcohol, and illicit drugs in the immediate environment also plays a role in adolescent problem behavior

Availability of weapons and substances makes it easier for youth to gain access to problem situations. In addition, it sets a normative standard for behavior that implies that high rates of violence and substance use are permissible. In addition, children who live in communities with these norms and practices are likely to be exposed to factors associated with increased availability or opportunity that further increase the risk for problem behaviors. For example, adults and older teens in these high-risk communities model problem behaviors for youth, and community sanctions for youth participation in these behaviors may be erratic. Although this area of research is new, exposure to community violence appears to relate to increased risk for aggression, antisocial behavior, and cigarette smoking in youth (Fick & Thomas, 1995; Gorman-Smith & Tolan, 1998; Miller, Wasserman, Neugebauer, Gorman-Smith, & Kamboukos, 1999).

Another community factor that relates to youth problem behaviors is the level of social organization within neighborhoods. A set of shared beliefs and norms or a coherent community identity reflects social organization. Neighborhoods with higher levels of mobility tend to have lower levels of neighborhood attachment and higher levels of social disorganization. Neighbors are less likely to look out for one another and less likely to feel that their behavior can contribute to the common good. This, in turn, increases the risk for youth violent outcomes (Sampson, Raudenbush, & Earls, 1997) and early pregnancy (Singh, 1986). In a large-scale study in Chicago, investigators found adults living in neighborhoods characterized by high residential mobility and concentrated poverty less likely to provide informal social controls on youth behavior. For example, they are less likely to monitor neighborhood children and to apply sanctions when they observe problem behaviors. Lower levels of informal social control, in turn, increased the likelihood of delinquency and aggression in youth (Sampson, 1997), consistent with findings we described earlier related to parental monitoring.

Studies concerning neighborhood risk factors for youth problem behaviors further highlight the interactive nature of neighborhood, economic, and family processes during adolescent development. Specifically, poverty predicts poor supervision and inconsistent discipline by parents, which, in turn, increase the risk for delinquent outcomes (Sampson & Laub, 1994). Neighborhood risk factors are also associated with the stress and mental health (e.g., depression and social isolation) of parents, which, in turn, have a deleterious impact on the child (McLoyd, 1990).

Economic Influences on Youth Development

Economic factors contribute to problem behaviors among teens. Lower neighborhood socioeconomic status is associated with an increase in adolescent criminal offending, drug and alcohol use, and risky sexual activity (Leventhal & Brooks-Gunn, 2000). Low occupational status of the adults in the neighborhood is associated with pregnancy outside marriage (Brooks-Gunn, Duncan, Klebanov, & Sealand, 1993), and neighborhood poverty is associated with sexual activity without contraceptive use (Ku, Sonenstein, & Pleck, 1993). Low neighborhood socioeconomic status is also related to increased delinquency in boys (e.g.,

Sampson & Groves, 1989), and youth who remain in low-income neighborhoods have higher levels of problem drinking and marijuana use than youth who move out of such neighborhoods (Briggs, 1997).

Economic factors, including both income and availability of resources, influence individual choices youth make. These factors also influence the communities in which the youth live. Here we consider two ways that economic factors may influence the development of youth behavior problems: (1) by influencing consumption of substances and (2) by influencing teen's allocation of time and effort among desirable and problematic activities.

The Economics of Consumption

Economic factors directly influence youth as they join the consumer market for tobacco, alcohol, and drugs. The adolescents' ability to pay, the cost of a particular substance, and the availability of a substance all influence youth consumption of alcohol, tobacco, and drugs. Such factors suggest means to intervene in youth substance consumption, even in the context of other social, physical, and psychological factors. Even if the youth wants to use an illegal substance, the inability to purchase it becomes a substantial barrier, especially in the initiation of substance use. Youth such as Michael, in our case study, find it easy to try substances, in part because they are readily available.

Economic analyses have shown that price affects youth consumption of tobacco, alcohol, and illicit drugs (e.g., Chaloupka, Grossman, & Tauras, 1997; Dee, 1999; Saffer & Grossman, 1987a). We discuss this empirical literature in more detail in Chapter 6, which reviews the impact of policy and economic changes on substance use among teens.

However, prices alone are not sufficient to explain individual differences in the behavior of youth exposed to similar market prices (e.g., because they live in the same neighborhood). For example, African American and white teens face similar prices for cigarettes, yet African American teens are less likely to smoke than are white teens, and African American teen smokers usually smoke different brands than white teen smokers do (DeCicca, Kenkel, & Mathios, 2000). Neither can price trends alone explain epidemiological patterns of youth risky behavior over time (DeCicca, Kenkel, & Mathios, 2002; Gruber, 2000).

A further element of youth consumer behavior is the availability of alcohol, tobacco, and other drugs. From an economic perspective, reducing the availability of a good increases the cost of obtaining it, either by making it more expensive or by requiring added effort to obtain it. For example, the minimum drinking age affects youthful consumption of alcohol in all states, even when there are differences in enforcement of this law (see review by Wagenaar & Toomey, 2000). In addition, decreasing youth access to sources of tobacco products, both by enforcing the legal age for tobacco purchase and by restricting certain sources such as vending machines, may affect levels of individual youth smoking and the initiation of smoking (Cox, Cox, & Moschis, 1990; Forster et al., 1997). Reliable data are not available to apply this perspective to illicit drugs. However, the evidence regarding alcohol and tobacco suggests that if drugs are readily available in the family, peer group, or neighborhood of a youth, the risk for individual drug initiation and regular use will increase.

Unfortunately, substances may be more available in precisely the neighborhoods that are high in other risk factors for substance use. Gruenewald, Millar, Ponicki, and Brinkley (2000) studied how alcohol outlet density varied with population growth across 144 neighborhoods in six communities. They found that alcohol outlets tended to become concentrated in the high-population-density, low-income, primarily minority communities—precisely the communities that host a number of additional risk factors for youth development. Again, risk factors—economic, social, community, psychological, and biological—travel in packs.

Time Allocation

As children move into adolescence, they begin to make important choices about how to allocate their time to different activities. They choose whether or not to stay in school and whether to do legal or illegal work. Many high-risk youth live in neighborhoods with depressed local labor markets where adult unemployment rates are many times the national average. Youth who face these poor earning prospects from legal work may perceive low returns on schooling, particularly if they have already done poorly in school. Consequently, they may drop out of school before graduation. In choosing between legal and illegal work activities, they may choose the option with the greatest payoff—unfortunately, in many neighborhoods that may mean choosing illegal activities such as drug dealing (Freeman, 1996).

STUDIES OF MULTIPLE PROBLEMS AMONG YOUTH

We have now followed the developmental pathway from conception to adolescence and have considered factors that predict more than one youth problem behavior. Of necessity, however, we base our discussion largely on studies examining only a single problem outcome. We found only a few studies that explicitly examined risk factors for multiple problem outcomes in youth. The findings of these studies have central relevance to understanding the development of children such as Michael and generally corroborate the factors we have underscored so far in this chapter.

The Oregon Research Institute Studies

Investigators at Oregon Research Institute (ORI) have done a series of studies that examined the relationships among problem behaviors and parent and peer influences on engaging in problem behavior. These studies consistently showed that antisocial behavior, academic failure, and tobacco, alcohol, and other drug use were sufficiently correlated to justify creating a single problem behavior construct (Ary, Duncan, Biglan, et al., 1999; Metzler, Biglan, Ary, & Li, 1998). Ary, Duncan, Duncan, et al. (1999) included a measure of high-risk sexual behavior and replicated the problem behavior construct. Barrera et al. (2001) found that a problem behavior construct consisting of antisocial behavior; academic failure; and tobacco, alcohol, and marijuana use was replicable across Caucasian, Hispanic, and Indian youth. Duncan et al. (1998) found the slopes for change in alcohol use, smoking, and marijuana use significantly intercorrelated over an 18-month period.

The studies consistently predicted the problem behavior construct from measures of family conflict, positive family relations, inadequate parental monitoring, and associations with deviant peers (Ary, Duncan, Biglan, et al., 1999; Barrera et al., 2001). Figure 4.1 presents the model tested by Ary, Duncan, Biglan, et al. (1999). As can be seen, in families in which family conflict is high, there are low levels of family involvement. In such families, parental monitoring is likely to be inadequate a year later, and poor monitoring correlates to greater association with deviant peers. Deviant peer association and poor monitoring predict problem behavior 6 months later. The model has been replicated across Caucasian, Hispanic, and Indian youth, with only minor variations, and Duncan et al. (1998) showed that increases in parent–child conflict and associations with peer deviance predict increasing levels of substance use over time.

Christchurch, New Zealand, Cohort Study

Fergusson, Horwood, and Lynskey (1994a) have examined factors associated with multiple problem outcomes in adolescents. Specifically, they examined the home environments of the small subsample of youth

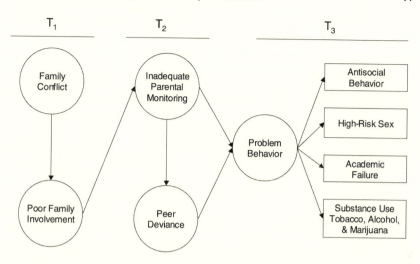

FIGURE 4.1. Model of adolescent problem behavior development. From Ary, Duncan, Biglan, Metzler, Noell, and Smolkowski (1999). Copyright 1999 by Kluwer Academic Publishers. Reprinted by permission.

(2.7%) in their birth cohort who evidenced substance use, early-onset sexual activity, alcohol abuse, conduct disorder, and police contacts for juvenile offending. Although selection criteria did not include associated internalizing disorders such as anxiety or depression, they noted that the multiple problem youth were also more likely than other youth in the sample to have mood disorders and to evidence suicidal ideation.

In the Christchurch study, multiple problem youth status was associated with dozens of family risk factors. These might include parental background (e.g., parent substance abuse, parent criminality, and low occupational status of parents), prenatal development (e.g., lack of prenatal care and maternal smoking during pregnancy), early childhood rearing conditions (e.g., less than 2 years preschool and low maternal emotional responsiveness), or family stability (e.g., multiple changes in school and residence and early parental separation). The total number of family risk factors was positively related to multiple problem behavior, with more than 20% of the youth with 19 or more risk factors evidencing a multiple problem outcome, compared to less than 1% of youth with six or fewer risk factors (replicating earlier work of Rutter, 1979). The results of this study suggest that family background factors are strongly associated with multiple problem outcomes in youth. Unfortunately, there was no direct comparison of family influences with one another or with peer, individual, and community influences in the prediction of multiple problem outcomes. Therefore, from the Christchurch study, we cannot assess the relative importance of risk factors from different sources.

Pittsburgh Youth Study

A more recent study of boys in Pittsburgh examined factors associated with multiple problem youth outcomes (Loeber et al., 1998a). In this study, Loeber and his colleagues examined the co-occurrence of the following problem behaviors: delinquency, substance use (including alcohol, drugs, and smoking), attention deficit problems, conduct problems, physical aggression, covert behavior (e.g., concealing and manipulating behaviors), depressed mood, and shy/withdrawn behavior. They assessed three samples, first, fourth, and seventh graders, and screened approximately 850 boys in each grade for behavior problems. Researchers oversampled boys with high rates of antisocial behavior for inclusion in the study so that each age/grade group contained approximately 250 antisocial boys and 250 controls.

Loeber and colleagues examined a large variety of individual, family, and community or macrolevel (e.g., bad neighborhood and low socioeconomic status) predictors. They also examined nested risks. That is, they asked whether most of the risks for one problem behavior were a subset of (nested in) the risks for a second problem behavior. Across all ages, the risk factors for substance use appeared nested in those for delinquency. Delinquent youth had the same risk factors as substance-using youth (primarily individual-level and family-level risks), but they also had an additional set of risk factors not shared by the substance-using youth (primarily macrolevel risks).

In a different type of analysis, they examined risk factors for multiproblem outcomes counting the number of problems that the boys had and then further analyzed data from boys with four or more problems as a group distinct from the rest. Hierarchical regressions revealed that lack of guilt, hyperactive–impulsivity–attention problems, low achievement, anxiety, parent anxiety or depression, poor parent–child communication, and parental stress were the best independent predictors of multiproblem status.

IMPLICATIONS FOR PREVENTION AND INTERVENTION

Our review of the etiological factors associated with youth tobacco smoking, alcohol misuse, drug misuse, serious antisocial behavior, and risky sexual behavior has several implications for prevention and inter-vention efforts, which we delineate here. In subsequent chapters, we turn our attention to selected prevention and intervention programs that may be relevant to multiproblem youth.

Common Etiologies

The common etiologies for diverse youth problem behaviors imply that prevention efforts that target such factors could help to prevent the en-tire spectrum of youth problems. It seems especially important to focus on early aggressive behavior and the factors that influence the develop-ment of such behavior. Studies of interventions that focus on aggressive behavior should evaluate the effects of the intervention on the entire range of youth problems (e.g., Lonczak, Abbott, Hawkins, Kosterman, & Catalano, 2002).

Multiple Pathways to Problem Behavior

There is no single developmental pathway to youth problem-behavior outcomes. Therefore, no intervention will have universal effects on the reduction of these behaviors. As both Wachs (2000) and Kellam (1990) have noted, we must attend not only to whether an intervention pro-duces better effects in the group that receives it than in a group that does not but also to which members of the treated group respond better and worse to the intervention. Depending on the targeted risk factors, the subgroup benefiting from the intervention may vary.

Timing of Interventions

Our developmental analysis also suggests that the timing of interven-tions is important—intervening earlier in the causal chain may be more effective because complex patterns have not built up over time. How-ever, interventions will also be needed that target problems that emerge in late childhood and adolescence despite our best efforts to prevent them.

On the other hand, the importance of risk factors in later childhood and adolescence suggests that behavioral outcomes are by no means pre-determined. Even genetic influences and impairments in brain develop-ment are malleable and responsive to positive environmental changes. Where and how to intervene will also be determined by the child's age, as somewhat different factors emerge and are implicated for children of different ages.

A Wealth of Possibilities for Intervention

The present review points to numerous ways that we can intervene to prevent the development of behavior problems. Individual characteristics of the child both influence and react to their macro- and microsocial environments, so we must design environments to nurture the assets that young people have and ameliorate characteristics that put them at risk for future problems. From infancy through adolescence, families influence youth development; thus, methods of supporting family nurturing of young people will be of value. Schools affect whether young people develop effective academic and social behavior or fail academically, whether peers reject them, and whether or not they join deviant peer groups. Peer groups can support prosocial behavior and skill development or they can contribute to problem behavior; the practices of families and schools are pivotal in ensuring that peer groups have a positive influence.

The economics and social organization of neighborhoods affect families and youth directly; if we foster economic well-being and social organization in neighborhoods, we may prevent many problems. The media contribute to aggressive behavior and other problems, although they could be a force for successful development.

The Generic Features of Supportive Environments

The evidence reviewed in this chapter also points to the key features needed in all youth environments (Biglan, 2003b). These environments must minimize the biological insults to youth that can result from physical trauma and psychological stressors. They must richly reinforce young peoples' desirable and skillful behavior and ensure that most of the environments for young people are rich in models and norms for positive behavior. Schools, families, playgrounds, and youth recreational settings should be places where effective teaching of skills occurs.

Parents, schools, and communities must also set limits on undesirable behavior, but they should do so through consistent use of negative consequences that are not harsh—and the use of much positive reinforcement. As children move into adolescence, effective monitoring is essential if parents and teachers are going to set limits and reinforce positive behavior. Young people also should be prevented from being in environments in which there are opportunities to experiment with misbehavior. It is especially clear that unsupervised after-school time among middle school students provides such opportunities (Richardson et al., 1989; Richardson et al., 1993).

As we will see in the next four chapters, there is a wealth of programs and policies that have been developed over the past 30 years that make use of these principles to improve the quality of one or more of the social fields for young people.

5

Prevention of Adolescent Problems through Interventions in the Preteen Years

In Chapter 1, we met Michael, a boy with serious problems that have threatened to derail his life by the age of 16. In Chapter 4, we learned that he had many of the risk factors that predict youth aggression, alcohol and drug misuse, smoking, and risky sexual behavior. Could Michael's adolescence have taken a different course if something had altered those risk factors when he was a child? At the age of 16, can anything help Michael get his life back on track and reduce the chances he will continue to have problems with criminal behavior, drugs, and alcohol?

The answer to both questions is yes. In Chapters 5–8, we review the effects of prevention and intervention programs on multiple behavior problems. In this chapter, we look at interventions directed toward children before their adolescence (defined here as beginning middle or junior high school). In Chapter 6, we review "universal" interventions—programs and policies designed to reduce the risk of one or more problem behaviors for all teens, regardless of their risk. In Chapter 7, we describe "selective" and "indicated" interventions. The selective interventions are designed for young people who can be selected as high risk on the basis of their having one or more risk factors associated with development of the behavior problems that are the focus of this book. Indicated interventions are for youth who already have problems. In Chapter 8, we describe community and statewide interventions.

In this chapter, we frequently describe specific programs or interventions, rather than discussing only general principles implied by successful interventions. By reviewing specific interventions, we identify approaches that might be implemented without starting from scratch. Many researchers have developed interventions with set materials and training procedures that enable others to replicate them; these technologies are becoming increasingly available to communities. In addition, highlighting specific interventions shown to be effective helps the reader see which of many approaches stands out from the pack. As we shall see, interventions that may seem quite similar often vary in their effectiveness. For example, not all school-based drug prevention programs work equally well. This is probably because most interventions have many components, only some of which may be the "active ingredients." Unfortunately, we do not yet know which specific active ingredients are necessary to produce change.

Although the focus is often on specific interventions to prevent or reduce serious adolescent problems, using this approach in isolation is too narrow. Some interventions—particularly policy interventions—do not lend themselves to easy identification as particular "programs." They are better viewed as strategies that hang together as a group. Similarly, the bulk of the evidence examining the effectiveness of some widely used approaches for handling problem behavior (e.g., boot camps) comes from meta-analyses of many programs of this generic type; no specific program has preeminence.

Because information on "what works" can come in many forms, we take a multipronged approach. First, we describe specific interventions shown to be effective at reducing or preventing one or more of the behavior problems on which we focus. We selected these interventions based on criteria described below and in subsequent chapters. Second, we draw from existing qualitative and quantitative reviews of programs and policies in order to make general statements about commonly used or potentially effective interventions. Third, we describe emerging patterns in the research literature that point toward future improvements in interventions to reduce the incidence and prevalence of the multiple behavior problems considered in this volume.

In this chapter, we review specific early interventions that well-conducted research evaluations indicate have been successful in reducing the later emergence of one or more of our focal adolescent behavior problems—antisocial behavior, smoking, risky sexual behavior, or alcohol or drug misuse or abuse. Our presentation follows the developmental phases covered in Chapter 4. We also mention other approaches that have had positive short-term effects, based on rigorous evaluation. The effects of many of these interventions are quite promising, but researchers have not yet gathered data on their longer-term impact when children who received these interventions become adolescents.

CRITERIA FOR IDENTIFYING EFFECTIVE INTERVENTIONS

Solid empirical evidence should form the basis for how communities, agencies, and individuals try to reduce the frequency and prevalence of youth behavior problems. At a minimum, this evidence should (1) provide substantial indication that the intervention can alter not just risk factors but also the youth problem behavior, and (2) be based on methodologically strong research. This is because adopting ineffective interventions cheats both the taxpayers whose money is wasted and the youth who might benefit from other, more effective, interventions.

A number of other organizations have sought to identify "model programs" (see Table 5.1 for descriptions of many of these efforts). Our approach borrows from the criteria used by many of these groups (see Table 5.2 for an overview of criteria these groups have used to select model programs). We adapted these criteria slightly as we considered different types of interventions, as described in subsequent chapters.

In selecting specific interventions shown to prevent the development of youth behavior for this chapter, we used the following criteria:

1. The researchers used at least one valid and reliable measure to measure the youth's problem behavior in adolescence.
2. Investigators measured at least one of the behavior problems of concern to us (antisocial behavior, drug/alcohol/tobacco use or misuse, risky sexual behavior).
3. Longitudinal studies indicated that the program prevented the development of one or more of these behavior problems after the child reached adolescence.
4. The data were analyzed using generally appropriate statistical techniques.
5. At least one study evaluating the effects of the program when children reached adolescence was a randomized controlled trial,[1] generally believed to be the strongest type of research design available for allowing results to be attributed to the intervention and not to associated uncontrolled factors.

---

[1]In a randomized controlled trial, participants in the study receive random assignment to the intervention of interest or to one or more control or comparison conditions. In some cases, the study began as a randomized controlled trial, but later follow-ups compromised the design. We describe these interventions if they met the rest of our criteria.

TABLE 5.1. Groups Identifying Model Programs for Youth

Program/author(s)	Sponsor	Purpose	Additional information
Blueprints Project	Center for the Study and Prevention of Violence (CSPV) and the states of Colorado and Pennsylvania	Identify model and promising programs for preventing violence	Center for the Study and Prevention of Violence, University of Colorado, Boulder, CO 80309; phone: 303-492-1032; fax: 303-443-3297; e-mail: *blueprints@colorado.edu*; website: *http://www.colorado.edu/research/cspv/blueprints*
Brestan & Eyberg (1998)	Division 12, American Psychological Association, Task Force on Effective Psychosocial Interventions	Identify efficacious treatments for conduct disorder in children and adolescents	
Center for Substance Abuse Prevention (CSAP)	Substance Abuse and Mental Health Services Administration (SAMHSA)	Provide a comprehensive list of effective youth substance abuse prevention programs, accessible via the Web	CSAP, Substance Abuse and Mental Health Services Administration; phone: 877-773-8546; e-mail: *modprog@samhsa.gov*; website: *http://www.samhsa.gov/centers/csap/modelprograms/.*
Chambless et al. (1996, 1998)	Division 12, American Psychological Association, Task Force on Psychological Interventions	Identify efficacious therapies for mental health problems	See: *http://pantheon.yale.edu/~tat22/est_docs.* *Click on tf2_1297.pdf*
Chambless & Hollon (1998)		Present guidelines to be used in evaluating the efficiency of psychological treatments	
Expert Panel on Safe, Disciplined, and Drug-Free Schools	U.S. Department of Education (DOE)	Review effectiveness of various school-based drug abuse and violence prevention programs, recommend to the Secretary of Education	1999 guidelines for submitting safe, disciplined, and drug-free schools programs for designation as promising or exemplary; website: *http://www.ed.gov/offices/OESE/SDFS/programs.html*

(continued)

TABLE 5.1. (*continued*)

Program/author(s)	Sponsor	Purpose	Additional information
Greenberg, Domitrovich, & Bumbarger (1999, 2001)	Center for Mental Health Services (CMHS), SAMHSA, U.S. Department of Health and Human Services	Identify programs that prevent symptoms of psychological disorders or reduce risk factors for those disorders; identify common characteristics of successful programs	
Kirby (2001)	National Campaign to Prevent Teen Pregnancy, Task Force on Effective Programs and Research	Review programs designed to prevent high-risk sexual behavior and teen pregnancy; make recommendations for successful implementation and evaluation of programs	
Mrazek & Brown (1999); Prevention Technologies, LLC	Invest in Kids Foundation, Toronto, Canada	Provide a literature review of outcomes of prevention and early intervention programs for young children	
Mrazek & Haggerty (1994)	Institute of Medicine Committee on Prevention of Mental Disorders	Develop criteria to identify programs that are promising in their ability to prevent mental disorders	
Sherman, Gottfredson, MacKenzie, Eck, Reuter, & Bushway (July 1998)	National Institute of Justice (NIJ)	Provide U.S. Congress with a comprehensive scientific review of what works in terms of crime prevention.	website: *http://www.preventingcrime.org*

TABLE 5.2. Scientific Criteria Used by Groups Evaluating Programs or Approaches for Preventing or Treating Youth Behavior Problems

Criteria	Blueprints	Brestan & Eyberg (1998)[a]	CSAP	Chambless et al. (1996)	Chambless & Hollon (1998)	U.S. DOE Expert Panel	Greenberg et al. (1999)	Kirby (2001)	Mrazek & Brown (1999)	Mrazek & Haggerty (1994)	Sherman et al. (1998)
Overall research design											
Comparison with no-treatment, alternative-treatment, or placebo control		×	×	×	×	×		×	×	×	×
Use of randomized controlled trial to evaluate intervention	×	×	×		×	×	×	×	×	×	×
Use of equivalent time-series design as alternative to randomized control design (RCD)					×			×	×	×	
Use of controlled single-case experiment as alternative to RCD									×		
Quasi-experimental design with appropriate comparison group as alternative to RCD				(9)	×				×		
Measures of potentially extraneous variables (physical health, personality, intelligence)							×	×		×	×
Selection bias threat: little difference between sample and target population			×								
Threats to internal validity		×	×	×		×					
Large enough sample								×			×
Follow-up	×	×	×	×	×	×	(1) ×	×	×	×	×
Dissemination capability (e.g., treatment manual or equivalent used, training available)											
Treatment implementation											
Adequate monitoring of intervention integrity	×		×					×	×	×	
Assessment of extent to which participants were exposed to intervention									×	×	
High rates of participant attendance at intervention sessions									×		
Effective engagement of target population						×					
Encouragement of use and application of skills; appropriate for multiple styles of learning						×					

(continued)

101

TABLE 5.2. (*continued*)

Criteria	Blueprints	Brestan & Eyberg (1998)[a]	CSAP	Chambless et al (1996)	Chambless & Hollon (1998)	U.S. DOE Expert Panel	Greenberg et al. (1999)	Kirby (2001)	Mrazek & Brown (1999)	Mrazek & Haggerty (1994)	Sherman et al. (1998)
Outcome assessment and data analysis											
Valid and reliable outcome measures assessing target of change	×	×	×		×	×		×	×		×
Data collection method reduces potential bias/demand characteristics (e.g., use of independent evaluators)			×		(3)	(2)			×	×	
Appropriate data analyses			×		×	×		×	×	×	
Consideration of side effects of intervention										×	
Data on/analysis of costs and benefit of intervention											
Resolution of conflicting results											
If conflicting evidence, preponderance supports treatment's superiority				×	×						
Applicability issues											
Target population clearly described		×	×	×	(4)	×	×			×	
Intervention appropriate to target population/setting (e.g., age, culture, language, SES, gender, ethnicity, developmental stage)						×					
Program application describes how program can be integrated into educational missions of schools											

Treatment effectiveness

Criterion									
Must affect measures of factors/behaviors targeted for change	×		×	×	×	×	×	×	×
Effects sustained at follow-up	×							×	
Low rates of attrition/missing data	×		×	×		×	×	×	×
Intervention superior to no intervention if compared to control	(8)		(8)	×		×		×	(5)
Intervention equal to alternative intervention with already established efficacy (if compared with such intervention)	×		×						
Intervention effects replicated	(6, 8)		(6, 8)	×		×	×	×	(6)
	×		×						
Results published in peer-reviewed journal						×		×	

Rationale for treatment

Criterion									
Based on clear theory/hypothesis, has operational relevance, based on literature reviews/previous research			×			×			(7)
Goals of program clearly stated/appropriate to target population				×		×	×		×
Program content and process appropriate to program goals						×			

General

Criterion									
Integrity: global rating of overall confidence can place in findings			×			×			×

Note. (1) Preferred but not required; (2) no testimonials, judgments based on clinical experience; (3) in replication; (4) required that target problem be documented in reliable and valid way; (5) also requires that there be sufficient power to detect moderate differences between treatments; (6) requires replication in independent evaluation setting; (7) evidence that risk/protective factor is related to disorder, precedes disorder, mechanism through which risk factor operates is specified; (8) required for "well-established" treatment but not for "probably efficacious" treatment; (9) permitted for "probably efficacious" treatment but not for "well-established" treatment.

[a]Brestan and Eyberg (1998) adopted the criteria of the APA Task Force described by Chambless et al. (1996, 1998) but applied additional criteria. These additional criteria are included in this table.

6. Effects of the program or policy were shown for a population like the one(s) for which it is likely to be adopted (gender, problem type, racial/ethnic groups, socioeconomic status, etc.).
7. Investigators described the intervention in sufficient detail that a community could replicate it.

We also attended to several things beyond the quality of research studies. First, we examined whether the intervention had the potential to affect multiproblem children. Sometimes we had to determine this by inference, as some studies did not assess multiple problems. Given the commonality of risk factors and the high correlation among these youth problem behaviors, however, it is likely that programs that successfully prevented one of these problems also prevented others. Second, we examined the potential for implementing and sustaining the intervention in diverse community settings. Researchers often evaluate interventions under almost ideal circumstances, with sufficient funding to hire, train, and closely supervise a highly motivated intervention staff. In addition, researchers may offer the interventions to "ideal" populations (e.g., those with circumscribed problems) who have many incentives for participating in the study. There is no guarantee that such interventions will work well when implemented with real-world youth in real-world schools, clinics, and communities. Finally, we attended to cost-effectiveness and cost-benefit information whenever it was available.

INTERVENTIONS FOR PRENATAL, PERINATAL, AND EARLY CHILDHOOD PERIODS

As we indicated in Chapter 4, many malleable risk factors for problematic development arise during the prenatal and early childhood periods. Low birthweight and perinatal complications predict the development of later problems among children. The mother's health habits and exposure to stress and conditions of poverty can affect the child directly and indirectly by disrupting the mother's physical and psychological health. As the child develops mobility, language, and social interaction, poor-quality interactions with the parent become particularly important risk factors and may be especially problematic for children prone to negative affect and overactivity.

Perhaps because the mother plays such a central role in the child's early life, effective interventions have focused on the mother's habits during pregnancy and skills in early parenting interactions with her children. Researchers used randomized controlled trials to evaluate two early intervention programs that produced positive effects on behavior in adolescence. One of the programs began during pregnancy and provided continued support and skills training for mothers and the children until the child was between 2 and 5 years of age. The other provided high-quality preschool education with substantial parent involvement.

The Olds Nurse Visitation Program

Risk Factors Targeted

David Olds developed a program that involved home visits by nurses during the mother's pregnancy and during the first 2 years of the child's life. The intervention focused on improving the outcomes of the pregnancy, the child's health and development, and the mother's subsequent development. Nurses attempted to encourage healthy behavior of the mother, such as quitting smoking. They supported mothers' appropriate childcare through advice giving, modeling, and approval. They also encouraged family planning, educational achievement, and participation in the work force; they linked mothers to services in the community; and they helped mothers obtain emotional and material support from family members and friends. In working with mothers, the nurses followed basic principles of behavior change, such as the importance of defining small measurable goals for behavior change and careful monitoring of change efforts from visit to visit. Nurses made an average of nine visits during pregnancy and 23 during the first 2 years of life, whenever feasible, with the same nurse visiting a family throughout the family's involvement in the program. Parents also received free sensory and developmental screening for their children at 12 and 24 months of age and free transportation to prenatal and well-baby care.

Evaluation

Olds, Henderson, Kitzman, et al. (1998) reported a randomized trial evaluating this program on high-risk mothers and their offspring when the children had reached the age of 15. Of the 400 mostly (89%) white women enrolled at the outset of the study, 47% were under 19 years old, 62% were unmarried, and 61% came from low socioeconomic families when the study began. Researchers used self-report and parent, teacher, and archival record data to assess criminal behavior, school suspensions, delinquent or sexual behavior, and substance use among the children of the mothers.

At age 15, children of mothers who were poor and unmarried and had received both pre- and postnatal nurse visitation had significantly fewer arrests, convictions, and violations of probation than did the offspring of poor unmarried women who did not receive any nurse visitation. They also reported fewer sexual partners, fewer cigarettes smoked per day, and fewer days on which they had consumed alcohol in the past 6 months. Parents of these children reported that their children had fewer behavior problems related to the use of alcohol and other drugs. Clearly, then, this program affected the development of a range of serious behavior problems. In addition, the program also showed numerous immediate benefits, including reductions in prenatal smoking, fewer preterm deliveries, fewer low-birthweight babies among young adolescent women, and lower rates of child abuse among poor unmarried mothers (Olds, 1988). Although researchers found these benefits only for the families in which the mother was unmarried and from a family of low socioeconomic status, these populations are particularly at risk for the development of behavior problems, and we should not view the specificity of results as a major problem with the intervention.

The largely white sample in Olds, Henderson, Kitzman, et al.'s (1998) study raises questions about the benefits of such a program for more ethnically and racially diverse populations. A subsequent randomized trial of the program assessed 743 mostly African American women (Kitzman et al., 2000) 3 years after the end of the program. Women who had received the home visitation program both before and up to 2 years after the birth had fewer subsequent pregnancies, fewer closely spaced pregnancies, longer intervals between the first and second births, and fewer months on Aid to Families with Dependent Children or food stamps than did the women who had not received the program. Given that these results parallel the findings in the same period for the initial study (Olds, Henderson, Kitzman, et al., 1998), there is some reason to believe that we may find similar long-term results when African American mothers receive the program.

Cost/Savings

Olds, Henderson, Phelps, Kitzman, and Hanks (1993) reported an analysis of effects of the program on government spending 2 years after the program had ended (4 years after the birth of the child) for participants in their first evaluation of the program. The analysis was restricted to the 89% of the sample who were white, apparently because the investigators felt that there were too few nonwhites to provide a reliable analysis. The average per-family cost of the program was $3,246 in 1980 dollars for the sample as a whole and $3,133 for the low-income portion of the sample. When the children were 4 years old, the estimated government savings was $1,772 for the whole sample and $3,498 for the low-income sample. Thus, 2 years after the program ended, it had produced a savings in government expenditures for low-income families but not for the sample as a whole.

Analysts made these estimates at a time at which government expenditures on welfare were probably higher than they are now. At the same time, the 15-year follow-up data indicating that the program prevented some crime and drug abuse suggest that the long-term cost benefit of the program may be considerably higher than these estimates, given the cost of crime and drug abuse that was described in Chapter 3 (Cohen, 1998). Aos, Phipps, Barnoski, and Loeb (2001) conducted cost–benefit analyses of the Olds program considering only outcomes related to crime. Considering both costs to taxpayers and costs incurred by victims, Aos et al. (2001) estimated that the Nurse Visitation Program would produce $3.06 in benefits for every dollar spent on it.[2]

Perry Preschool Project

Risk Factors Targeted

The High/Scope Perry Preschool program attempted to improve academic readiness in children with low IQs from economically disadvantaged families. Children began 1 to 2 years of half-day, 5-day/week preschool beginning at age 3 or 4. Preschool activities were largely child-directed with adult support. In addition, teachers made 90-minute home visits to parents each week to involve parents in their children's education.

Evaluation

A sample of 123 3- and 4-year-old African American children with IQ scores between 60 and 90 from low-income families (49% on welfare, 47% from single-parent households) were randomly assigned to either the Perry Preschool or a no-preschool group. Researchers followed these children regularly through age 27 with remarkably little attrition (Clarke & Campbell, 1998; Schweinhart, Barnes, & Weikart, 1993). Also remarkable are findings that show consistently lower rates of juvenile and adult crimes, including drug-related, among the youth who attended the Perry Preschool (Yoshikawa, 1995). Effects on chronic criminal offending were particularly noteworthy for males: 12% of the Perry Preschool

---

[2]Aos et al. (2001) calculated benefits using only taxpayer costs (i.e., only what it would cost the taxpayer to deal with the problem per se). This provided a conservative estimate of costs, because it did not take into account the costs borne by crime victims. Here we use cost estimates based on both taxpayer costs and costs associated with victimization.

group had been arrested five or more times by age 27, compared with 49% of the control males. Benefits went beyond reducing problem behaviors. Compared to controls, children from the preschool program had higher incomes as young adults, were more likely to own their own homes (36 vs. 13%), and were less likely to have ever been on welfare (20 vs. 41%). Fifty-seven percent of women in the program gave birth out of wedlock compared to 80% of those in control condition (*http://www.highscope.org/research/RESPER.HTM*; *http://www.highscope.org/research/Perry%20fact%20sheet.htm*).

Cost/Savings

Evaluators of the program estimated that the cost of the program was $12,356 per participant, with a cost savings of $88,432 (estimates in 1992 dollars: see *http://www.highscope.org/research/Perry4.ppt*). These savings came from criminal justice and victim costs accrued by controls but not by the Perry Preschool sample, as well as special education and welfare savings. Perry Preschool participants also contributed more in tax revenues because of their higher incomes. A more recent evaluation (Barnett, 2000) reached similar conclusions: In 1995 dollars, Barnett estimated the cost of the program to be $13,184 and the benefits to be $115,238, or $9.74 of benefits for every dollar spent.[3] In evaluating these figures, it is important to note that they take into account various outcomes in the young adult lives of the participants as well as costs and benefits beyond those associated with crime accrued while they were children and adolescents. Aos et al. (2001) calculated the benefit in terms of crime-related outcomes only to be $5.70/dollar spent.

General Comments on Early Childhood Interventions

Two specific early interventions evaluated with sufficient rigor found positive effects on child outcomes in adolescence. The Olds Nurse Visitation Program focused on early intervention to promote maternal health before the birth of the child and attended to maternal adjustment following the birth of the child. In terms of the basic mechanism of risk discussed in Chapters 1 and 4, this program probably worked by getting the child off to a good biological start, by reducing stressors for the

---

[3]We rely heavily on Aos and colleagues' in-depth economic analyses of many of the approaches we describe in this book. Aos et al. (2001) based the data on savings on Washington State estimates of cost of incarceration, recidivism, etc. Although Aos et al. (2001) estimated benefits based on estimated longer-term effects of interventions, they looked only at crime-related benefits. Programs that prevented other negative outcomes (e.g., pregnancy) would have additional economic benefits not reflected in Aos et al.'s calculations.

mother and the child, and by building maternal and—to a lesser extent—child skills during the child's early years. The Perry Preschool Project focused on school readiness but did not include maternal health components. The project started later in the child's development and its general focus was on building the child's academic skills.

Unfortunately, published reports of these interventions do not provide data on treatment components, treatment processes, or the extent to which nurses and other program personnel faithfully implemented the treatment components (called treatment integrity). As a result, we could not examine relationships between the types of services families actually received and outcomes. This information is particularly important for programs with many components that participants could access or decline.

This issue is also important because programs that often seem similar have had differing results. For example, Olds and Kitzman (1993) reviewed 31 home visiting programs previously evaluated in randomized controlled trials. Outcomes of these programs (based on data usually collected when children were 5 years of age or younger) were variable: Some produced positive effects on child behavior while others found no effects. Their review also indicated that programs that employed professionals generally produced better outcomes than programs in which paraprofessionals provided the services. For example, the providers of Olds's original program were nurses who themselves had children and who displayed considerable life experience and wisdom, according to the program developers (Olds, 1988). Their professional training and experience may have been critical to the success of the program.

The same mixed results are true of preschool programs. Although the Perry Preschool Project produced striking results, we cannot say the same of other, similar interventions. For example, the Abecedarian project in North Carolina randomly assigned 111 high-risk African American infants to preschool intervention that began in infancy and lasted through age 5, or to a no-preschool control group. Researchers randomly assigned half of each group to receive follow-up intervention when they began school. Although the program produced many lasting positive effects on academic outcomes, treatment and control samples did not differ on indicators of crime and delinquency assessed when youth were between the ages of 18 and 24 (Clarke & Campbell, 1998).

Surprisingly, despite a wealth of information on academic outcomes associated with Head Start and other state-funded preschool programs (e.g., Barnett, 1995; Gilliam & Zigler, 2000), virtually no studies have examined whether Head Start reduces the risk of developing multiple behavior problems in adolescence (Zigler & Styfco, 2001). In one promising exception, Oden, Schweinhart, Weikart, Marcus, and Xie (2000) compared criminal records in two states of 22-year-olds who had received Head Start with records of adults who had not had a preschool experience. The findings indicated that generally authorities arrested fewer girls who participated in Head Start than they arrested comparison girls (5 vs. 15%). In another set of analyses, Oden et al. (2000) also compared records of children who had received the High/Scope curriculum with those who received the "standard" Head Start curriculum. Those who received the High/Scope program as children had half the conviction rate when they were young adults compared to those who received "standard" Head Start.

Other interventions besides preschool programs warrant more long-term evaluation for their potential to prevent serious problems in adolescence. For example, parent training—one widely used method for reducing noncompliant behavior in preschoolers—has been subject to no long-term follow-up of children involved in randomized trials. These programs generally teach parents more effective ways of directing their child's activities, responding positively to positive behavior, and disciplining the child's problem behavior in effective, nonabusive ways. Examining whether these programs reduce noncompliance and early aggression is particularly important because, as we indicated in Chapter 4, these behaviors are early warning signs that, in some children, foreshadow the development of serious problems in the teen years.

Some versions of parent training have produced impressive immediate reductions in child misbehavior in the home among young children and have replicated these findings with preschool children who are referred to mental health professionals for noncompliant behavior. These approaches have used randomized controlled trials and have shown sustained improvement to children at short-term follow-up, a likely prerequisite for longer-term effects. One such program is Forehand and colleagues' approach, documented in the book *Helping the Noncompliant Child* (Forehand & McMahon, 1981; McMahon & Forehand, 2003). A closely related approach is parent–child interaction therapy (Schuhmann, Foote, Eyberg, Boggs, & Algina, 1998). Although Forehand and Long (1988) conducted a 7½-year follow-up of a small sample of children they had treated and found no evidence of more behavior problems than would be expected in the general population, they did not follow a comparable untreated group. The promising findings of these approaches for preschoolers certainly warrant long-term follow-up with larger samples and control groups to assess their preventive impact on adolescent behavior problems.

INTERVENTIONS FOR SCHOOL-AGE CHILDREN

As the child enters school, new risk factors come into play. Coercive parenting characterized by harsh, inconsistent discipline promotes aggressive and noncompliant behavior at home and at school. Disruptive behavior at school can both lead to and exacerbate academic problems, so the child falls behind in learning core academic skills such as reading and arithmetic. Aggression and poor social skills in general can alienate the child's peers, leading to social ostracism and rejection by prosocial peers and propelling the child toward associations with other rejected children who share similar risk profiles. Effective interventions for this age group generally address one or more of these areas.

Good Behavior Game

Risk Factors Targeted

Barrish, Saunders, and Wold (1969) designed the Good Behavior Game to reduce disruptive behavior and increase task-oriented behavior in elementary classroom settings, thereby decreasing the early aggression and noncompliant behaviors that are often precursors of later problem behaviors in adolescence. The program provides a structure for the teacher to provide consistent positive consequences for positive behavior and appropriate noncoercive negative consequences for problem behavior. The game involves dividing the class into two teams, each of which receives a reward if its members have fewer than a specified number of disruptive behaviors. The rewards can be tangible (e.g., candy) or can involve free time (e.g., additional recess). Typically, participants play the game for a short period—as little as 10 minutes—and the period expands as classroom behavior improves.

Evaluation

Embry (2000) reviewed 13 studies that evaluated immediate effects of the Good Behavior Game using interrupted time-series experiments in which investigators alternatively implemented and withdrew the game. These experiments consistently showed that the game substantially reduced daily rates of disruptive behavior with age groups ranging from preschool (Swiezy, Matson, & Box, 1992) through sixth grade (Harris & Sherman, 1973). The game produced similar effects with special education students (Grandy, Madsen, & De Mersseman, 1973) and adolescents labeled "emotionally disturbed" (Salend, Reynolds, & Coyle, 1989). Researchers replicated the results in Germany (Huber, 1979) and in the Sudan (Saigh & Umar, 1983).

The long-term effects of the Good Behavior Game are quite impressive. Kellam, Ling, et al. (1998) followed up with children who had received the Good Behavior Game in a randomized controlled trial in first and second grades. Nineteen public elementary schools and their teachers were randomly assigned either to implement this program or not during first and second grades. The game significantly reduced aggressive behavior in first grade (Dolan et al., 1993). Even in sixth grade, the effects of the program were still detectable: Teachers rated boys who had received the Good Behavior Game in first grade as significantly less aggressive than boys in the control groups (Kellam, Mayer, et al., 1998). Moreover, boys who had received the intervention were significantly less likely to be smoking at age 14 (26 vs. 33% for controls; Kellam & Anthony, 1998).

Investigators have not examined the effects of the Good Behavior Game specifically on the development of multiple concurrent problems. However, the fact that delinquency, smoking, and substance use outcomes were all better in the group that received the Good Behavior Game than in the control group supports the possibility that this intervention may affect children who might develop multiple concurrent difficulties. In addition, this intervention was relatively straightforward in comparison to other strategies and involved intervention solely with children's classroom behavior. That a circumscribed intervention could have effects that persisted into adolescence speaks to the possibility that classroom management strategies that specifically address discipline problems early in a child's school life can have dramatic effects on the child's later development.

Cost/Savings

To our knowledge, no one has performed cost/benefit analyses of the Good Behavior Game. However, given the relatively circumscribed nature of the intervention, it is likely to cost less to implement than many of the more extensive interventions reviewed here.

Montreal Longitudinal Experimental Study

Risk Factors Targeted

The Montreal Longitudinal Experimental Study attempted to reduce children's problem behavior by addressing three risk factors for problem behavior: (1) family interactions, particularly parental consequences for positive and negative child behavior; (2) children's social skills for interacting with peers; and (3) children's cognitive skills for thinking through problem situations. The latter two interventions should, at least in theory, prevent the peer rejection that often results from aggressive and disruptive behavior and teach impulsive children to take a more thoughtful and less reactive approach to interpersonal problems. Family intervention consisted of an average of 17.4 family sessions held every other week in which the caseworker taught parents to monitor their child's behavior, reinforce positive child behavior, and manage discipline effectively and nonabusively. School intervention consisted of seven small group sessions involving participants and prosocial peers in which a professional taught prosocial skills to the boys using coaching, peer modeling, role playing, and reinforcement contingencies. In the second year of the project, the professional taught 10 sessions of problem-solving and self-control skills.

Evaluation

Tremblay, Pagani-Kurtz, Masse, Vitaro, and Pihl (1995) evaluated the effects of their 2-year intervention with kindergarten boys selected from an inner-city sample that had been selected based on low parent education (14 years or less), use of French as a first language, and high teacher ratings of disruptive behavior. Boys were randomly assigned to an intervention, attention-control (which involved intensive observational and research study but no intervention), or treatment-as-usual control condition. Tremblay et al. (1995) obtained yearly follow-up data on self-reported delinquency and on juvenile court records when the boys reached ages 10–15. Treated boys consistently reported significantly less delinquency than control boys did over the same time. The number of boys who had been charged, arrested, and found guilty of a crime by age 15 did not differ significantly in the treatment and control conditions, but the total number in both conditions combined who met these criteria was small (13 of 166 participants). Researchers did not assess other problem behaviors.

This research program represents an impressive effort in several ways. First, investigators gathered data from almost all participants in the study, regardless of the amount of intervention they received. However, one-third of those offered intervention declined to participate further and researchers did not evaluate the differences between participants and nonparticipants. They also did not follow nonparticipants over time. Second, they selected the population carefully for high-risk status, based on kindergarten screening for aggression and disruptive behavior. Third, the authors included an attention-control as well as a treatment-as-usual control group. These two conditions were equivalent at follow-up, allowing a more conclusive attribution of findings to the intervention. Given the long-term effects of this program, it warrants replication of the intervention, with additional, diverse populations.

Cost/Savings

To our knowledge, no one has conducted cost/benefit analyses of this program.

Linking Interests of Families and Teachers

Risk Factors Targeted

Like the Montreal Longitudinal Experimental Study, Linking the Interests of Families and Teachers (LIFT) addressed parent–child management and children's skills for interacting with peers as risk factors for later problem behavior. LIFT also included interventions designed to provide positive consequences for appropriate peer interactions on the playground, which should presumably help children generalize the skills they learn in social skills training to real-life situations. LIFT staff members also taught parents skills for improving their communication with their children, which becomes increasing important as children approach adolescence.

Evaluation

Reid, Eddy, Fetrow, and Stoolmiller (1999) evaluated LIFT in a randomized controlled trial over 3 years. They assigned each intervention school at random to provide the program to first or fifth graders. Investigators invited all families in the relevant grade to participate, and 85% of them agreed to do so. The total sample consisted of 382 students in the program schools and 289 in the control schools. At 3-year follow-up, the study had lost only 3% of the sample.

Postintervention comparisons between treatment and control families showed that the program children were less aggressive on the playground. Teachers perceived them more positively. In addition, their parents were less hostile toward them during problem-solving discussions.

Particularly relevant here are the 3-year follow-up data for fifth graders. Children who had been involved in the program had less association with deviant peers, lower likelihood of a first arrest, and less initiation of alcohol and marijuana use than did fifth graders not receiving the program (Eddy, Reid, & Fetrow, 2000). Importantly, these effects were found regardless of the level of problem behavior initially exhibited by the children, implying that children most at risk to develop multiple behavior problems benefited as much as children with fewer risk factors. Fifth graders in control schools were 1.8 times more likely to be using alcohol, 1.5 times more likely to have tried marijuana, and 2.4 times more likely to have been arrested than fifth graders who received LIFT. Longer-term follow-ups are clearly necessary, but the fact that LIFT delayed the initiation of more than one problem behavior among fifth graders suggests that it may have the potential to influence children at risk for developing multiple problems when they reach adolescence.

A number of aspects of the LIFT evaluation were particularly positive. The LIFT group paid particular attention to specifying the intervention and to assuring that staff delivered the program properly. They also formally assessed how well participants implemented the program. Another impressive feature of their work was the use of observational data to show actual behavior changes in both child and parent.

Cost/Savings

Unfortunately, cost-benefit analyses of LIFT are not available. Nonetheless, the program warrants replication with additional diverse populations of children. The fact that both LIFT and the Montreal study produced similar results with similar interventions suggests that interventions that address parent and teacher consequences for positive and negative child behavior and that promote positive interactions between children may interrupt some of the family and peer processes that promote problem behaviors.

Seattle Social Development Program

Risk Factors Targeted

The Seattle Social Development Program (SSDP) provided teacher training plus social skills and problem-solving training for elementary schoolchildren and their parents in the interest of preventing drug use. Like LIFT and the Montreal Study, the SSDP specifically addressed risk factors associated with parent discipline, poor peer relations and peer influence, and poor problem solving and impulsivity. Unlike these programs, however, the intervention continued throughout elementary school and provided some focus on academic skills, another risk factor for the development of behavior problems in adolescence.

Teachers in first-grade classrooms delivered a problem-solving curriculum that taught children to think through alternatives to problem situations. In addition, professional staff provided voluntary parent training classes offered each year of the project. When the children were in first and second grades, the seven-session parent training program taught parents to pinpoint positive and negative child behavior and to provide appropriate consequences for each using modeling, role plays and feedback, and homework assignments (Hawkins, von Cleve, & Catalano, 1991). When the children were in second and third grades, staff provided a four-session program designed to teach parents good ways of helping their children in reading and arithmetic.

For children in fifth and sixth grades, staff provided a five-session program designed specifically to reduce the likelihood that the child would initiate drug use. The program established a family policy on drugs and alcohol, helped parents teach their children skills for resisting peer influence, and worked on skills to reduce family conflict and create new roles for children in the family as they matured (O' Donnell, Hawkins, Catalano, Abbott, & Day, 1995). In addition, teachers provided four hours of refusal skills training to sixth-grade children. Children learned to recognize problematic situations and to generate positive alternatives for staying out of trouble and maintaining their friendships.

SSDP also included extensive teacher training that addressed factors that could promote disruptive behavior in the classroom. When the children were in first through fourth grades, project staff trained teachers in ways to manage child behavior in the classroom by establishing classroom routines and clear expectations, giving clear instructions, using encouragement and praise, and minimizing the impact of minor disruptive behavior. Project staff also trained teachers in interactive teaching, which involves close monitoring of children's progress toward specific learning objectives. In the spring, teachers received training in cooperative learning strategies in which children of differing skills worked together on academic tasks, often earning team rewards. Project staff and principals (who had also received training) observed each teacher and provided feedback about once every 3 weeks (O'Donnell et al., 1995).

Evaluation

Hawkins et al. (1992) evaluated the effects of this program by comparing children who had received the program during all of elementary school, those who received the program only in fifth and sixth grades, and those who did not receive the program. When children reached the fifth grade, additional schools joined the study, some of which received the last 2 years of the intervention and others that joined the control/comparison sample (O'Donnell et al., 1995), thus changing the study design from a randomized controlled trial to a quasi-experimental study.

A high percentage of those children enrolled in the study in first grade were eligible for free lunch (about 85%) and about half lived in single-parent households. About 46% were white, 32% black, 15%

Asian, and the remainder from other ethnic/racial groups (Hawkins, von Cleve, & Catalano, 1991). The ethnically diverse group of children added to the study in grade 5 came from high-crime neighborhoods (Williams, Ayers, Abbott, Hawkins, & Catalano, 1999).

Hawkins and colleagues evaluated the effects of their intervention when the children were in grade 2 (Hawkins, Abbott, Catalano, & Gillmore, 1991), and at the beginning of grade 5 (Hawkins et al., 1992) when they also examined effects for a low-income (highest-risk) sub-sample (O'Donnell et al., 1995). Of greatest interest is the follow-up when the children were 18 years of age, when researchers assessed life-time crime, substance use, and sexual activity data (Hawkins, Catalano, Kosterman, Abbott, & Hill, 1999). Analyses revealed no significant differences on substance use, delinquency, or sexual behavior between those who received the intervention only in grades 5 and 6 and the controls. In contrast, the full intervention produced significantly fewer reports (compared to controls) of lifetime violence (48 vs. 60%), sexual intercourse (72 vs. 83%), and (for working- and middle-class youth only) pregnancy (5 vs. 21%). Measures of drug, alcohol, and cigarette use were unaffected by the intervention.

A subsequent follow-up when participants were 21 years old (Lonczak et al., 2002) indicated that, compared to controls, those who received the full intervention had fewer sexual partners. Females receiving the intervention were less likely to become pregnant (38 vs. 56%) and less likely to have a birth before age 21 (23 vs. 40%). Single individuals who received the intervention were more likely than those who did not to use condoms during their last intercourse (60 vs. 44%). Finally, African Americans in the intervention condition had lower rates of sexually transmitted disease (7%), compared to controls (34%).

A number of methodological issues temper evaluation of these impressive results. One positive feature of the research is that observational data collected by the researchers when the children were second graders indicated that experimental teachers used the procedures they had learned significantly more than the control group teachers did (Hawkins, von Cleve, & Catalano, 1991). Apparently, this effect replicated for 4 of the remaining 5 years of the study (O'Donnell et al., 1995). However, no other treatment integrity data addressed the adequacy with which investigators implemented various components of the intervention. Second, attrition over the course of the study was considerable, with analyses conducted for those who completed intervention, not for the entire population initially enrolled in the study. This may have biased the findings in favor of the intervention group. Third, although the authors compared those participants who did not contribute data to those who did in several of their analyses, often they did not start with the en-

tire sample but, rather, with only the subset of participants who provided data at later points in the study. Fourth, researchers apparently
created virtually all the measures in these studies for the study, with no
published data examining their reliability and validity.

Fifth, shifting from a true experimental to a quasi-experimental design creates particular problems in interpreting the results. One key issue
in this kind of study is conducting analyses to see if the groups are equivalent before treatment. Surprisingly, although Hawkins and colleagues
(Hawkins et al., 1999) tested differences between control and full intervention participants on various demographic variables and found no
differences, they did not examine the partial treatment group in the same
way. Nor did they look at earlier indicators of possible group non-
equivalence, especially on variables, such as aggression, known to predict later outcomes. As a result, one cannot be sure that the groups were
similar at the outset of the study.

Cost/Savings

Aos et al. (2001) evaluated the cost and benefits of the SSDP. Their
data indicate that $4.25 of benefits accrued (based on both criminal
justice and crime victim benefits) for every dollar spent on the program.

General Comments on Interventions for School-Age Children

The effective preventive interventions for school-age children all address
similar risk factors using similar interventions. All, with the exception of
the Good Behavior Game, were multicomponent and emphasized parent
training, social or problem-solving training for children, and classroom
management interventions. Thus, they focus on two general mechanisms: promoting adults' effective and appropriate use of positive and
negative consequences for child behavior, and building the child's social
and cognitive skills.

Other evidence supports the long-term positive outcomes of building positive competencies among children, teachers, and families, although not with randomized controlled trials. The Positive Action
program is a comprehensive K–12 program that includes content on self-
concept, social–emotional learning, and social and self-management
skills for the prevention of negative behaviors and the promotion of positive behaviors and school performance. The elementary school program
includes classroom curricula taught for 15–20 minutes almost every day,
together with schoolwide climate change and family components designed to improve parenting skills and parent–child interactions. All

teachers and staff in a school are trained how to identify and reinforce positive behaviors.

Flay, Allred, and Ordway (2001) and Flay and Allred (2003) have conducted three evaluations of the program using "school report card" data. In three districts where substantial numbers of schools had used the program for multiple years, Flay and his colleagues matched program schools with control schools based on student mobility, percentage of those receiving free/reduced lunch, and ethnic distribution—three major predictors of school-level achievement and disciplinary referrals. In all three districts, schools with the Positive Action program demonstrated higher student achievement on standardized tests and reduced levels of behavior requiring disciplinary referrals. In middle schools and high schools, students who had received Positive Action during elementary school evidenced improved student behavior (e.g., drug use, violence, disrespect, and property crime), involvement in school (attendance/absenteeism, drop out), and achievement (standardized test scores for reading and math). There was a clear relationship between the amount of intervention students had received and problem reduction in adolescence. One important finding was that schools with higher-risk students benefited most. It is hoped these impressive results will be replicated in a randomized controlled trial that is currently underway.

Other types of interventions for school-age children are worth noting as well. As with preschool interventions, a number of approaches aimed particularly at aggressive youngsters have good track records in producing immediate reductions in aggressive behavior in randomized controlled trials. Because aggression in childhood is reasonably stable and increases the child's risk for continued problems, these programs have the potential to prevent more serious difficulties in the adolescent years. Investigators have not yet assessed the long-term impact of interventions to reduce childhood aggression by following treated children into adolescence and comparing them to control samples, however.

Several parent training approaches for aggressive children have produced positive findings in randomized controlled trials and are prime candidates for longer-term follow-up. One is the Incredible Years program (Webster-Stratton, 1981, 1982). A second is the Positive Parenting Program, developed in Australia and known as Triple-P (Sanders, 1999; Sanders, Markie-Dadds, Tully, & Bor, 2000). Triple-P is particularly interesting in that practitioners can implement it with different intensities; thus it has the potential to be quite useful for different populations and settings, if researchers can establish its long-term efficacy in preventing adolescent problems. A related but more intensive program is problem-solving skills training, a clinic-based intervention that teaches aggressive children to think through problem situations. It has produced good effects on aggressive behavior when accompanied by parent training (Kazdin, Siegel, & Bass, 1992).

Even more intensive is Fast Track, a prevention approach that involves comprehensive intervention addressing developmental precursors of serious aggressive behavior. Interventions are delivered systematically between the time children enter 1st grade and when they complete the 10th grade. Fast Track is particularly interesting because it involves both general classroom interventions (which all children in the classroom receive) to promote self-control and social skills and more intensive interventions, including parent training and academic tutoring for children identified as particularly high in aggressive behavior. The Conduct Problems Prevention Research Group (1999a, 1999b, 2002) has published data on the effects of Fast Track from a large randomized controlled trial involving four sites across the United States. At the end of first and third grades, several measures of aggression indicated that high-risk children in the Fast Track program were less aggressive than their counterparts who had not been part of Fast Track. Ongoing research will examine whether these effects translate into fewer serious problems in the teenage years—important outcomes to assess in light of the intensive (and presumably costly) nature of this program.

Fast Track, unlike many other prevention programs, focuses on academic skills as well as on the child's social skills and behavior. Very little research has examined whether improvements in academic instruction can prevent adolescent behavior problems. Given that early academic failure is a significant risk factor for the serious behavior problems that concern us in this volume, it is quite possible that teaching children to read and master academic tasks would have a preventive effect. Although much research has assessed the effects of various instructional strategies on achievement (White, 1988), we are aware of only one study that has shown the benefit of instruction on social behavior. Kellam, Mayer, et al. (1998) found that the implementation of research-based instructional practices in first grade led to gains in achievement for boys that, in turn, led to lower teacher ratings of aggressive behavior. Girls who received the instruction were also less likely to become aggressive, but only if they were higher achieving at outset and gained in achievement over the year.

Finally, we have yet to establish the essential components of interventions that produce positive results. The fact that the Good Behavior Game produced such positive findings in the absence of other intervention components particularly raises questions about whether other components are essential to the preventive effects. Which components are necessary and sufficient at different ages would also be important to establish.

SUMMARY AND RECOMMENDATIONS

The approaches just reviewed indicate that various interventions implemented across childhood have the potential to prevent youth behavior problems that would otherwise emerge in adolescence. Effective approaches that begin when the mother is pregnant and continue after the baby is born focus initially on the mother's health and on other risk factors that contribute to healthy biological development of the fetus and newborn. These approaches also seek to reduce the environmental stressors that may make mothers more prone to interact in maladaptive ways with their infants and toddlers.

As children enter school, effective interventions focus on parenting, especially around discipline issues, and teacher training in managing classroom misbehavior and promoting prosocial and other adaptive behavior. These curricula often also teach problem-solving and social skills to children in the interest of promoting thoughtful responses to problems, improved social skills, and peer acceptance. Interventions delivered through middle childhood tend to be generic in the sense that they target key social and maternal health risk factors in ways not specifically linked to delinquency, substance use, or risky sexual behavior, although many focus at least in part on reducing aggression, noncompliance, and disruptive behavior. Not surprisingly, then, these programs often evaluate their long-term impact on various problem outcomes, most often showing that they affect more than one problem behavior. These results are particularly impressive because a decade or more may have passed between participating in the program and assessing the outcomes in the adolescent years. Clearly, these programs must put at least some children on more positive tracks toward better outcomes. Many of these programs are quite cost effective as well.

The programs varied in the extent to which they examined serious behavior problems, particularly risky sexual behavior, and drug and alcohol misuse or abuse (as opposed to drug use). Risky sexual behavior is important to examine because of its links with several of the behavior problems that prevention programs explicitly target. Drug and alcohol abuse are important to evaluate because we cannot be sure that use of alcohol and other drugs necessarily leads to abuse of these substances (Biglan, Flay, & Foster, 2003). Although delaying the onset of experimentation with drugs and alcohol is a positive first step in preventing possible later abuse, looking specifically at prevention of abuse is important as well.

Related to this is the general need to go beyond statistical significance in data analyses to look at the incidence and prevalence of meaningful outcomes—such as drug abuse or pregnancy or acquiring a

RESEARCH DIRECTIONS

- Replicate randomized controlled trials of interventions shown to be effective in preventing adolescent problems.

- Develop cost-effective methods for promoting, tracking, and maintaining intervention integrity.

- Evaluate the outcomes of early prevention on the entire range of risk factors and adolescent problem behaviors.

- Evaluate the economic costs and benefits of intervention strategies, and do so in ways that consistently track the costs of all problem behaviors prevented.

- Link changes on risk factors to prevention outcomes in the interest of expanding understanding of (1) which risk factors must be altered to change developmental outcomes, and (2) the degree to which risk factors must be affected to produce meaningful changes in the emergence of later problems.

- Study who does and does not benefit from prevention efforts to provide a foundation for the next generation of prevention efforts, with particular attention to the interaction between biological predispositions for the development of problems and environmental alterations that can prevent those predispositions from flowering into problems.

- Fund long-term follow-up of evaluations of interventions that have proven effective at reducing risk factors and behavioral precursors to adolescent problems.

- Study methods of engaging and retaining families in prevention efforts, with particular attention to underserved and difficult-to-engage populations.

sexually transmitted disease—in the populations researchers study. This is crucial in particular for interventions attempting to reduce risk factors for these outcomes. It is not enough to reduce the risk factor; we must also show that serious problem behaviors are affected as well.

At the same time, we should not underestimate the importance of what may seem at first glance to be small differences between a treated and a control group. For example, consider the finding cited earlier that 5% of girls who had been in Head Start were arrested by they time they reached the age of 22, compared to 15% of those who had not attended preschool (Oden et al., 2000). This means that three times the number of girls was arrested in the comparison group than in the Head Start group.

In a population of 500,000 females, this translates into a difference between 25,000 and 75,000 girls having at least one arrest. Multiply this by the economic cost of each arrest and the difference becomes even more pronounced. Even small differences can have large economic and social impacts when we consider entire communities.

Evaluation of a range of outcomes (i.e., arrests and substance abuse and smoking and risky sexual behavior) is also necessary to estimate costs versus benefits of these programs. The benefit of programs that reduce a full range of problems is obviously greater than the benefit of programs that reduce only one among a host of negative outcomes. Related to this is the need to conduct cost–benefit analyses in a more consistent and systematic way across studies. Aos, Phipps, Barnoski, and Lieb's (1999) report provides one example of how practitioners can do this. This approach, however, looked only at outcomes on delinquent behavior and not on the other behavior problems that concern us here. If these programs affect multiple behavior problems, many of the dollar figures reported here likely underestimate the actual economic effects of prevention programs.

In addition, as Barnett's (2000) analysis of the Perry Preschool program indicates, other outcomes that accrue as children become successful adults further increase the financial savings seen when prevention approaches are effective. Until we apply consistent methods to economic analyses of program costs and benefits in ways that take into account effects on multiple serious behavior problems, assessed in comparable ways over comparable time intervals, we (1) cannot directly compare interventions with each other on economic indicators, and (2) will likely underestimate the economic benefits of effective prevention.

No studies reviewed here specifically addressed whether the programs prevented the emergence of multiple behavior problems. Similarly, only a few examined whether some subgroups of children benefited more than others. Related to this is a need to document carefully those who do and do not participate in interventions to establish whether the intervention is missing those most at risk. This kind of research is essential because—despite our best efforts and some positive effects—our interventions are not powerful enough to change the destinies of all children exposed to risk factors for the development of youth behavior problems. We must therefore not only implement programs that work but also study why they do not always work, so we can create the next generation of prevention programs that build on the lessons learned from the best we have tested so far.

In addition, we must address practical issues in program delivery. Programs that began many years ago often were not characterized by the careful attention to treatment integrity and specificity that we demand of scientists studying interventions today. It is important to describe methods of ensuring that practitioners, teachers, and others implement interventions in ways that are true to the program, because ensuring widespread, faithful implementation of these programs will be a challenge.

Greater discussion of how to make sure programs are implemented with fidelity is particularly important for settings in which practitioners try to replicate programs developed and tested under ideal circumstances. Often the developer of the intervention oversaw highly trained, motivated staff. In less ideal circumstances, staff may resist change and lack the necessary training to implement new interventions faithfully. Even skilled practitioners, teachers, and other implementers of interventions may need training to learn programs with which they are unfamiliar. In addition, the lessons learned from decades of research on teaching people new skills are straightforward: Simply providing written material is unlikely to result in changes in staff behavior. Hands-on training in which people practice the skills and receive feedback is much more likely to be effective. Furthermore, plans to implement new programs must include methods that will enhance the likelihood that staff members' interventions will continue with integrity over time. This in turn requires the intervention setting to support and reinforce appropriate intervention efforts.

It should be clear by now that selecting interventions with good track records is only one step necessary for obtaining positive outcomes for youth. Other areas closely associated with intervention success involve determining the conditions under which treatment effects accrue. That is, one must ask if the intervention works, for whom it does work, and under what conditions it works (e.g., does it require intense supervision?). Good prevention research in each of these areas is sorely needed.

Technologies for engaging families, schools, and community organizations in effective interventions also warrant a closer look and better elaboration to ensure that interventions reach those who can benefit from them. Providers must focus on engaging the consumer. The adage "If you build it they will come" does not apply to current mental health and prevention services. A major bane of mental health practice is the often high rates of premature termination. Of particular relevance is the finding that multiproblem youth (e.g., substance-abusing delinquents) have some of the highest rates of treatment dropout and premature termination (Stark, 1992). This is also true for ethnic minorities. For example, ethnic minorities underuse mental health services (Atkinson & Gim, 1989; Sue & Morishima, 1982). These minorities also tend to terminate treatment prematurely (Armbruster & Fallon, 1994; Sue, 1977; Vernon & Roberts, 1982), which has raised concern by advocacy groups that mental health services are failing to meet the mental health needs of eth-

RECOMMENDATIONS FOR POLICIES FOSTERING EFFECTIVE PREVENTION

- Provide a range of empirically based, accessible services for families during pregnancy, infancy, and the school years.

- Select evidence-based treatments whenever possible to address key risk factors for the development of multiple behavior problems.

- Adopt or build evidence-based interventions that address maternal health during pregnancy, reduced maternal stress and improved maternal skill building while the child is young, and access to high-quality preschool education that includes parental involvement when the child is very young.

- Adopt or build evidence-based interventions that focus on effective, noncoercive parent and teacher disciplinary strategies for young children, particularly as they enter school.

- Adopt or incorporate into school programs approaches that build children's interpersonal skills and promote adults' use of effective disciplinary skills and positive consequences.

- Make evidence-based interventions available in schools, mental health agencies, and community centers (e.g., churches) to parents of children who show early patterns of disruptive, aggressive behavior.

- Create service delivery systems that engage and retain parents who can benefit most from prevention efforts.

- Implement evidence-based strategies in ways that are faithful to the program that had positive effects and monitor prevention integrity.

- Evaluate outcomes regularly using reliable and valid measures of child outcomes and of risk factors. The key to effective prevention lies in results.

nic minorities (Brondino et al., 1997; Drotar, Stein, & Perrin, 1995; Tarnowski, 1991). Given the stark reality that youth residing in some ethnic communities have higher than average prevalence rates of multiple problem behaviors, ignoring consumer engagement will undermine our prevention efforts.

Finally, investigators have not yet rigorously tested many interventions for their long-term impacts. Indeed, one striking aspect of this literature is how few studies have evaluated the long-term impact of interventions with children. This is particularly true of interventions to reduce aggression that are delivered in mental health settings and that have proven effective in the short and medium term. Similarly, researchers have repeatedly evaluated medication interventions designed to reduce impulsivity (e.g., Ritalin)—a risk factor for many problem behaviors with children diagnosed with attention-deficit/hyperactivity disorder—that have had beneficial effects on disruptive and inattentive behavior. However, to our knowledge, they have neither followed these samples into adolescence nor compared them to randomly assigned control groups. This is crucial for looking at the long-term impact of these interventions on children when they reach the critical adolescent years. Such long-term follow-up evaluations are costly, but important, to do so that policymakers can make informed choices about how to use often scarce resources. Interventions that have produced positive short-term follow-up results on child aggression in high-quality research are particularly good candidates for long-term follow-up investigations because they have produced such clear effects on a known precursor of later problems.

Longitudinal evaluations of the effects of policy interventions on adolescent problem behavior are particularly scarce. In addition, many attempts at prevention lack evaluation. Yet, these may be as—or more—effective than the approaches presented here. Without comparative data, however, we will never know their real benefits or costs. In addition, the cost of an ineffective intervention that continues due to political or other pressures in the absence of evaluation is high, because it robs children of the chance to have experiences that might really make a difference in their lives.

Clearly, more work remains. At the same time, solid evidence suggests that many interventions can change the course of some children's lives. Communities with high rates of problem behaviors would do well to consider adopting these approaches as their standard practice, then using these as standards to compare future policies and programs.

6

Prevention Practices Targeting
All Adolescents

When Michael became an adolescent, he increasingly associated with friends who drank, smoked, and offered him various drugs. Drugs and alcohol were readily available in his neighborhood. As he continued to increase his use of drugs and alcohol, he became even more distant from his mother and disengaged from school. These many risk factors at the individual and community level collectively increased the chances that Michael would move from what was a troubled boy into a teen with serious behavior problems. Moreover, nothing stood in the way of these developments. What could have helped deter Michael from his increasingly detrimental behavior as he reached adolescence?

In this chapter, we describe prevention practices designed to reach all adolescents that might have helped Michael once he became an adolescent. Such interventions are commonly labeled *universal*, because they are intended to affect adolescents without regard to the level of risk that the adolescents show. Unlike the interventions reviewed in the previous chapter, these approaches begin when children enter adolescence, the period when problems most often begin with smoking, drug and alcohol use, serious delinquency, and risky sexual behavior. Most are designed to prevent the initiation of problem behaviors.

Universal prevention approaches with solid histories of success fall into three general groups. The first are those programs focused on family and school influences on youth development. The second group consists of media campaigns that use persuasion to reduce youth motivation to engage in problem behaviors or to persuade adults to alter the environment for young people. The third group consists of efforts to modify the community environment through laws and regulations that reduce influences and opportunities to engage in problem behavior.

FAMILY-FOCUSED INTERVENTIONS

Family interventions designed to prevent drug use and related problem behavior focus on promoting effective parenting practices, improving family communication and parental involvement with their children, and providing young people with skills for dealing with peer pressure. Two programs meet our criteria for rigorous assessment and document that they help families through the sometimes difficult transitions that take place between elementary school and middle school. Both focus primarily on parent use of consequences and monitoring as mechanisms for preventing behavior problems. They also teach children skills for resisting peer pressure.

Iowa Strengthening Families Program

Risk Factors Targeted

The Iowa Strengthening Families Program (ISFP) is a seven-session intervention that focuses primarily on improving parental use of consequences and on building better relationship skills in both parents and their children. Parents learn skills for making their expectations clear, using appropriate discipline practices, managing their own and their children's emotional reactions, and communicating with their children. Youth learn similar skills—how to manage their emotions, respond to discipline, and communicate more clearly. In addition, they learn skills for dealing with peer pressure and stress. In part or all of each session, parents and young people practice communicating with each other.

Evaluation

Spoth, Redmond, and Lepper (1999) evaluated ISFP in a randomized controlled trial in which families of sixth-grade students in 33 schools in small Iowa communities received (1) the Strengthening Families Program, (2) Preparing for the Drug Free Years (reviewed later), or (3) no intervention. Most families were dual parent (85%) and white (98%).

At 2-year follow-up, alcohol consumption differed significantly among ISFP teens versus those in the control condition (Spoth et al., 1999). Whereas 30% of adolescents in the control condition had begun use of tobacco, alcohol, or other drugs between Year 01 and Year 02 follow-ups, only 15% of the adolescents in the ISFP condition did so. Spoth and colleagues also reported that scores on the Alcohol Initiation Index were significantly lower for ISFP adolescents than for control adolescents at both 1- and 2-year posttreatment assessments. Moreover, the proportion of young people who initiated alcohol use was lower for the ISFP condition at both times.

Because binge drinking is one indicator of alcohol misuse, the number of young people who reported having been drunk is of particular interest. Among control youngsters, 19.1% reported having ever been drunk at 2-year follow-up, while only 9.8% of the ISFP young people did so. Spoth, Redmond, and Shin (2000) also reported that the proportion of young people who had ever drunk alcohol, drank it without permission, had been drunk, had smoked cigarettes, or had smoked marijuana was lower for the ISFP group than for the control group. Rates of alcohol and cigarette use in the past month were also significantly lower for the ISFP condition than for the control condition.

In addition to reporting lower drug, tobacco, and alcohol use, adolescents whose families received ISFP reported significantly less aggressive and destructive behavior in 10th grade than did the adolescents who had not been in the program (Spoth et al., 2000). For example, 7.9% of those in the control condition reported breaking into a building, whereas only 2% of the ISFP youth did so. In addition, observations of interactions between mothers and teens who had been in the program indicated less hostility than in the interactions of mother–teen pairs that had not been in the program.

The fact that the program affected a variety of problem indicators suggests that it may help to reduce the number of children who develop multiple behavior problems, although researchers did not analyze the data with this specific question in mind. At the same time, only about 51% of the 1,309 families of sixth graders recruited for the study participated in pretesting. This likely overestimates the number who would be involved in similar programs in the community, given that most research studies of this sort make serious efforts to recruit and enroll families in order to fulfill their promises to the funding agencies. This issue is not unique to ISFP and underscores the need for communities to adopt a range of effective interventions and policies in the interest of reaching youth and families who do not choose to enroll in voluntary programs such as ISFP. Finally, whether this intervention would produce the same effects in more diverse urban communities is an empirical question.

Cost/Savings

Spoth, Guyll, and Day (2002) estimated that the accumulated lifetime cost of preventing a single case of alcohol use disorder was $121,878 (discounting future avoided costs by 3% per year). Based on the number of young people who (due to the program) did not get drunk, they estimated that the program could reduce the later cost of alcoholism by $9.78 for every $1 invested in it. The net benefit per participating family was $6,039. This analysis does not include benefits associated with the effect the program has in lowering aggressive behavior (Spoth et al., 2000). Of course, Spoth and colleagues based the estimate on the assumption that one long-term outcome will be to prevent alcohol abuse, something Spoth and colleagues have not yet assessed. Nonetheless, the potential savings from this program may be substantial.

Preparing for the Drug-Free Years

Risk Factors Targeted

Preparing for the Drug-Free Years (PDFY) is a five-session program that helps parents and their middle school children prepare for early adolescence, when children are susceptible to developing drug or other behavioral problems. For the majority of the program, four out of five sessions, the intervention involves only the parents. The program encourages parents to use consequences and persuasion effectively and to monitor children's behavior. Parents receive information about risk factors for drug use, including family management problems, family drug use, alienation and rebelliousness, peer drug use, and early use of drugs or alcohol. They learn how to conduct family meetings that involve their children, as well as how to communicate their expectations to their children that they will not use alcohol, tobacco, and other drugs. Parents are encouraged to monitor their children's behavior to be sure they meet parental expectations and to provide consequences for adherence to or violation of those expectations. The program teaches parents and children a five-step approach for teens to use in resisting peer influences to use drugs. Parents also learn skills for expressing and controlling anger and ways to teach these skills to their children.

Evaluation

Spoth, Redmond, and Shin (2001) evaluated the program in the same study that evaluated ISFP (described in the previous section). By 2-year follow-up, 30% of control adolescents but only 12% of PDFY adolescents had initiated some sort of substance use. In addition, 50% of control adolescents who had been using alcohol and/or tobacco at 1-year follow-up began to use marijuana, whereas only 23% of those in the PDFY condition progressed to marijuana use. By 10th grade, the proportion of adolescents using alcohol in the past month was significantly lower for adolescents in the PDFY condition than for those in the control condition (Spoth, Redmond, & Shin, 1998).

Cost/Savings

Spoth et al. (2002) estimated that PDFY could produce $5.96 in reduced cost of later alcoholism for every dollar spent on the program, a net benefit of $2,747 for each participating family.

Family-Focused Programs on Risky Sexual Behavior

The two family-focused programs described earlier produced positive results at delaying and reducing drug, tobacco, and alcohol use. Other family-focused programs have been less successful in preventing high-risk sexual behavior. Kirby (2000) reviewed these programs, two of which involved randomized controlled trials. Neither those programs nor the less carefully evaluated ones had significant benefit in reducing high-risk sexual behavior. The programs typically attempted to increase parent–child communication about sexual behavior. The rationale for them was that few parents communicate with their children about sexual matters and lack of communication correlates to engagement in sexual behavior (Meschke, Bartholomae, & Zentall, 2000).

Focusing on parent–child communication about sex in essence relies on persuasion as a mechanism of preventing problem behaviors. Persuasion on its own has not been effective in preventing drug use either (Tobler et al., 2000). Persuasion (especially by parents) may be less important than helping parents set limits on activities that lead to diverse problem behaviors, including high-risk sexual behavior. Indeed, most of the mechanisms involved in promoting other problem behaviors (e.g., monitoring, opportunities, norms, and consequences) are also involved in the development of risky sexual behavior. For example, young people whose friends are experimenting with risky behavior are more likely to engage in high-risk sexual behavior (e.g., Metzler, Biglan, Noell, Ary, & Ochs, 2000). Yet, none of the programs Kirby (2000) reviewed focused on increasing parents' monitoring or setting limits on their child's involvement with deviant peers.

Programs such as the Iowa Strengthening Families Project that encourage parents to do a more effective job of limit setting might be more effective in preventing risky sexual behavior than ones that focus only on encouraging communication. Supplementing programs such as IFSP with components that specifically address risky sexual behavior should make these interventions even stronger.

SCHOOL PRACTICES AND PROGRAMS

Researchers over the last 30 years have identified a number of programs and practices that middle and high schools could adopt to prevent diverse adolescent problem behaviors. In this section, we describe classroom-based curricula and schoolwide practices shown to prevent one or more problems.

Preventing Aggressive Behavior

Given the extensive evidence about effective behavior management techniques in elementary schools, it is surprising how seldom researchers have investigated the use of such techniques as ways of preventing problems in middle and high school settings. Behavior management generally involves using positive and negative consequences effectively and sometimes includes strategies for arranging the environment to reduce opportunities for problem behavior.

We found only one randomized controlled trial examining the value of behavior management techniques that included junior high schools. Mayer, Butterworth, Nafpaktitis, and Sulzer-Azaroff (1983) randomly assigned 20 schools to receive a behavior management intervention either immediately or after a delay of 1 or 2 years; one school dropped out of each condition. Investigators selected two teachers in each school to be model teachers who would initially implement the practices and they selected two other teachers for observation who would not receive consultation. They chose six students who were low in reading achievement from the classrooms of the latter teachers so they could assess the effects of the intervention on student performance. Mayer et al. (1993) employed a series of workshop and consultations to assist principals and model teachers in implementing practices that would increase reinforcement for specific targeted appropriate student behaviors. In addition to a focus on increasing positive reinforcement, the workshops and consultations covered the deleterious side effects of punishment and worked on increasing the use of response costs, time-out, and antivandalism programs.

The intervention led to significantly lower costs associated with vandalism than were found in the delayed intervention schools. When they implemented the intervention in the second year in the delayed-intervention schools, it again led to significant reductions in their vandalism costs. These benefits generally continued in the third year of study. Observations of model teachers indicated that they increased their rates of praise, particularly those who used praise infrequently at the start of the intervention. Students in immediate-intervention schools had significantly greater decreases in off-task behavior than did those in delayed-intervention schools, though the decrease was greater in elementary schools than in junior high schools. In a related but not as well-controlled study, Mayer et al. (1993) also found that an intervention to increase teachers' positive reinforcement and decrease their disapproval was associated with decreased high school dropout rates and increased on-task behavior of poorly performing students. Although vandalism and dropping out of school are not specifically the behaviors on which we focus in this book, vandalism is a form of antisocial behavior and school dropout is related to aggressive social behavior. Together these findings suggest the possible value of the Mayer et al. (1983) intervention for preventing other problem behavior.

At least two other reports suggest the value of specifying a small number of clear rules and increasing positive reinforcement for desirable behavior in middle schools (Horner, Sugai, Lewis-Palmer, & Todd, 2001; Metzler, Biglan, Rusby, & Sprague, 2001; Taylor-Greene et al., 1997). Both involve quasi-experimental designs, however. Each has shown that effective schoolwide implementation of the approach called Effective Behavior Support led to significant reductions in discipline referrals. The study by Metzler et al. (2001) also showed that Effective Behavior Support reduced student reports of victimization.

Curricula to Prevent Substance Use

Over the last 25 years, investigators have developed and evaluated a sizable number of school-based substance abuse prevention programs. Although the effect of these programs has generally not been large, the programs have confirmed the value of preventing tobacco, alcohol, and other substance use.

Meta-Analyses

The best evidence about the effects of these programs comes from meta-analyses. Tobler et al.'s (2000) meta-analysis of 207 evaluations published between 1978 and 1998 identified two types of programs with clear benefit. *Social influence programs* rely principally on skill building, persuasion, and norm-setting mechanisms of behavior change. They typically inform students about peer and media influences to use drugs and the negative consequences of their use. They counter the perception that use is widespread and provide modeling and role-play practice of skills for resisting peer influences to use drugs. *Comprehensive life skills programs* include the features of social influence programs and teach additional skills like problem solving, assertiveness, decision making, coping, and goal setting. Tobler et al. (2000) labeled these two types of programs interactive, as they involve extensive interaction between teachers and students and among students.

An important finding of Tobler et al.'s analysis was that these types of programs had a significantly greater impact than did noninteractive programs (which involved didactic presentations designed to affect self-esteem and/or knowledge, attitudes, and values about substance use). Indeed, noninteractive programs generally did not have a significant impact on any form of substance use. The message is clear: Relying on information or persuasion alone is unlikely to affect teen behavior. Additional skill building that involves rehearsal and engagement by teens seems to be required to produce changes in substance use.

The effectiveness of social influence and comprehensive life skills programs is quite robust. Researchers found effects both when they analyzed all available studies and when they evaluated only the studies with sound experimental designs. They were equally effective for white middle-class and other populations. Tobler et al. (2000) analyzed effects on specific substances separately and found that these two types of programs prevented tobacco, alcohol, and other substance use. Programs of these types were beneficial when delivered at the elementary, intermediate, or high school levels. They also had beneficial effects for youth with all levels of prior use of substances—nonuse, experimentation, and abuse.

Some of the most effective and most carefully evaluated programs focus only on a single substance (e.g., Emshoff & Moeti, 1986; Sussman, Dent, Burton, Stacy, & Flay, 1995). The Tobler et al. (2000) meta-analysis therefore examined whether social influence and comprehensive life skills programs that target multiple substances are less effective in preventing alcohol and tobacco use than programs that target only tobacco or alcohol. For tobacco, they found that programs that targeted only tobacco use had a significantly greater impact on its use than did programs targeting all substance, although the latter programs did have significant benefit (effect size .17 vs. .10 standard deviations). Alcohol-specific and multisubstance programs were equally effective in preventing alcohol use.

Tobler et al. (2000) found that studies involving larger sample sizes quite consistently had smaller effects on substance use and suggested two possible explanations of this finding. First, many of the larger studies were more recent. In recent years, all schools have been under pressure to implement prevention programs, due to the Safe and Drug Free Schools program. Thus, because students in comparison conditions most likely received some sort of antidrug programming, it may have been harder for these more recent studies to show effects. Second, it may be harder to assure a program's implementation when it is in a large number of schools. If this is the case, it points to the difficulty of achieving preventive effects when good programs are widely implemented.

Tobler et al. (2000) focused on outcomes within a year of the pretest evaluation. However, preliminary additional analyses suggest that the effect sizes increased over time in large-scale evaluations of interactive programs (Michael Roona, personal communication, April 10, 2001). These increased effect sizes could occur because follow-ups capture the effects of longer programs delivered over more years. It could be that the effects of the programs become more evident as adolescents mature and encounter more peer influence to use substances. Smaller-scale evaluations of interactive programs did not find the pattern of increasing effect sizes over time.

A concern in evaluating school-based programs is that their effects on illicit substance use may not translate into the prevention of drug abuse. In general, the studies show that these programs prevent marijuana use. Whether preventing marijuana use prevents the development of drug abuse or dependence is not clear. It could be that these programs discourage lower-risk youth from experimenting with marijuana but have no effect on multiproblem youth who, as was shown in earlier chapters, are at greatest risk to develop serious drug abuse problems. One study (Botvin, Baker, Dusenbury, Botvin, & Diaz, 1995) reported positive effects of a comprehensive life skills program (Life Skills Training) on use of illicit drugs other than marijuana at 6-year follow-up. These results provide the strongest evidence to date that curricular-based prevention programs may prevent the use of illicit drugs, although they fall short of documenting the prevention of drug abuse. However, this is only one study, and its results may not be typical of those produced by other interventions.

Too many randomized trials have evaluated programs for adolescents to describe all of them here, and the Tobler et al. (2000) meta-analysis provides a good overview of what the most effective of these had in common. Two widely studied programs, however, do warrant description. The first, Life Skills Training, is one of the few interventions evaluated in more than one randomized trial. The second, Drug Abuse Resistance Education (DARE), is notable both because it has been widely adopted and because evaluations have generally shown it to be ineffective.

Life Skills Training

Life Skills Training (LST) is probably the most extensively evaluated school-based prevention program developed to date. Designed to begin in seventh grade, LST teaches social and problem-solving skills that focus on decision making, resisting media influences, coping with negative affect, managing one's own behavior, communicating effectively with others, behaving appropriately in situations that require assertiveness, and resisting peer pressure to smoke or use drugs or alcohol. Youth also receive information about consequences and social acceptability of drug and/or tobacco use. Thus, the intervention focuses on altering social norms and provides extensive teen skill building. The intervention typically takes 15 sessions that include instruction, modeling, role plays and feedback, and between-session tasks to complete. Booster sessions (10 in eighth grade and 5 in ninth grade) supplement the initial intervention delivered in seventh grade (Botvin, 1996).

Botvin and colleagues have conducted a number of randomized experimental evaluations of LST with different populations. Posttest analyses during the year of intervention generally capture 70–90% of the original sample. These analyses have indicated that, relative to control conditions, LST reduced reports of cigarette use in the past month and the number of new smokers. Effects were found with white suburban middle-class and urban, multiethnic, and predominantly Hispanic samples (Botvin, Dusenbury, Baker, James-Ortiz, & Kerner, 1989; Botvin, Batson, et al., 1989). Some evidence suggests that effects are more likely with youth who have not yet initiated smoking than with the much smaller number who already started by seventh grade (Botvin, Renick, & Baker, 1983).

Two studies also found that LST produced long-term effects on use of alcohol, marijuana, and other drug use. Botvin et al. (1992) found that LST produced significantly less heavy drinking than the control conditions 6 months after the intervention. In an even more impressive follow-up, Botvin et al. (1995) assessed a large, mostly middle-class, white sample and found that treatment affected reports of cigarette smoking, getting drunk, and poly-drug use 6 years after the intervention, suggesting that LST may prevent some of the serious problems that characterize multiproblem youth. We located no information on costs relative to benefits for this program. A further follow-up with 447 individuals contacted 6½ years after the initial pretest indicated that the program prevented the use of "illicit" drugs other than marijuana (Botvin et al., 2000).

Although a number of randomized trials demonstrated the value of the program, not all versions of LST have produced significant effects.

Botvin, Baker, Renick, Filazzola, and Botvin (1984), for example, showed that only peer-led, not teacher-led, LST produced better results among experimental than control participants. Follow-up data indicated that the experimental group continued to do better than controls only if they received booster sessions from peers (Botvin, Baker, Dusenbury, Botvin, & Filazzola, 1993).

Furthermore, the teacher-led groups that received booster sessions reported significantly *more,* not *less,* alcohol use at 1-year follow-up. This iatrogenic effect disappeared when the authors examined data from only those youth whose teachers implemented the program with the greatest consistency. Implementation was assessed through observation data collected in teachers' classrooms that documented how much of the curriculum teachers actually implemented. For this high implementation group, girls (but not boys) exposed to LST showed less drug use than did controls (Botvin, Baker, Filazzola, & Botvin, 1990). The authors indicated that the negative effects on alcohol use in the teacher-led condition may have been due to some teachers failing to present the program correctly and, in some cases, discussing alcohol use with "a wink and smile."

A number of other studies also demonstrate the importance of implementing LST with fidelity. In these studies, youth who received a well-implemented intervention showed significant (or marginally significant) prevention effects, but youth with poor intervention implementation did not (Botvin, Dusenbury, et al., 1989; Tortu & Botvin, 1989). Effects were much stronger in groups with high treatment integrity than in the experimental sample as a whole (Botvin et al., 1995), and the degree of treatment integrity was related to positive outcomes (Botvin et al., 1992).

Please note that many of the just reviewed analyses are based on a subsample that received 60% or more of the program. Although it is important to look at the effects of variations in treatment delivery or receipt, once we look at a subgroup, we no longer have a randomized trial or an efficacy trial. The fact that only 60% of the sample received all the intervention is important information for ultimate effectiveness in the real world.

In any case, findings showing that incomplete delivery of the program undermines its outcome underscore the importance of assessing and ensuring high-quality implementation of interventions. Further, these findings show that one cannot simply assume that the program will be effective once adopted and widely implemented. The findings of Botvin, Baker, Dusenbury, Tortu, and Botvin (1990) that inadequate implementation can actually induce higher rates of drug use are particularly disturbing. The mechanisms underlying these effects warrant further investigation.

Drug Abuse Resistance Education

DARE is probably the most widely used school-based substance use prevention program. Police officers in upper elementary school classes conduct the program. DARE was begun in 1984 by the Los Angeles Police Department and by 1994 it had been adopted by about 50% of the school districts in the nation (Ennett, Tobler, Ringwalt, & Flewelling, 1994). In 1986, the federal Drug-Free Schools and Communities Act specifically named the program as one to disseminate. Unfortunately, repeated evaluations have not found the program to be effective. Ennett et al. (1994) did a meta-analysis of eight methodologically rigorous short-term controlled evaluations of DARE. They reported that the average size of the effect on drug use was .06 standard deviation, which is smaller than other school-based approaches. Similarly, the meta-analysis by Tobler et al. (2000) showed that DARE and DARE-like programs had an average effect size of only .05 across 17 evaluations. Considering only the nine studies that employed sound experimental designs, the effect size was only .03 and was not statistically significant.

Conclusions

Our review of the evidence leads to several conclusions. First, some school-based programs that address social influences to use substances have small but significant effects in preventing the use of tobacco, alcohol, or marijuana. These programs sensitize students to peer and media influences to use substances, correct misperceptions about the prevalence of substance use among peers, and make peer norms for nonuse salient. Although effects have been found for both genders and for diverse ethnic groups, and are reliably found as much as a year after their delivery, effects have proven difficult to sustain through 12th grade.

In contrast, comprehensive life skills programs such as LST have a larger and more long-lasting impact on substance use. These programs supplement curricula that attempt to change norms with more generic social skills training, such as assertiveness, active listening, and decision-making skills. Although the effects of these programs are greater than are those for social influence programs, they are modest, typically averaging about .2 standard deviation units 1 year after the intervention. Investigators have found that these programs have a preventive effect with both genders and for diverse ethnic groups. They have also found preventive effects for tobacco, alcohol, and other drugs. Researchers observed effects when students are in 12th grade, even when the program ended in 8th grade. Furthermore, LST in particular has documented an effect in preventing drug abuse—not just drug use—at 12th grade.

Prevention programs without interactions between teachers and students or among students do not appear to prevent tobacco, alcohol, or other drug use. These more didactic programs involve one or more of the following: imparting knowledge about substances, self-esteem building, decisions/values/attitudes, and some social skills training (e.g., assertiveness).

Although the effect of school-based programs has generally not been large, there is definite evidence of the value of these programs in preventing tobacco, alcohol, and other substance use. The optimal approach to preventing substance use might include, but not be limited to, a comprehensive life skills program such as LST. We discuss this issue more fully in later chapters on comprehensive community intervention strategies.

Finally, implementation integrity is crucial. Even with extensive training, program implementers might deviate from the essential components of the program, and these deviations may weaken the effects of the program.

Classroom-Based Programs Targeting Sexual Behavior

In the last decade, evaluations of school-based curricula to prevent high-risk sexual behavior have begun to accumulate, although many of them failed to employ random assignment to intervention and comparison conditions. We rely on Kirby's (2001) review of these interventions. He evaluated three different types of school-based prevention programs. The first type consists of the abstinence-only programs (which emphasize abstinence as the only acceptable strategy to prevent pregnancy, STDs, and HIV infections). The second are the sexuality education programs (which address pregnancy, HIV, and STDs and discuss both abstinence and birth control/disease prevention). The third types are HIV education programs (such as sexuality education, but focused solely on HIV and STDs). Because most of the HIV education programs involved high-risk samples likely to be already sexually active, we will review those programs in Chapter 7. Only two studies used randomized controlled trials to evaluate abstinence curricula (Jemmott, Jemmott, & Fong, 1998; Kirby, Korpi, Barth, & Cagampang, 1995). Jemmott et al.'s (1998) abstinence curriculum implemented with sixth and seventh grades delayed initiation of sex but did not affect frequency of sex. Kirby et al.'s (1995) classroom-based program with seventh and eighth graders found no evidence that the program delayed the initiation of sex, but it did increase the use of condoms or birth control pills and decreased the number of sex partners.

Eight of the sexual education programs used randomized controlled designs. Three of these prevented initiation of sex at the first post-treatment assessment, but the effects were gender-specific. Two programs delayed boys' (but not girls') initiation of sex (Coyle, Kirby, Marin, Gomez, & Gregorich, 2000; Eisen, Zellman, & McAlister, 1990) and one delayed it for girls but not for boys (Aarons et al., 2000). Each of these programs taught teens about social pressures to have sex and provided training in assertive or refusal skills. However, a fourth program (Moberg & Piper, 1998) found that a more comprehensive program that included refusal skills training in grade 6 had no effect on initiation at grade 8 but actually increased initiation of intercourse in 9th and 10th grade. This finding was unusual, however: Most programs found either no effects or positive effects

Only one program reduced the frequency of sex, and only for boys (Coyle et al., 2000). However, another similar program increased it. Three other programs did not affect frequency of sex.

Surprisingly few programs assessed use of condoms (three studies) and other forms of contraception (five studies). Of those that did, the results again were mixed, with some studies reporting improvements, others reporting no change, and one reporting that girls who received the intervention as virgins and then initiated sex after the intervention were less likely to use contraception than girls in the comparison group (Eisen et al., 1990).

A major controversy in the sex education area has been whether sex education encourages young people to have sex. Of the 20 sexual education programs that evaluated this outcome (both randomized trials and quasi-experimental studies), 1 hastened initiation of sex, but 12 had no effect and 7 decreased the likelihood of young people starting to have sex. None of the HIV programs hastened initiation, while 3 delayed it and 6 had no impact.

In sum, although there is little evidence that classroom-based sexual education programs will increase young people's sexual involvement, evidence that these programs can prevent risky sexual behavior is mixed. Although some approaches have had positive findings, no single program has had benefits replicated in two randomized controlled trials. Programs also frequently lack evaluations of long-term or follow-up effects. Moreover, two of the programs reported deleterious effects. Further research seems needed before curricula are ready for dissemination to schools that do not experimentally evaluate them.

MEDIA CAMPAIGNS

Because youth have so much exposure to television and other media, these media provide a logical vehicle for trying for prevention and pro-

POLICY RECOMMENDATIONS: SCHOOL- AND FAMILY-FOCUSED
PROGRAMS

- The universal interventions most extensively evaluated are
  classroom-based programs to prevent tobacco, alcohol, and other
  drug use. Each middle school should be required to have a program
  shown in multiple studies to prevent substance use. Because we
  can expect no program to be effective in the absence of monitoring,
  schools should continuously monitor the fidelity of implementation
  and youth substance use in middle school.

- Middle and high schools should (1) have systems for monitoring the
  level of problem behavior, (2) promulgate a *small number* of clear
  rules specifying desired behavior in all school settings, (3) provide
  direct instruction in rule following, and (4) provide high levels of
  positive reinforcement for rule following.

- There has been insufficient research on universal interventions
  targeting parenting skills to justify a policy favoring their widespread
  adoption. Policy in this area should require simply that *if* a group
  implements a parenting or family intervention, it should also
  evaluate its effects.

motion of positive development. However, evidence is quite limited. Few
investigators have conducted well-controlled, experimental evaluations
of media campaigns and those that have been have done produced
mixed results.

Media might be used three ways to affect adolescent behavior. First,
a media campaign might attempt to directly influence young people's
behavior via persuasion, communication of norms, or modeling of skills.
Second, the campaign might direct their efforts toward convincing
parents, teachers, and coaches to influence teen's behavior. Third, a
campaign might help to advocate a policy known to affect behavior,
such as an increased tax or an ordinance regarding access to tobacco and
alcohol (Wallack & Dorfman, 1996; Wallack, Dorfman, Jernigan, &
Themba, 1993). Most of the empirical evaluations of campaigns have
focused on the first strategy. A few have examined media effects on parents. We are aware only of case studies of the use of media to affect policy, though this strategy may be particularly valuable.

Media Campaigns Directed at Youth

Giesbrecht and Grube (2003) reviewed research on the effects of media
designed to reduce alcohol use or its related problems. The types of

media they reviewed included public service announcements, news coverage of alcohol issues, and counteradvertising. They cited a single study of the effects of public services announcements about drinking during pregnancy that showed increased awareness of the dangers of drinking while pregnant. However, the study did not have a control group that did not receive the media. The study suggests that news coverage could have an effect on both individual drinking behavior and public policy-making, but there seem to be no experimental evaluations of the effects of news coverage.

Counteradvertising—designed to directly offset the persuasive appeal of advertising for a product—includes warning labels on alcohol containers and in advertisements. Giesbrecht and Grube (2003) cite only one experimental evaluation of the effects of warning labels. Snyder and Blood (1992) apparently randomly assigned college students to see six different advertisements for alcoholic products, either with or without the U.S. Surgeon General's warning. The warnings had no effect on perceptions of the risk of drinking; they actually made products more attractive. MacKinnon, Pentz, and Stacy (1993), in a national survey of youth, found increases in self-reported awareness of, exposure to, and memory of the labels after they were required but found no substantial changes in alcohol use or beliefs about the risks targeted by the warning.

Derzon and Lipsey (2002) did a meta-analysis of 72 evaluations of media campaigns designed to discourage adolescent substance use. The analyses included studies of antitobacco campaigns. Unfortunately, most of the studies merely involved a comparison of levels of reported substance use before and after the campaign. Therefore, their basic measure of effect was the pre- to postcampaign difference. They compared the size of the pre–post change for samples exposed to the campaign with the changes for samples not exposed to a campaign. They found small, but reliable changes after media campaigns in young people's knowledge, attitudes, and behavior concerning substance use. They estimated that effects of the size they obtained would translate into a reduction of alcohol use from 53 to 51% of the population of adolescents, while for tobacco use the reduction would be from 37 to 35% and for marijuana use from 24 to 22.5%. These are certainly not big changes. However, Derzon and Lipsey (2001) cite evidence that a 2% annual reduction in the smoking rate in the United States would result in 5.5 million fewer smokers by the year 2010.

Flynn, Worden, and colleagues (Flynn et al., 1994, 1997; Worden et al., 1988) evaluated a media campaign designed to deter smoking initiation. A series of 13 spots was created to increase knowledge and attitudes favorable to nonsmoking, model skills for resisting peer pressures to smoke, and enhance young people's perception that social norms were favorable to their not smoking. Four communities were involved in the evaluation—two in Montana and two in the northeastern United States. The investigators matched communities in pairs according to census data and further matched study samples by selecting schools within the communities that were comparable in parent income. Two of the communities received a school-based prevention program, while the other two received the same intervention as well as the media campaign. Over a 4-year period, TV spots aired at times and on stations earlier evaluated as reaching a large proportion of the target audience.

A sample of 5,458 students received assessment in grades 4–6 and 4,670 of them (865) received a second assessment when they were in grades 10–12. Flynn et al. (1994) reported that, when students were in grades 10–12, those exposed to the media campaign were less likely to have smoked in the previous week than those who received only the school-based program. The results were unchanged in a subsequent analysis that corrected for the effects of the students' clustering in only four communities (Murray, Moskowitz, & Dent, 1996). A further analysis of the data indicated that the campaign was specifically effective with higher-risk students (those who, at pretest, indicated that they had ever had a cigarette or who had two or more friends or family members who smoked).

This study provides the strongest evidence that a media campaign can affect adolescent smoking. However, at least two other studies evaluated media campaigns in randomized trials, but did not find effects on adolescent smoking.

Bauman and colleagues (Bauman et al., 1988; Bauman, LaPrelle, Brown, Koch, & Padgett, 1991) randomly assigned media markets in the southeastern United States to receive one of three media campaigns or no campaign. One campaign used radio only and focused on expected health and social consequences of smoking. A second used the same radio spots but added a contest in which young people wrote about why they would not smoke. The third campaign added television to the radio and contest components. Surveys of 12- to 14-year-olds from communities in each condition did not indicate that any of the campaigns affected smoking behavior.

Flay et al. (1988) compared the effectiveness of (1) a school-based social resistance curriculum alone, (2) that curriculum plus television programming designed to parallel the classroom program, (3) the television intervention alone, and (4) two control conditions. The program targeted seventh-grade students. In Los Angeles, investigators randomly assigned 28 schools to either of the two conditions and in San Diego an additional 12 schools received either the curriculum or no intervention. Follow-up assessments in grades 7, 8, 9, and 12 did not find that the media affected adolescent smoking.

One recent study provides evidence of the effects of television spots in reducing adolescent marijuana use. Palmgreen, Donohew, Lorch, Hoyle, and Stephenson (2002) developed five television spots, each of which was designed to be appealing to sensation-seeking youth (i.e., youth who are highly motivated to participate in exciting activities); the spots were high in novelty, drama, surprise, and emotional appeal. Each depicted a negative consequence of marijuana use, such as harm to relationships, loss of motivation, or impaired judgment. Biglan, Ary, and Wagenaar (2000) evaluated the effects of a 4-month campaign in an interrupted time-series experiment in which each of two Kentucky counties received the intervention at different times. Monthly for 32 months, 100 students from grades 7–10 in each county took part in telephone interviews concerning their marijuana use in the past month. Thus, for each county, there were monthly estimates of the prevalence of marijuana use. After 8 months of baseline data collection, the 4-month campaign started in one county. It stopped for 8 months and then started in both counties. Each time the campaign went into effect, self-reported marijuana use went down significantly. Researchers observed the effect only for high sensation-seeking young people; low sensation seekers seldom reported marijuana use.

We have been unable to find any studies evaluating media campaigns designed to affect antisocial behavior. Few studies have evaluated media campaigns to reduce risky sexual behavior among teens, either, with most of these oriented toward HIV prevention (see Rotheram-Borus, O'Keefe, Kracker, & Foo, 2000) and testing (e.g., Futterman et al., 2001) activities. In Switzerland, however, a 10-year national program was associated with increased condom use among youth, and other countries have similarly implemented effective media campaigns addressing HIV risk (see Rotheram-Borus et al., 2000, for review). As Rotheram-Borus et al. point out, media coverage of sexual matters— particularly when directed toward adolescents—is quite controversial and is likely to meet with resistance in the United States. This resistance conflicts directly with the need for broad-scale and effective interventions to prevent high-risk sexual behavior among adolescent populations most at risk.

Media Directed at Parents

Investigators have designed several media campaigns to influence parents. Perhaps the most ambitious is one by the Office of National Drug Control Policy (ONDCP). ONDCP is conducting a national media campaign involving TV, radio, and print ads encouraging parents and other adults to praise and reward appropriate behavior, monitor young people's behavior, make rules about substance use, and enforce those rules

(Kelder, Maibach, Worden, Biglan, & Levitt, 2000). These ads are noteworthy because they use persuasion to get parents to employ two of the mechanisms consistently linked to the absence of problem teen behavior—consistent use of consequences and monitoring. Although ONDCP is currently evaluating the effects of the campaign through cross-sectional and longitudinal samples of parents and young people, the design of the evaluation does not involve a randomized controlled trial. It is therefore impossible to definitively rule out alternative explanations of any effects on parents or adolescents. We are not aware of any experimental evaluations of the efficacy of such campaigns, despite their popularity.

There is some evidence that parenting practices can be affected by newsletters about parenting that emphasize the same mechanisms for preventing problem behaviors described in the Office of Drug Control ads (Riley, Meinhardt, Nelson, Salisbury, & Winnett, 1991; Sanders, 1996; Sanders, Montgomery, & Brechman-Toussaint, 2000). For example, in a randomized trial, Bogenschneider and Stone (1997) randomly assigned parents of 9th–12th graders to receive or not to receive a series of newsletters advocating parental monitoring, limit setting on children's alcohol use, and networking with other parents. Parents who received the letters reported increased monitoring compared to control parents. Homework assignments that children complete with parental assistance also can prompt parent–child interactions designed to influence nutritional habits (Crockett, Mullis, Perry, & Luepker, 1989; Perry et al., 1988), smoking (Biglan, Ary, Yudelson, 1996; Holder, Perry, & Pirie, 1988), and alcohol use (Perry et al., 1996; Williams et al., 1995). In a similar vein, Derzon and Lipsey (2001) assessed the effects of media campaigns targeting parents and concluded that these campaigns were generally associated with positive changes in parent–child interactions.

These studies suggest that direct mail and parent–child homework activities are viable methods of influencing parenting practices, but the strategy requires more research to develop its potential. In addition, whether the changed parenting practices result in decreases in serious behavior problems also requires further study.

Media to Affect Policy and Its Implementation

Another potential for mass media is its use to increase public interest in and support of public policy strategies that can, in turn, affect youth problem behavior. Wallack and colleagues term the purposeful use of the news media to advance policy change as "media advocacy" (Wallack et al., 1993). Media advocacy involves getting news and editorial coverage that increases public support for a policy, regulation, or practice. The advocacy effort may frame the issue in a way that puts a specific policy in a favorable light. Alternatively, it may try to increase public demand for some type of change. For example, efforts to pass an ordinance requiring tobacco vendors to be licensed might be framed in terms of the value of licensure for preventing young people from getting addicted to tobacco and ultimately dying of a tobacco related illness (e.g., "About 3000 teens start smoking each day and 1000 of them will eventually die of a smoking related illness").

Media advocacy changes the environment that influences behavior rather than the motivation of individuals to engage in the behavior (Holder & Treno, 1997). Thus, many media advocacy efforts encourage policies that limit teens' opportunities to engage in problem behavior rather than try to persuade teens not to engage in the behavior. For example, until recently, preventing adolescent tobacco use was seen as a matter of influencing individual adolescents to resist influences to use tobacco through school-based programs, media campaigns, and so on. Only in the last 10 years have tobacco marketing practices and easy access to tobacco received attention for their roles in tobacco use.

The effectiveness of media advocacy is difficult to assess. Media coverage of the smoking problem has undoubtedly aided the substantial progress made in tobacco control in the United States (Biglan & Taylor, 2000). Evidence from a quasi-experimental comparison of New Zealand communities found a relationship between media advocacy and increased support for enforcement of laws regarding alcohol use (Stewart & Casswell, 1993). Similarly, in a quasi-experimental evaluation, Barber and Grichting (1990) found that an Australian media campaign led to increased support for restrictive antidrinking and antismoking legislation. Holder and Treno (1997) found a statistically significant effect of local news coverage of alcohol issues on public awareness of alcohol trauma and support for policy strategies. News coverage of law enforcement against driving under the influence of alcohol significantly increased perceived risk of arrest and decreased drinking and driving. This behavioral change contributed to a 10% reduction in alcohol-involved crashes, comparing experimental with comparison communities (Holder et al., 2000).

Clearly, the media can influence changes in behavior in many different ways. The content of the message, the medium delivering it, the duration and scope of a media campaign, and the population targeted by the message all can vary widely. It is likely that all are implicated in the effectiveness of various media strategies at preventing and reducing problem behavior among adolescents. Given the pervasiveness and reach of various media, more research is clearly warranted on how to use the media effectively to promote positive practices and policies. Ideally, more studies would involve true experiments or use time series analyses to permit stronger cause–effect statements about different sorts of media-based interventions.

If such research establishes the value of media for influencing youth problems, it will become necessary to study how to influence the practices of major media organizations (Biglan, 1995).

POLICIES TO AFFECT ADOLESCENT PROBLEM BEHAVIORS

In this section, we describe policies that affect one or more adolescent problem behaviors. A policy is a rule, regulation, or law that has an impact on the social, economic, or geographic environment affecting behavior. Those in the alcohol and tobacco fields have done the best research on these strategies. However, we discuss the potential of these strategies for preventing other problems.

We examine four types of policies shown to help prevent problem behaviors. Some policies affect the *price* of engaging in the behavior, which relates both to opportunities to engage in the behavior and the immediate dollar cost (or consequences) of so doing. Related policies that do not involve price affect the *opportunity* to engage in the behavior by making the means for doing so less available. Policies may also increase the *certainty of consequences* for engaging in a behavior. For tobacco and alcohol, policies may affect adolescents' *exposure to advertising* that tries to persuade teens to use these substances.

Advocates of policy research make the compelling argument that policy strategies can significantly alter environmental support of problem behaviors. If effective policies were in place to reduce the opportunities and incentives to engage in problem behaviors, those policies would make it less necessary to motivate individual youth not to engage in these behaviors and to motivate parents to engage in effective parenting practices. And because neither youth-focused nor parent-focused programs are anywhere near 100% effective in reaching and motivating youth and parents, policies that alter community environment for problem behavior are an essential component of efforts to prevent youth problems (Holder, 1998; Levy, Friend, Holder, & Carmona, 2001; Wagenaar, Murray, & Toomey, 2000).

Before turning to our review, a few words about research that evaluates policies are in order. Investigators rarely evaluate broad-scale policy interventions with randomized control designs because it is difficult or impossible to undertake randomized controlled trials. With interventions such as increasing cigarette and alcohol taxation and implementing drunk driving laws, the political process, not random assignment, determines whether individuals in a certain jurisdiction on a given

RESEARCH RECOMMENDATIONS REGARDING POLICIES

- We need research to develop and evaluate policies to reduce antisocial and risky sexual behavior among adolescents. This requires viewing antisocial behavior (such as violence) as reflecting a larger social context (e.g., encouraging or discouraging violence or increasing access to condoms to reduce risk of HIV exposure during intercourse). Policy approaches make the most sense when viewed independent of judgment or moral admonishments. Rather, with a public health approach to violence or HIV exposure, the concern is to reduce risks associated with such behavior rather than judging the behavior per se.

- Studies should look specifically at the effects of policies on adolescent behavior and particularly at whether policies affect the behavior of multiproblem youth. This research would examine how universal strategies (those designed to affect all youth) can specifically reduce the harm associated with the behaviors of youth engaging in multirisk behaviors.

- Policy studies should look at effects on both initiation and reduction of problem behavior.

- We need experimental evaluations of strategies for getting policies adopted and effectively implemented. Here we are concerned with understanding the processes that increase the chances that communities will adopt evidence-based policy strategies and will enforce and implement those strategies in order to maximize effects.

date are subject to high or low taxes, tough or lenient drunk driving laws, and so on. However, it is often possible to examine the effects of policies on repeated measures of a relevant outcome that have been obtained over an extended period. One example is the number of car crashes each month in a given jurisdiction. Such interrupted time-series designs can provide strong evidence about the effects of a new policy, especially when the data are available for many time points and are available from jurisdictions that did not change their policy (Biglan, Ary, & Wagenaar, 2000).

In this section, we look principally at studies that evaluated the effects of policies on adolescent problem behavior. We gave most weight to those policies examined by using more than one research approach (e.g., using both cross-sectional and longitudinal data). In addition, we paid closest attention to studies that took steps to rule out alternative hypotheses for any intervention-related behavioral change the researcher found.

Affecting Price of Substances

Increasing the price of tobacco and alcohol decreases their use. Policies affecting cost also may be relevant to influencing other adolescent behaviors, though research is generally lacking.

Economists assess the effect of price on consumption in terms of *price elasticity*. Price elasticity is a measure of change in demand relative to changes in price. As price increases, demand declines, and vice versa. Economists typically measure elasticity as the percentage of change in demand per 1% change in price. For example, if price increases 10% and the price elasticity is −1.00, then demand will decline by 10%. Zero elasticity would mean no change in demand as price changes.

Tobacco Use

Table 6.1 summarizes studies of the effects of price on adolescent smoking. Except for the Wasserman study (Wasserman, Manning, Newhouse, & Winkler, 1991), these studies looked separately at the effect of price on adolescents taking up smoking (participation) and on the number of cigarettes they consume (amount smoked). More than half of the effect of price was on whether or not adolescents took up smoking.

In a recent analysis, Chaloupka, Tauras, and Grossman (1997) concluded that a conservative estimate of the effect of cigarette prices on adolescent price elasticity is −1.0. That is, for every percent increase in the price one can expect a corresponding percent decrease in adolescent demand. They also concluded that price affected high school students' demand for smokeless tobacco. The total price elasticity was −0.6 (−0.4 for taking up chewing and −0.2 for amount consumed).

In a recent study (not included in Table 6.1), Chaloupka and Pacula (2000) used nationally representative data from the 1994 *Monitoring the Future* study surveys of students in grades 8, 10, and 12 and paired each student's self-reported tobacco use with information about his or her state's tobacco-control laws. Using advanced statistical modeling techniques and controlling for other variables, they found evidence of substantial price elasticity. However, the effects of price varied according to gender and race. Males were significantly more responsive to price than females were and black males were more responsive to price than any other group was.

Thus, the best available data suggest that increases in price reduce the number of new smokers as well as the rate at which teens who already smoke use tobacco. Furthermore, price elasticity is greater for adolescents than for adults (Lewit & Coate, 1982).

TABLE 6.1. Studies of Price Elasticity That Included Adolescents

Study	Methods	Age group	Price elasticity
Lewit, Coate, & Grossman (1981)	1966–1970 U.S. Health Exam Survey data, linear	Teens 12–19 years	−1.44; −1.2 P
Wasserman, Manning, Newhouse, & Winkler (1991)	1970–1985 National Health Interview Survey data, poisson	Adults Teens	−0.23 −0.89, NS
Chaloupka & Wechsler (1997)	1993 college survey	College students	−1.11; −0.53 P
Chaloupka & Grossman (1996)	1992–1994 *Monitoring the Future* project, log, two-part models	8th, 10th, and 12th graders	−1.3; −0.67 P
Evans & Farrelly (1997)	1987 National Interview Survey data, probit and ordinary least squares, two-part models	18–24 years 25–39 years 40+ years	−0.58 P; NS; A −0.43 P; −0.33 A NS; P; −0.50 A
Chaloupka, Grossman, & Tauras (1997)	1992–1994 *Monitoring the Future* project, log, two-part models, smokeless tobacco	8th, 10th, and 12th graders	−0.59; −0.43 P
Lewit, Hyland, Kerrebrock, & Cummings (1997)	1990, 1992 Community Intervention Trial, logistic regression	9th graders	−0.87 P
Chaloupka et al. (1997)	1994 *Monitoring the Future* project, log, two-part models	8th, 10th, and 12th graders	−1.19; −0.62 P; −0.57 A
Evans & Huang (1998)	1977–1992 *Monitoring the Future* project, log, two-part models	12th graders	−0.20 to −0.50

Note. NS, not significant; NR, not relevant (not included in the equation or not reported); P, elasticity for participation; A, elasticity for the amount smoked per smoker.

150

Alcohol Use and Alcohol-Related Problems

Numerous studies show that raising the cost of alcohol has beneficial effects (Cook & Tauchen, 1982; Levy & Sheflin, 1983; Ornstein & Levy, 1983; Saffer & Grossman, 1987a, 1987b). Coate and Grossman (1988) found that as the price of beer went up, the frequency of adolescent beer consumption went down. Other studies have found similar relationships (Grossman & Chaloupka, 1997; Grossman, Chaloupka, Saffer, & Laixuthai, 1995; Grossman, Coate, & Arluck, 1987). As described with tobacco, the effect of price on consumption is greater for young people than it is for adults.

Even more important, youth who drink weekly or are heavy drinkers (typically defined as five or more drinks per occasion) are *more* price-sensitive than are other youth (Coate & Grossman, 1988), suggesting that price may particularly affect multiproblem youth. The differential price sensitivity of youth and of heavy drinking youth makes sense because youth have less disposable income than adults and heavier-drinking youth must advance more of their disposable income to purchase alcohol when the price rises.

Laixuthai and Chaloupka (1993) estimated that if the price of beer (the beverage of choice of youth) were indexed to inflation, then overall youthful drinking over any past year would have been reduced by 9% and youthful heavy drinking would have been reduced by 20%. Pacula's (1998) analysis of data from the U.S. National Longitudinal Survey of Youth indicated that doubling the tax on beer would reduce alcohol consumption among young people between three and six percent.

Other policy factors influence the effect of price on consumption, however. For example, Malmquist (1948) and Huitfeld and Jorner (1972) showed that in Sweden, when restrictions on the availability of alcohol increased, the influence of changes in prices and income on consumption decreased. Gruenewald, Ponicki, and Holder (1993) replicated this finding with U.S. data.

Alcohol price also affects drunk driving and alcohol-related crashes and fatalities. Several studies examined the impact of higher alcoholic beverage taxes or prices on drinking and driving among youth and/or young adults (Chaloupka & Laixuthai, 1997; Chaloupka, Saffer, & Grossman, 1993; Dee, 1999; Kenkel, 1993; Ruhm, 1996; Saffer & Grossman, 1987a, 1987b). As with the research on consumption, these studies generally, but not always, conclude that tax- or price-induced reductions in drinking and driving among younger populations would be larger than those inducements would be among adults. For example, Kenkel (1993) used data from the 1985 National Health Interview survey to estimate the impact of alcoholic beverage prices on self-reported drinking and driving. His estimates imply that a 10% increase in the price of alcoholic beverages would reduce the probability of drinking and driving by over 7% among all men and by over 8% among all women, but that there would be a reductions of almost 13% among young men and over 21% among young women.

Cook (1981) investigated the short-term effects of changes in liquor taxes on the auto accident death rates and found that fatalities declined as taxes increased. Similarly, Saffer and Grossman (1987a) estimate that a 100% increase in the real beer tax (approximately $1.50 per case) would reduce highway mortality by 27% among 18- to 20-year-old drivers. Other estimates suggest that a 15% decline in traffic fatalities among this age group would result from simply increasing the excise tax on alcohol at the rate of inflation (Saffer & Grossman, 1987a).

Increasing the cost of alcohol products also may have an effect on violent and nonviolent crime among all age groups (Cook, 1981; Markowitz, 2000a, 2000b, 2000c; Sloan, Reilly, & Schenzler, 1994). Using data from the Core Alcohol and Drug Surveys of College Students, Grossman and Markowitz (in press) concluded that higher beer prices could make significant reductions in several areas. It could reduce the number of college students (1) getting in trouble with the police or college authorities, (2) damaging property or pulling a fire alarm, (3) getting into an argument or a fight, and (4) being a victim or perpetrator of sexual coercion. Similarly, Markowitz (2000b) examined the impact of beer prices on violent behavior among teens using data from the YRBS and concluded that higher beer taxes would reduce the likelihood of teens getting into fights. Evidence also suggests that higher alcoholic beverage taxes and prices would lower child abuse and other violence toward children—problems that contribute to the development of adolescent problem behaviors (Markowitz, 2000b; Markowitz & Grossman, 1998).

Consumption of Other Drugs

Just as it does with alcohol and cigarettes, retail price affects the demand for other drugs. Pacula, Grossman, Chaloupka, O'Malley, and Johnston (2001) provide evidence from *Monitoring the Future* that the price of marijuana affects adolescent marijuana consumption. They obtained data on marijuana prices and potency from the Drug Enforcement Administration for local communities and related it to the prevalence in those communities of youth marijuana use. They estimated that the price elasticity for use of marijuana in the last 30 days ranged from −0.002 to −0.69. This means that a 10% increase in the cost of marijuana could produce as much as a 6.9% decrease in the number of youth who used in the last month. The study did not indicate whether the effect was more or less strong depending on how many other problem behaviors the young person was engaging in.

Because drugs are illegal, the only current means to increase price is by reducing the supply. Rydell and Everingham (1994) present a model-based policy analysis of alternative methods of controlling cocaine use in the United States. The study focuses on ways to intervene in the supply and demand processes to mitigate the cocaine problem. They note that the proportion of people who use cocaine has gone down in recent years. However, the total consumption of cocaine has not declined. They attribute this to a reduction in the number of occasional users and an increase in heavy users who consume cocaine at a rate approximately eight times that of light users. Thus, the trend in consumption by heavy users roughly cancels the downward trend in consumption by light users.

Rydell and Everingham (1994) examined the value of four interventions: source-country control, interdiction, domestic enforcement, and treatment of heavy users. The first three programs focus on supply control and the fourth is a demand control program. They concluded that money spent on supply control programs increases the cost to producers of supplying the cocaine. Further, they found that supply costs increase as producers replace seized product and assets, compensate drug traffickers for the risk of arrest and imprisonment, and devote resources to avoiding seizures and arrests. The producers and suppliers pass these price increases on to consumers, who then decrease consumption.

Summary

The strong and consistent findings regarding the effects of price on tobacco, alcohol, and other drug use are in keeping with numerous other studies showing the effect of various kinds of costs on human behavior. Increasing taxes on these products is an important method for reducing consumption of these products and the associated problems substance use produces. Efforts to increase the price of illicit drugs through interdiction would appear to affect their use, although it is not clear that this will affect drug abuse. These efforts may affect only occasional users.

Systematic examination of ways to influence other desirable and undesirable behaviors through manipulation of prices is called for in light of the evidence just reviewed. Further research could examine whether increasing the costs of undesirable behaviors *and* decreasing the costs of desirable behaviors will influence the frequency of those behaviors and the number of young people who engage in them. For example, decreasing the cost of condoms may increase their use. Decreasing the cost of recreational activities that promote prosocial behavior should increase participation in them. Increasing the cost of weapons should decrease the number of young people who carry them.

Affecting Availability and Opportunity

A behavior is more likely to occur when the means to engage in it are readily available and opportunities for doing so are abundant. Reducing the availability of tobacco and alcohol clearly reduces the opportunities to consume them. Although some evidence suggests that policies limiting opportunity can prevent other problems, less research is available.

Access to Tobacco

Until recently, cigarettes and smokeless tobacco have been readily available to young people in the United States, despite the fact that sales to those under 18 are illegal in all 50 states and in the District of Columbia. In survey data, most youths say they can easily obtain cigarettes if they choose (Cummings, Sciandra, Pechacek, Orlandi, & Lynn, 1992). Researchers who study the success of purchase attempts reach the same conclusions. Jason, Ji, Anes, and Birkhead (1991) surveyed Woodbridge, Illinois tobacco outlets and found that between 60 and 80% of underage purchase attempts were successful. Forster, Hourigan, and McGovern (1992) found in Minnesota that 12- to 15-year-old male and female confederates could purchase cigarettes in 53% of over-the-counter attempts and 79% of attempts to purchase from vending machines. DiFranza and Tye (1990) estimated that in 1988, more than 3 million Americans under 18 consumed almost 1 billion packs of cigarettes and 26 million containers of smokeless tobacco, generating approximately 3% of tobacco industry profits in that year.

Boys and younger adolescents may have more difficulty than girls and older adolescents do in purchasing tobacco over the counter (CDC, 1996; Forster, Hourigan, & McGovern, 1992; Forster et al., 1997; O'Grady, Asbridge, & Abernathy, 1999). Younger smokers are more likely than older smokers are to cite vending machines as their primary source of cigarettes (CDC, 1996; Forster et al., 1997). Retail outlets with self-service displays are more likely to sell cigarettes to underage youth than outlets keeping tobacco behind the counter (Cummings, Hyland, Saunders-Martin, & Perla, 1997; Wildey, Woodruff, Pampalone, & Conway, 1995).

Researchers have evaluated several strategies for reducing illegal sales of tobacco to young people. Attempts to simply educate merchants about the law have limited impact (Feighery, Altman, & Shaffer, 1991). Similarly, vendors participating in voluntary industry-sponsored programs may be as likely to make illegal sales as nonparticipants are (DiFranza, Savageau, & Aisquith, 1996).

Increased law enforcement does appear to reduce sales to young people. Jason et al. (1991) found that when enforcement intensified through warning letters and citations, the sales rate to underage buyers in one Illinois community fell to 35% in the first 3 months and below 5% within 6 months. Hinds (1992) surveyed 10th-grade students before and after implementation of a local ordinance designed to prevent tobacco sales to minors. The proportion of students who reported having to supply proof of age when they attempted to purchase tobacco increased significantly (from 29.3 to 61.5%). Tobacco use declined from 25.3 to 19.7% overall, with a statistically significant decline from 26.4 to 11.5% among girls. Similarly, Landrine, Klonoff, and Reina-Patton (2000) found that sales to minors by 72 California tobacco outlets decreased significantly after the implementation of a California law increased enforcement. Rigotti et al. (1997) found similar results in a Massachusetts study.

The results have not been completely consistent, however. Forster et al. (1998) randomly assigned seven Minnesota communities to receive a community-organizing campaign to strengthen ordinances against selling tobacco to young people and to increase enforcement. Seven additional communities were in the control condition. Each intervention community passed a comprehensive access ordinance. In intervention communities, rates of illegal sales went from 38.8% in 1993 to 4.9% in 1996. However, in control communities, sales also declined, from 41.9 to 11.5%. Although sales rates dropped more in intervention communities, the difference was not statistically significant.

Because enforcement of laws is so critical, a few studies have investigated specific consequences for vendors who either break or obey the laws prohibiting tobacco sales to minors. Forster, Hourigan, and McGovern (1992) found in Minnesota that over-the-counter sales of cigarettes significantly reduced following a statewide increase in the penalty for tobacco sales to minors. However, this increase did not affect vending machine sales.

Rewarding clerks and stores for not selling tobacco to young people can reduce illegal sales. Biglan and colleagues (Biglan et al., 1995; Biglan, Ary, Koehn, et al., 1996) evaluated a strategy in which young people gave gift certificates and public recognition to clerks who refused to sell to minors; they gave reminders about the law to those willing to sell to them. Biglan et al. (1995) evaluated the interventions using a series of multiple baseline experiments in which they repeatedly measured sales rates in each of eight communities and introduced the program in one or two communities at a time. Sales rates dropped when they introduced the program in a community but not at other times. The average proportion of outlets willing to sell reduced from 57% at baseline to 22% following program introduction.

Embry and colleagues recently replicated these effects in Wyoming, where they helped to implement the program statewide. In the 4 years before the program, the rates of sales were 41, 29, 45, and 55% respectively. The rate reduced to less than 10% in 3 consecutive years after onset of the reward program (Embry, 2000).

Given the ease with which teens can purchase cigarettes from vending machines, some have tested the value of locking devices. Forster, Hourigan, and Kelder (1992) assessed youth purchases from a random sample of vending machines before and after implementation of electronic locks. Minors' ability to purchase cigarettes from vending machines dropped from 86% at baseline to 36% at 3 months. However, it rose to 48% at 1 year. The authors concluded that locking devices are not as effective as vending machine bans and require additional enforcement to ensure compliance with the law.

A critical question is whether reducing sales actually contributes to reducing adolescent smoking. Fichtenberg and Glantz (2002) did a meta-analysis of studies of the effects of access reduction efforts on the prevalence of adolescent smoking. They did not find that access reduction led to fewer young people smoking. These findings are not entirely surprising in light of the fact that friends and family are also sources of tobacco. The data of Forster et al. (1997) indicate that youth reported more difficulties getting cigarettes from over-the-counter outlets and vending machines than from friends and family. Reducing adolescent tobacco use may require constricting the flow of cigarettes to youth from such social sources as well as from commercial outlets.

In sum, stepped-up enforcement of laws against sales to minors can reduce adolescent access to tobacco, as can a program of rewards to clerks for not selling. Given that considerable resources go into access reduction, further study of the effects of access reduction on smoking prevalence should be a high priority. It would be premature to curtail these efforts, however, as doing so would undermine the strong norms established in recent years against youth tobacco use.

Availability of Alcohol

One tried and true way of restricting availability of alcohol is the establishment of a minimum drinking age. In the 1980s, all U.S. states were required to adopt 21 as the minimum age for all alcoholic beverages. The U.S. General Accounting Office (GAO; 1987) reviewed 32 published research studies both before and after the law changed. It concluded that there was solid evidence that increasing the minimum age for purchasing alcohol reduced the number of alcohol-involved traffic crashes for those under the age of 21.

These and more recent studies uniformly show that increasing the minimum drinking age significantly decreases self-reported drinking by young people, the number of fatal traffic crashes, and the number of arrests for driving under the influence of alcohol (DUI). In the most comprehensive review to date, Wagenaar and Toomey (2000) analyzed all published studies on the drinking age from 1960 to 1999, totaling 132 documents. They coded eight key variables for each study. The variables included the jurisdiction (i.e., state or province) studied, specific outcome measures analyzed (e.g., self-reported drinking and car crash fatalities), and whether the study was specific to college student populations. In addition, they rated each study on three indicators of methodological quality. Forty-eight of the studies examined the effects of changes in the drinking age on alcohol consumption, using 78 alcohol-consumption measures (e.g., sales figures and self-reported drinking). There was a significant reduction in youth alcohol use on 45% of the 78 measures.

Wagenaar and Toomey (2000) found 57 published studies that assessed the effects of changes in the legal minimum drinking age on indicators of drunken driving and traffic crashes. They analyzed 102 crash-outcome measures (e.g., fatal crashes, drunken-driving crashes, and self-reported driving-after-drinking). Of the 102 analyses, over 50% found that raising the drinking age reduced crashes and lowering it raised the crash rate. Only two found a positive relationship between the legal drinking age and traffic crashes. Of the 95 analyses including comparison groups, 50 (53%) found a statistically significant effect of changing the drinking age on car crashes. Most of these analyses (92%) employed probability samples or a complete census of the relevant population, increasing the likely generalizability of these findings to the general population. In agreement with Wagenaar and Toomey's (2000) analyses, the National Highway Traffic Safety Administration estimated that a drinking age of 21 reduced traffic fatalities by 846 deaths in 1997 and has prevented 17,359 deaths since 1975 (National Highway Traffic Safety Administration, 1998).

Wagenaar and Toomey (2000) analyzed 24 published studies that assessed the effects of changes made in the legal minimum drinking age on indicators of other health and social problem outcomes such as suicide, homicide, or vandalism. Sixteen percent of these studies showed lower problem levels among adolescents when the drinking age was higher. When they analyzed the 23 studies of higher methodological quality, they found that 35% showed that a higher minimum drinking age was associated with lower rates of other problems. Their analysis of the evidence led them to conclude that compared to a wide range of other programs and efforts to reduce drinking among high school students, college students, and other teenagers, increasing the legal age for purchase and consumption of alcohol to 21 appears to have been the most effective strategy.

If the law is not enforced, no one benefits from a higher drinking age. Despite higher minimum drinking age laws, young people can and do purchase alcohol (e.g., Forster et al., 1994; Forster, Murray, Wolfson, & Wagenaar, 1995; Grube, 1997; Preusser & Williams, 1992). Such sales result from low and inconsistent levels of enforcement (Wagenaar & Wolfson, 1994, 1995). As with tobacco sales, good enforcement of laws matters. Even moderate increases in enforcement can reduce sales of alcohol to minors by as much as 35 to 40%, especially when combined with media and other community and policy activities (Grube, 1997; Wagenaar et al., 2000).

Studies have shown that a number of other policies relevant to access to alcohol affect alcohol consumption and alcohol-related problems. However, there are fewer studies of their impact on adolescents. For example, the number and concentration of alcohol retail outlets may affect consumption (Colon, 1982). Gruenewald et al. (1993) conducted a time-series cross-sectional analysis of alcohol consumption and density of alcohol outlets over 50 U.S. states. The results indicated that a 10% reduction in the density of alcohol outlets would reduce consumption of spirits from 1–3% and consumption of wine by 4%. However, Gruenewald et al. (2000) did not find a significant relationship between consumption and the density of outlets in neighborhoods. At this date, no studies have examined specifically the impact of outlet density on adolescents' use of alcohol, though there is no reason to believe that regulations that affect density would affect adolescents less than they do adults. In fact, given that many adolescents do not have regular access to automobiles, they may be even *more* affected than adults are.

Licensing alcohol outlets can restrict the number or density of outlets in a given area, the hours of sale, the types of beverages, and the size of beverage containers. Several U.S. studies have investigated the effects of privatizing wine sales and eliminating state monopolies on retail sales of distilled spirits (e.g., Holder & Wagenaar, 1990; Wagenaar & Holder 1995). These studies found an increase in overall consumption but did not analyze consumption by young people. Valli (1998) reported that when medium-strength beer was available in grocery stores in a township in Finland, drinking among 13- to 17-year-olds increased. Minors were better able to purchase than when sales had been restricted to state stores.

Reducing the days and times of alcohol sales restricts the opportunities for alcohol purchasing and is a common strategy for reducing drinking-related problems, although in recent years such restrictions have been loosened in many countries (e.g., Drummond, 2000). Smith (1990) found the introduction of Sunday alcohol sales in Victoria, Australia was related to increased traffic crashes. However, these results could be contaminated by other effects on Sunday sales and nonequivalent distribution of crashes over days of the week (see Gruenewald, 1991). Reducing the hours of sale is associated with decreases in drinking and drinking problems (e.g., Gray, Saggers, Atkinson, Sputore, & Bourbon, 2000) and with reductions in hospital admissions and arrests for alcohol-related causes. In one of the few studies focusing on youth, Baker, Johnson, Voas, and Lange (2000) found that temporary bans on the sales of alcohol from midnight Friday through 10 A.M. on Monday due to federal elections reduced cross-border drinking by young Americans in Mexico. In particular, the early closing on Friday night was associated with a 35% reduction in the number of pedestrians crossing the border and a reduction in the number of those with blood alcohol content (BAC) of 0.08 or higher.

In sum, changes in licensing provisions that substantially reduce hours of service may have a significant impact on drinking and drinking-related problems overall. The evidence that such changes affect young people is more limited as most evaluations have focused on the total drinking population.

Keg registration laws require purchasers of kegs of beer to complete forms linking names to numbers on kegs. Keg registration primarily is a tool for prosecuting adults who supply alcohol to young people at parties and those establishments that rent to underage persons. Keg registration laws have become increasingly popular in local communities in the United States. Unfortunately, no studies have examined the effectiveness of these laws in reducing adolescents' access to alcohol.

Many other methods reduce opportunities to drink or to drink and drive. Efforts to promote responsible beverage service or sales (RBS) involve the creation of clear policies (e.g., requiring clerks or servers to check identification for all customers appearing to be under the age of 30 years) and training in their implementation (e.g., teaching clerks and servers to recognize altered or false identification). Saltz and Hennessy (Saltz, 1989; Saltz & Hennessy, 1990a, 1990b) demonstrated that server training is most effective when coupled with a change in actual serving policy and practices of a bar or restaurant. RBS has been found to reduce the number of intoxicated patrons leaving a bar (e.g., Dresser &

Gliksman, 1998; Gliksman et al., 1993; Saltz, 1987, 1989) and reduce the number of car crashes (e.g., Holder & Wagenaar, 1994). However, it is not clear that RBS interventions can reduce minors' use of alcohol. Establishments with firm and clear policies (e.g., checking ID for all patrons who appear under the age of 30) and a system for monitoring staff compliance are less likely to sell alcohol to minors (Wolfson, Toomey, Forster, et al., 1996; Wolfson, Toomey, Murray, et al., 1996). However, Grube (1997) found that voluntary clerk and manager training had a negligible effect on sales to minors beyond the effects of increased enforcement. Similarly, a study in Australia found that even after training, employers rarely checked the age of customers in bars, although decreases in the number of intoxicated patrons were observed (Lang, Stockwell, Rydon, & Beel, 1996, 1998). These results mirror those found for tobacco sales to minors and suggest that enforcement rather than education per se may be key.

Availability of Illicit Drugs

The U.S. government steadily increased its annual drug control budget from $2.8 billion in 1986 to $12 billion in 1992, allocating approximately 70% to support drug enforcement efforts and 30% to prevention and treatment. Although policies for reducing drug supply are in place, limited data have illustrated the extent to which these strategies reduce drug use, particularly among adolescents.

A report by the U.S. GAO (1993) identified the major pro and con arguments regarding drug law enforcement and the alternative approaches most often discussed. Supporters of an enforcement emphasis claim that law enforcement activities in recent years have led to substantial drug seizures and to the arrest, prosecution, and punishment of many drug traffickers and users. Supporters are content that these seizures and arrests have reduced the availability and use of illegal drugs, both directly and through deterrence. They also claim that the connection between illegal drugs and crime is so strong that an intense law enforcement response to drugs has been necessary. Advocates of alternative strategies suggest that the federal strategy, with its emphasis on enforcement, has not made a serious dent in the nation's continuing drug problem. Although the GAO report identifies a range of approaches that do not involve enforcement, it presents no evidence regarding their effectiveness.

DiNardo (1993) examined the relationship between drug law enforcement and the price and use of cocaine, using data from the Drug Enforcement Administration's (DEA) System to Retrieve Information from Drug Evidence (STRIDE) and Monitoring the Future (MTF). The data covered the years 1977–1987. He found no evidence that regional and time variations in DEA seizures of cocaine, among both adults and adolescents, related to variation in either the demand or price of cocaine.

A study undertaken by the U.S. Congress House Subcommittee on Crime (International Drug Supply, 1993) investigated the effectiveness of strategies to reduce the supply of drugs in the United States and the wisdom of readjusting the proportion of funds given to supply-and-demand efforts to combat illegal drug use. The study noted that interdiction programs failed to prevent the rapid growth of cocaine imports in the 1980s and that imports seem to have stabilized at historically high levels, notwithstanding a significant growth in late 1980s interdiction expenditures.

Caulkins, Crawford, and Reuter (1993) presented a computer simulation of the smuggling and interdiction of illicit drugs that specifically allowed for adaptation across routes and modes (air, land, sea). The authors took into account (1) the existence of a "backstop" technology (smuggling small shipments over land), (2) the low cost incurred by smugglers as a function of the fraction of all routes on which the interdiction rate is increased, and (3) the reality that not all smuggling costs are caused by interdiction. With these factors in mind, they concluded that increasing interdiction would be unlikely to have a substantial impact on U.S. cocaine consumption.

Access to Weapons

Brewer, Hawkins, Catalano, and Neckerman (1995) reviewed evidence on various strategies for reducing access to or availability of guns. They concluded that laws restricting the sale and purchase of guns have prevented gun-related crime. For example, a law in the District of Columbia required registration of all firearms and prohibited sales to those other than the military and police. The implementation of the law was associated with a significant reduction in firearm homicides. Not all studies have shown such effects, however, perhaps because of limited enforcement of such laws. Brewer et al. (1995) also described studies of three laws that regulated the place and manner of carrying firearms. Such laws prohibit carrying concealed weapons or require the carrying of a firearm owner identification card when carrying a weapon. The evidence for the value of these laws was not conclusive.

Crime Prevention through Environmental Design

A movement in the crime prevention field seeks to redesign environments by changing physical settings to make crime harder to commit and easier to detect. For example, better locks can make it more difficult to break into a building. Designers can make entrances to buildings more readily visible from a distance through improved lighting and the removal of physical obstacles. They can make public spaces safer and more orderly by improved lighting and a reduction of graffiti or litter. The theory is that these small reminders of deviant behavior encourage other acts of deviance (Kelling & Coles, 1996).

Casteel and Peek-Asa (2000) reviewed 16 studies of the value of Crime Prevention through Environmental Design (CPTED) approaches to reducing robbery in workplace settings. The studies looked at whether environmental redesign helped to reduce robbery. Multicomponent programs of environmental redesign reduced robbery rates from 30 to 84%. However, single-component approaches were not uniformly successful.

Researchers have not examined whether these approaches specifically reduce crime among juvenile offenders. Nonetheless, these findings suggest that future research should evaluate policies that encourage environmental redesign.

Access to Health Care and Condoms

A few investigations have explored whether making access to health care makes risky sexual behavior less likely among adolescents. Most of these have explored the effect of having free reproductive health care at school or at a facility close to school. These sites provide birth control and HIV-related counseling and some dispense contraceptives as well (Kirby, 2000, 2001; Rotheram-Borus et al., 2000). To our knowledge, none have been evaluated with randomized controlled trials. Kirby (2001) reviewed these interventions and concluded that having these services available did not increase sexual activity. However, services also were not consistently associated with decreases in sexual activity and pregnancy rates and with increases in contraceptive use.

Studies evaluating the effects of easy access to condoms (e.g., via vending machines or baskets in schools) have been similarly plagued by methodological weaknesses and inconsistent findings with regard to sexual activity and condom use. None has been associated with increased reports of sexual behavior, however (Kirby, 2001). As Rotheram-Borus (2000) notes, this policy strategy is controversial when implemented in school settings because—although a majority of parents in opinion polls believe students should be able to obtain condoms through their schools (Rotherman-Borus et al., 2000)—some believe that the intervention implicitly condones sexual activity by teens and therefore find the intervention morally unacceptable. A Massachusetts policy dealt with this concern by recommending that school districts consider providing condoms as part of their HIV prevention efforts, allowing communities to determine their own stance on this issue. About a third of the districts elected to make condoms available (Rotheram-Borus, 2000).

Increasing the Certainty of Detection

Basic research on human and animal behavior shows that a behavior can be decreased when immediate, meaningful, nonabusive negative consequences reliably follow such behavior (Biglan, 1995). Consistent with this evidence, policy researchers have explored the effects of various ways of increasing the certainty that a negative consequence would follow use or problematic use of a substance.

Drinking and Driving

Policies that discourage drinking and driving can reduce alcohol-related crashes and the injury and death that result from them. Whether such policies reduce intoxication per se (i.e., affect consumption rates) as well as reduce the rates of driving when intoxicated is not as clear.

Random breath testing (RBT) involves extensive and continuous random stops of drivers who are required to take a breath test to establish their BAC. Tests of RBT in Australia (Homel, 1986, 1990), Canada (Mercer, 1985), and Great Britain (Ross, 1988a, 1988b) indicate that it reduces car crashes. For example, in Australia, RBT resulted in a 24% reduction in nighttime crashes, especially in metropolitan areas (e.g., Cameron, Cavallo, & Sullivan, 1992; Cameron, Diamantopolou, Mullan, Dyte, & Gantzer, 1997; Drummond, Sullivan, & Cavallo, 1992).

Both enforcement and public awareness are necessary for the success of these programs. Moore, Barker, Ryan, and McLean (1993) found that males and those under 30 years of age believe it unlikely that they will face arrest for drinking and driving, despite RBT programs. However, the perceived likelihood of apprehension increased with exposure to RBT, notably when that exposure was recent. Ross (1982) pointed out that the threat of enforcement, or public expectation of detainment and/or arrest, might have more influence than actual enforcement. However, increased public expectations of arrest must be reinforced with actual increased enforcement to have sustained effect (Hingson, Howland, & Levenson, 1988; Vingilis & Coultes, 1990; Zador, Lund, Fields, & Weinberg, 1989).

Individual U.S. states implement sobriety checkpoints, a limited version of RBT, under prescribed circumstances. These frequently involve prenotification about the time and place of their implementation. Even under these restricted circumstances, some evidence suggests that they reduce drinking and driving and related traffic crashes. Evaluation of a Tennessee checkpoint program (Lacey, Jones, & Smith, 1999), for example, showed a 20% decrease in alcohol-related fatal crashes and a 6% reduction in single-vehicle nighttime crashes. These effects were observable 21 months after implementation of the program. Similarly, an evaluation of checkpoint programs in four California communities indicated that they decreased alcohol-involved injury and fatal crashes by between 9 and 40%, depending on the community (Stuster & Blowers, 1995). Investigators observed no significant changes in non-alcohol-involved crashes or in a comparison community. Surprisingly, the degree of success of the programs was the same regardless of low or high staffing levels or whether officers used mobile units or stationary checkpoints. Public awareness and publicity, however, were important mediators of effectiveness. No studies have analyzed the effects of these strategies on youth drinking and driving, but there is no reason to believe that this age group of drinking drivers would react any differently to such policies.

Per se laws specify the blood alcohol level or concentration at which a driver is legally impaired (i.e., the level at which a driver can be arrested and charged with drinking and driving). Zero-tolerance laws set lower BAC limits for underage drivers. Usually this limit is set at the minimum easily and reliably detected by breath testing equipment (i.e., .01–.02 BAC). Zero-tolerance laws also commonly invoke other penalties such as automatic license revocation. An analysis of the effect of zero-tolerance laws in the first 12 states enacting them found a 20% relative reduction in the proportion of single-vehicle nighttime (SVN) fatal crashes among drivers under 21, compared with nearby states that did not pass zero-tolerance laws (Hingson, Heeren, & Winter, 1994; Martin, Grube, Voas, Baker, & Hingson, 1996).

Zwerling and Jones (1999) reviewed six studies of the impact of zero tolerance. All studies showed that the policy reduced injuries and crashes attributed to youthful drivers. In three of the studies, the reductions were not statistically significant, but this may have resulted from a lack of statistical power. Empirical studies conducted more recently have provided additional evidence for the effectiveness of zero-tolerance laws. A study of all 50 states and the District of Columbia in the United States found a net decrease of 24% in the number of young drivers with positive BACs due to the implementation of zero-tolerance laws (Voas, Tippetts, & Fell, 1999). Similarly, a 19% reduction in self-reported driving after any drinking and a 24% reduction in driving after five or more drinks was found using *Monitoring the Future* survey data from 30 states (Wagenaar, O'Malley, & LaFond, 2001).

Scientists have identified differences in enforcement of zero-tolerance laws as a key issue in understanding why some programs are less successful than others are (Ferguson, Fields, & Voas, 2000). Young people's awareness of the law also makes a difference (Hingson et al., 1994). License revocation is one type of punishment shown to be effective in reducing repeated incidents of drinking and driving and as a major deterrent to youthful drinkers who drive. Ross found that the threat of loss of one's drivers license can deter drinking and driving by persons previously convicted of driving under the influence (Ross, 1991). In addition, 38 states have adopted laws permitting license revocation without court action in order to prevent traffic crashes caused by unsafe driving practices, including driving with a BAC over the legal limit (Hingson, Heeren, & Winter, 1996; Hingson, McGovern et al., 1996). These laws were associated with a 5–9% decline in nighttime fatal crashes in some studies (Hingson, 1993).

School alcohol policy is another area in which increasing the certainty of detection and punishment has been tried. About 45% of elementary, middle/junior high, and senior high schools in the United States have explicit policies prohibiting alcohol use on campus and at school functions and, in some cases, any possession of alcohol by students (Modzeleski, Small, & Kann, 1999). Although students report that school policies are a deterrent to drinking (Grimes & Swisher, 1989), formal evaluations of such policies are rare.

Certainty of Consequences and Tobacco Use

There is little evidence on whether increasing the certainty of negative consequences for tobacco use will reduce youth use. Some states have made it illegal for young people to possess tobacco and that might be seen as a means of making it more likely that tobacco use will lead to negative consequences. A recent experimental evaluation showed that combining the enforcement of possession laws and access reduction efforts leads to a significant reduction in the prevalence of adolescent smoking (Jason, Berk, Schnopp-Wyatt, & Talbot, 1999). However, it is unlikely that in most places these laws are being enforced sufficiently to change young people's perception that there will be negative consequences for tobacco use.

School policies to restrict smoking have some empirical support. Pentz et al. (1989) examined the impact of school smoking policies on more than 4,000 adolescents in 23 schools in California. The schools' written smoking policies were evaluated on whether they banned smoking on school grounds, restricted students leaving school grounds, banned smoking near school, and included education on smoking prevention. Schools that had policies in all these areas and emphasized prevention and cessation had significantly lower smoking rates than did schools with fewer policies. Similarly, Elder et al. (1996) evaluated 96 schools in four states and reported that implementation and enforcement of school policies are crucial parts of a school-based intervention. Further, educators must tailor these implementations to political and regional factors affecting a specific school district. However, we know of no studies in which researchers experimentally manipulated school policies in an effort to see whether strong antitobacco school policies alone can reduce adolescent smoking.

Certainty of Detection and Other Problem Behaviors

Brewer et al. (1995) reviewed the effects of various policing strategies, including increasing motor patrol and police helicopter surveillance, community policing, and silent alarms when robberies occur. All these could potentially reduce crime through increased likelihood of detection. Brewer et al. (1995) concluded that intensified patrol strategies during times and in areas that crimes were most likely to occur generally reduced or prevented serious crime. Community policing had mixed results on crime, but different community policing interventions had different components, so it is difficult to compare them directly. Silent alarms resulted in more arrests but not fewer incidents of robberies. It is not clear, however, whether these evaluations focused on adolescent crime or all crime, regardless of the age of the criminal.

In any case, we need to be cautious about encouraging widespread efforts to increase surveillance and consequences for adolescent problem behavior. First, given society's overreliance on punitive practices, we need to distinguish between practices to increase detection and consequences versus those that pertain to the severity of the consequences. Across a wide variety of human and animal behaviors, results show that it is not necessary to impose severe negative consequences in order to discourage a behavior. Instead, the frequency with which a mild negative consequence follows the behavior is pivotal (Biglan, 1995). Indeed, research on parenting shows that children's aggressive and disruptive behavior is more likely when parents use harsh and inconsistently applied punishment (Patterson et al., 1992). The evidence reviewed here does not imply that we should increase the penalties for drinking and driving. Rather, we should increase the certainty of detection so that small negative consequences more reliably follow unwanted behavior.

Second, unbridled pursuit of surveillance policies could produce a negative set about young people that would undermine efforts to establish more nurturing environments for their development. One could readily imagine increasing the surveillance of young people in the interest of detecting early and minor occurrences of problem sexual behavior, antisocial behavior, and substance use. However, such procedures would probably also increase the perception that young people engage in a lot of problem behavior. In addition, it could increase the amount of punishment that they receive. Mayer, Gensheimer, Davidson, and Gottschalk (1986) have documented how schools that invest heavily in punishment-oriented approaches to managing young people's behavior have higher rates of vandalism and other misbehavior.

Third, there is a risk that policies designed to crack down on minor crime will increase police misconduct. Certainly, events such as the Diallo shooting in New York (Flynn, 1999) should make us cautious about encouraging aggressive tactics toward crime without an assurance that we will also protect civil liberties. Perhaps the proper balance would be to introduce policies designed to increase detection of a problem behavior only in conjunction with careful evaluations of its positive and negative effects and to retain that policy only if evaluation showed that its benefits outweighed its risks.

Restrictions on Advertising

Restrictions on advertising seek to limit exposure to children and teens of those materials attempting to sell cigarettes and alcohol. In other words, restrictions seek to limit youth's exposure to material designed specifically to persuade consumers to use substances that are illegal for teens to purchase.

Cigarette Advertising

Despite extensive and sophisticated denials from the tobacco companies, it is apparent that they have systematically been marketing cigarettes to those under 18 (e.g., Biglan, 2001; Pierce & Gilpin, 1995). Wakefield, Flay, Nichter, and Giovino (2003) reviewed evidence about advertising of cigarettes. They concluded that partial bans on advertising did not reduce consumption of cigarettes, but that totally banning cigarette advertising would affect consumption. The so-called Master Settlement Agreement between the states and the tobacco companies requires that tobacco companies not market to young people. But, in the most recent year for which data are available, they spent $9.7 billion on marketing—an increase of about $2 billion from the previous year—and several studies show that they continue to advertise to and reach those under 18 (Chung et al., 2002; King, Siegel, Celebucki, & Connolly, 1998).

Alcohol Advertising

Policies that restrict advertising of alcohol to young people could conceivably affect consumption. Survey studies consistently find small, but significant, relationships between awareness of and liking of alcohol advertising and adolescents' drinking beliefs and behaviors (e.g., Casswell & Zhang, 1998; Connolly, Casswell, Zhang, & Silva, 1994; Grube, Madden, & Friese, 1996; Grube & Wallack, 1994; Wyllie, Zhang, & Casswell, 1998). Although a few econometric studies have shown positive relationships between advertising expenditures and overall consumption or alcohol-related mortality (e.g., Saffer, 1997), most are negative or mixed in their findings (Duffy, 1995; Nelson & Moran, 1995). However, Saffer and Chaloupka (2000) have pointed out that most studies examine relationships between minor variation in advertising expenditures and consumption. Such studies are inadequate for estimating the effects that substantial reductions in advertising might have. To our knowledge, no studies have investigated the specific effects of advertising restrictions on youth drinking or associated problems.

THE VALUE OF POLICY

Policy strategies make a unique contribution to prevention of adolescent problem behaviors because they affect environmental influences more than family, school, and media interventions do. Policies have a potentially longer effective life than prevention programs requiring maintenance and annual funding. Even when the potential effectiveness of any policy decays over time due to lower compliance or lowered enforcement, policies continue to have some sustaining effect. Policies may also provide cheaper ways to prevent problems than those afforded by school, family, or media-based approaches. For example, policies that reduce adolescents' access to alcohol or tobacco products may be less costly than communitywide campaigns to discourage young people from using alcohol or cigarettes. In addition, as noted previously, policies that increase the costs and reduce the opportunities for engaging in problem behaviors may make it unnecessary to motivate young people not to engage in these behaviors.

At the same time, environmental strategies face at least two difficulties. First, they are often controversial and thus politically difficult to implement, especially for alcohol and tobacco, which are legal retail products. Without public support and a strong political force, these strategies will not succeed. Second, policy strategies, especially those conducted at the community level, often do not provide the level of

POLICY RECOMMENDATIONS REGARDING POLICIES

- Studies of compliance are essential for policies. Policies to limit teens' access to opportunities for problem behavior or to increase surveillance by youth and adults (to lower opportunities for such behavior) should examine mechanisms to ensure compliance by those implementing the policy. This means we must increase our understanding of how implemented policies have increased potential to reduce harm associated with youth multiproblem behavior.

- We need research that periodically examines the effectiveness of policy enforcement and possible misuse of policies. In many countries, policies are often lightly disguised efforts to punish youth for undesired or "immoral" behavior rather than to reduce the public health harm associated with such behavior. Therefore, research should be required that assesses effects of policy strategies in terms of their actual reduction of harm. Such monitoring and surveillance will help to discontinue policies that have no effects (other than to increase punishment of youth).

immediate public satisfaction and personal reward to program staff that educational or service strategies provide. This can mean that environmentally focused policy strategies may not be as attractive to community members, especially volunteers. Finally, policies—like other universal prevention efforts—do not reduce problem behaviors to zero. For example, fatalities due to teenage drunk driving will not be eliminated. Nonetheless, policies provide important ingredients, often overlooked by prevention scientists, who focus on intervening with individuals.

THE VALUE OF FEDERAL POLICIES

Local and state groups have designed and implemented most policies evaluated to date. In contrast, federal policymaking has the potential for much broader influence by encouraging states to adopt research-based programs and policies and then providing adequate incentives for those states and communities to comply with the policy.

One example of federal policy with wide-ranging impact is the "Synar Amendment," introduced by Rep. Mike Synar (D-Okla.) and attached to the legislation that provided block grants to states for alcohol and drug services. The amendment required the USDHHS to withhold a percentage of these block funds from any state that did not systematically assess and reduce illegal sales of tobacco to young people ("Substance abuse prevention. . . ," 1993). As a result, each state was required to undertake a survey of attempts by underage youth to purchase tobacco, in random and scientifically valid samples of tobacco outlets within the state. The USDHHS had to preapprove a sampling plan as a valid and reliable survey design. Once a base of sales was established, each state had to demonstrate yearly via a new survey, using the same sampling plan, that it was reducing tobacco sales rates to underage youth. As a result, tobacco sales to minors are declining in most states (see Synar website, *http://www.samhsa.gov/centers/csap/SYNAR/01synartable.html*).

A second example is the federal requirement that states must increase the drinking age to 21 years for all alcoholic beverages (beer, wine, and spirits) or risk losing federal highway construction funds. Because of the requirement, by 1984 all 50 states had a minimum drinking age of 21. As noted earlier, studies uniformly show that increasing the minimum drinking age significantly decreased the number of fatal traffic crashes for youth and the number of arrests for DUI. Finally, in 1998, the federal government, through its highway construction funds, provided special incentives of additional funds to states that enacted a zero-tolerance law that set lower legal limits for BAC on young drivers. As reviewed previously, such laws have reduced auto crashes and injuries. As research clarifies the programs and policies that will foster successful youth development, we should implement federal policies that encourage states to adopt such research-based practices.

SUMMARY AND RECOMMENDATIONS

This chapter has enumerated a broad array of "universal" strategies for preventing the development of adolescent problem behaviors that have been experimentally evaluated. Universal strategies target all of the young people in a population.

Family interventions such as the ISFP and PDFY improve parent–child communication and parental monitoring and limit setting; they appear to be cost-effective methods of preventing substance use. Family-focused interventions to prevent risky sexual behavior have not produced such results, perhaps because they fail to enhance general parental limit-setting skills.

Universal school interventions appear to be of value for reducing aggressive behavior, but, despite substantial evidence of the value of behavior management techniques in elementary schools, we found only one experimental evaluation in high school; it found significant reductions in vandalism. School-based curricula to prevent substance abuse that focus on enhancing a broad array of life-skills have a well-established, albeit modest effect in preventing substance use. However, the widely used DARE project has not been shown to prevent substance use. Less research has been done on curricula to prevent high-risk sexual behavior. Although there is little evidence that such programs increase the initiation of sexual activity, evidence that they prevent risky sexual behavior is mixed and their widespread dissemination would seem to be premature.

There is some evidence from meta-analyses of nonexperimental studies suggesting that media campaigns could prevent youthful substance use. However, we could find only one randomized controlled trial and one interrupted time-series experiment supporting this conclusion. Given the amount of money being put into such strategies, the lack of experimental research is inexcusable. Media campaigns are also being used to try to promote more effective parenting. However, the evidence for their value is even more meager than it is for youth campaigns. Media may also be used to advocate for needed policies and programs. Evidence of the value of media is lacking.

Policies can have the potential to produce a widespread effect at a low cost. Their effects are usually evaluated through interrupted time series designs. We reviewed four types of policies that appear to have preventive effects: increasing the price of engaging in the behavior, reducing the opportunity to engage in the behavior, increasing the certainty of consequences for engaging in the behavior, and, in the case of tobacco and alcohol use, restricting advertising that promotes the behavior.

7

Interventions Targeting Adolescents with Behavior Problems

No matter how widespread our prevention efforts, they will not reach every child in every family. Communitywide efforts to reduce the incidence and prevalence of serious behavior problems must therefore also provide interventions for teens like Michael, who develop serious behavior problems despite our best prevention efforts.

Prevention scientists take two different approaches to these interventions. *Selected* interventions target a subset of youth with identified risk factors that make them more likely than the general population to develop a particular problem.[1] *Indicated* interventions target youth who already evidence the problem.

In this chapter, we discuss interventions for adolescents already exhibiting serious behavior problems. We describe specific programs that (1) met the criteria for sound evaluations described in Chapter 5, and (2) replicated their effects in two or more randomized trials. We draw primarily from literature on indicated interventions, although we also ex-

---

[1]The difference between universal and selected interventions is often a matter of degree—a *universal* intervention directed toward everyone in a low-income community may in fact be selected if low income puts the community youth at risk for the problem being prevented. Further, investigators often examine the effects of universal interventions by looking at general populations of teenagers and at children identified as at risk. Thus, they examine both universal and selected or indicated levels of analysis.

amine selected interventions when we believe the population is likely to contain a large number of teens exhibiting the targeted problem behavior. We also examine reviews of the literature evaluating how well general types of intervention (e.g., wilderness camps and family intervention) succeed.

We begin by reviewing interventions, including pharmacotherapy, to reduce delinquent behavior and antisocial behavior. We also examine juvenile justice policies that have had varying levels of success, some of which may even be harmful. We then turn to literature regarding treatment of substance misuse, risky sexual behavior, and smoking.

One important note: The interventions we review here virtually always target a single problem, despite the compelling evidence that many youth who behave in seriously antisocial ways, such as Michael, are likely to be misusing drugs, tobacco, or alcohol as well as engaging in risky sexual behavior. Research provides little information about the extent to which interventions addressing one set of problems, such as delinquency, alter related problems, such as risky sexual behavior. Nor do we know the extent to which related problems interfere with interventions addressing specific problem areas. Finally, in most cases we infer that the populations of the studies we review below are likely to be teens with multiple problem behaviors, although rarely do authors of the studies specify this.

INTERVENTIONS FOR DELINQUENCY AND ANTISOCIAL BEHAVIOR

A number of reviews have focused on interventions for juvenile delinquency in general. Lipsey and Wilson (1998) conducted a meta-analysis based on about 200 studies examining the effect of a variety of juvenile justice system treatments on recidivism among offenders who had evidenced aggression or serious behavior problems in the past. Specifically, they focused studies of previously recidivistic or aggressive samples referred by the juvenile justice system. These juvenile offenders were mostly male and white, and were on average 14–17 years of age. Lipsey and Wilson reported that researchers had randomly assigned offenders to treatment conditions in about 50% of the studies (treatment and comparison groups were matched in the others). Control/comparison group youth received either institutionalization or probation ("treatment as usual" by the juvenile justice system), depending on which was more appropriate for the type of intervention being evaluated.

The results of this meta-analysis showed that treatment programs in the juvenile justice system (as a whole) reduced recidivism. However, the effect was not large. The researchers described it as "equivalent to the difference between a 44% recidivism rate for treated juveniles and a 50% rate for the untreated control group" (Lipsey & Wilson, 1998, p. 318). Importantly, there was a great deal of variation in effects of juvenile justice system interventions in separate studies. This variation occurred based on type of assignment to experimental groups (with random assignment associated with a lower effect), attrition (higher attrition, smaller effect), type of outcome measure (arrest rates were associated with larger effect sizes than were measures of court contacts or parole violations), and sample size (larger samples, smaller effects).

Lipsey and Wilson also examined whether different types of programs differed in their effects. We should treat the results with caution because Lipsey and Wilson do not describe the criteria used to code interventions into different categories, nor do they indicate the reliability of this coding. In fact, although they were able to label one set of interventions "family counseling," two highly effective family interventions (described later) were not included in this category, underscoring our concerns. It is also not clear what time frame the recidivism measures covered and whether effects were immediate or more long-term.

Lipsey and Wilson (1998) examined the relative effect of different types of interventions separately for institutionalized and noninstitutionalized offenders. They reported that the most effective types of treatments for noninstitutionalized offenders were programs that focused specifically on delinquent behavior (e.g., interpersonal skill treatment), programs that improved parental discipline, and individual counseling. Multicomponent treatments and restitution programs also proved effective with these offenders. Less specific approaches (e.g. advocacy/casework, employment-related interventions, or interventions classified as "group" and "family" counseling) had more mixed results.

Importantly, some programs were ineffective with noninstitutionalized offenders. Those included vocational programs (without a job component), wilderness programs, and shock incarceration. In general, treatment was most effective when the population included offenders who had committed offenses of a more serious nature (e.g., violent crimes against persons). Studies indicating that some of the youth might not have received the complete treatment found poorer outcomes.

Treatment programs found to be the most effective for institutionalized offenders were quite similar to those that were effective for noninstitutionalized youth, with the most effective programs (e.g., interpersonal skills training and teaching family home programs) either emphasizing teen competencies and adult consequences for antisocial behavior or containing multiple components. Individual and group counseling with institutionalized offenders had mixed results. Milieu therapy, wilderness/challenge programs, drug abstinence, and employment-related programs showed no evidence of effectiveness with these institutionalized juveniles. Greater monitoring to ensure that youth received the intended intervention was also associated with better effects.

Although meta-analyses such as this are useful, most underscore the point that different treatments produce different effects. For example, Lipsey and Wilson's analyses suggest that different family interventions may differ in their impact. Simply intervening with a family will not necessarily do the job. The content of the intervention with the family matters. Key ingredients may reside within the extent to which interventions address the mechanisms promoting problem behavior in the first place—factors such as parental monitoring, opportunities for deviant and prosocial behavior, skills, life stressors, and consequences. In the next part of this chapter, we review specific interventions shown to be effective with noninstitutionalized juvenile offenders in more than one randomized controlled trial. We then review other approaches to aggressive behavior, including treatment using medications and other juvenile justice approaches. We also summarize evaluations of approaches that may in fact be harmful—increasing rather than decreasing delinquent behavior.

Functional Family Therapy

Risk Factors Targeted

Functional family therapy (FFT; Alexander et al., 1998) is a family treatment for delinquent teens that focuses principally on family communication, rules, and consequences as risk factors for delinquent behavior. Trained therapists deliver the intervention weekly. Initially, therapists meet with parents and the teen and assess the teen's difficulties and family members' responses to those problems. The therapist formulates a conceptualization of difficulties by looking particularly at patterns of interactions among family members. During this stage of treatment, the therapist also works to reframe the problems in nonblaming ways to engage the family, reduce negativity and blaming, and decrease resistance to participating in family treatment. Then the therapist moves into developing here-and-now plans with the family to use strategies for altering their interactions. These strategies may involve altering consequences for the problem(s), negotiating alternative ways of structuring family life, and communicating in better ways with other family members.

Evaluation

Alexander and colleagues evaluated FFT in the 1970s and 1980s. In a randomized controlled trial, Alexander and Parsons (1973) found that male and female teens between ages 13 and 16 who had been court-referred for behavioral offenses showed less recidivism 6–18 months after FFT than after client-centered therapy, an eclectic psychodynamic treatment, or no formal treatment program. The groups did not differ significantly in the most serious criminal offenses. At 2½–3½ years after treatment, however, significantly fewer siblings of families who participated in FFT had been involved with the juvenile court, relative to the other groups (Klein, Alexander, & Parsons, 1977). A subsequent study with 21 adolescents and their families showed similar recidivism rates (Alexander, Barton, Schiavo, & Parsons, 1976). A third study with similar recidivism rates was one in which trained paraprofessionals worked with 27 teens and their families (Barton, Alexander, Waldron, Turner, & Warburton, 1985). Improvement in family communication after treatment was associated with greater improvements in delinquency outcomes (Alexander & Parsons, 1973; Alexander et al., 1976).

A fourth study (also reported in Barton et al., 1985) with teens who had been incarcerated for serious and repeated delinquent behavior also showed significantly lower recidivism than a comparison sample during the 15 months following about 30 hours of FFT coupled with supportive services (e.g., school placement and job training) immediately after their release from jail. Unfortunately, teens received referrals to FFT based on workers' judgments that they were entering a home environment with at least minimal commitment to maintaining the teen, but researchers did not select the comparison participants in a similar fashion. This raised the possibility that the teens receiving FFT were already more likely to succeed than the comparison teens. Nonetheless, the results are impressive, as this was likely a multiproblem population with histories of serious delinquent behavior.

Finally, Waldron, Slesnick, Brody, Turner, and Peterson (2001) conducted a randomized trial that compared FFT—alone or in combination with individual cognitive-behavioral therapy—with a group intervention and with cognitive-behavioral therapy alone. Teens were referred to treatment for marijuana abuse. Results on marijuana use indicated that FFT and the combined intervention produced significant declines at 4 months after treatment began, but only the combined intervention maintained these changes at 7 months. Both FFT treatments, however, produced declines in the percentage of teens who changed from "heavy" to "minimal" use at both 4- and 7-month follow-ups. The treatments did not differ in their effects on parent reports of aggressive and disruptive behavior or on reports of family conflict; all groups declined significantly over time.

Clearly, FFT has had promising results, but the extent to which it affects multiproblem adolescents is unknown. In addition, many early studies did not address treatment integrity issues. This is particularly important because FFT is a flexible intervention, and this adaptability may make treatment integrity harder to determine, establish, and sustain. Applicability to diverse samples is also unclear.

Cost/Savings

Aos et al. (1999) provided cost-benefit analyses of FFT when used to treat delinquency. Considering benefits both to the crime victim and in terms of criminal justice savings, FFT saves about $11 for every $1 spent on the intervention.

Multisystemic Therapy

Risk Factors Targeted

Multisystemic therapy (MST) is an intensive family- and community-based treatment for youth exhibiting serious clinical problems, including violence, substance abuse, and severe emotional disturbance. Henggeler and colleagues describe the multisystemic approach in detail (Henggeler, Schoenwald, Borduin, Rowland, & Cunningham, 1998). MST targets the known correlates of antisocial behavior in the major contexts of adolescent development (i.e., individual, family, peer, school, and community). Consistent with family systems (e.g., Haley, 1976; Minuchin, 1974) and social ecological (Bronfenbrenner, 1979) conceptualizations of behavior, MST views youth as nested within a complex of interconnected systems (i.e., individual, family, peer, school, community) that can have direct and/or indirect influences on child and family functioning. Consequently, changing a youth's social ecology from one that supports antisocial behavior to one that supports prosocial behavior may require interventions in each system or a combination of systems. Typical MST goals include improving caregiver disciplinary practices, enhancing family affective bonds and decreasing family conflict and hostility, decreasing youth association with deviant peers and increasing their association with prosocial peers, improving school performance, engaging youth in prosocial recreational activities, and developing indigenous supports for the family to help manage current and future problems.

MST therapists provide services in the youth's natural ecology (e.g., home, school, and community), treat youth and their families for 4–6 months, target children at risk for out-of-home placement, provide services to meet the unique needs of each family member, and provide culturally competent services (i.e., based on the family's values, beliefs, and culture). In addition, MST therapists carry low caseloads (two to six families), are available 24 hours per day, 7 days a week, and provide a comprehensive array of services to meet the multiple needs of each family.

Evaluation

To date, researchers have published the results of eight randomized clinical trials of MST, with more than 850 families participating. These clinical trials have targeted violent and chronic juvenile offenders (three trials), substance-abusing or dependent juvenile offenders (one trial), inner-city delinquents (one trial), juvenile sexual offenders (one trial), youths presenting in a psychiatric emergency (one trial), and maltreating families (one trial). In addition, randomized trials including more than 2,000 youths and families are currently in progress across numerous sites in North America and Europe. Youth have ranged in age from 7–15 years (mean = 13.7); most were male (mean = 78%, range = 65–100%) and African American (mean = 54%, range = 37–81%), with a large percentage of Caucasians (mean = 46%, range = 19–70%). In addition, this intervention explicitly assessed the presence of multiple problems in participants. For example, Henggeler, Pickrel, and Brondino (1999), in a study of 118 substance-abusing and dependent juvenile offenders (60% poly-substance abusers), found that 72% of the participants met criteria according to the third edition, revised of *Diagnostic and Statistical Manual of Mental Disorders* (DSM-III-R; American Psychiatric Association, 1987) for one or more psychiatric diagnoses. In addition, substance-abusing and dependent offenders averaged 2.9 previous arrests and 33% had at least one out-of-home placement.

Across trials, in comparison to control groups that received the usual services offered in the community, MST has consistently produced decreased drug use, decreased long-term rates of rearrest (declines of 25–70%), decreased self-reported criminal offending, and decreased days (47–65% declines) in out-of-home placements (Thornton, Craft, Dahlberg, Lynch, & Baer, 2000). MST has also consistently produced significant improvements in family relations and functioning, school attendance, and psychiatric functioning. Youth, family, or therapist characteristics have not influenced these outcomes. MST has also proven to be family-friendly, as evidenced by significantly higher consumer satisfaction ratings than comparison conditions, and 97 and 98% treatment completion rates in recent studies (Henggeler, Pickrel, Brondino, & Crouch, 1996; Henggeler et al., 1999).

A great deal of evidence supports the effectiveness of MST with multiproblem youth. It is one of the first interventions developed in a university setting to explore its utility in community settings. In at least two clinical trials, however, intervention effects were relatively weak (Henggeler, Melton, Brondino, Scherer, & Hanley, 1997; Henggeler et al., 1999; Henggeler, Rowland, et al., 1997). These weak effects were associated with problems implementing the program with fidelity. However, the developers of MST have well-developed dissemination and training strategies for groups wishing to adopt MST. These strategies address fidelity issues. In addition, Henggeler and colleagues have operationalized MST through adherence to nine treatment principles that serve as the clinical foundation for MST. These principles guide the selection of interventions rather than dictate that all families receive exactly the same procedures. This makes the intervention flexible but also requires considerable clinical judgment, which may make effects more variable and dependent on the practitioner's skills.

In addition, to be delivered with treatment integrity, MST requires that therapists carry low caseloads and receive regular supervision from MST-trained supervisors. It also requires that agencies restructure caseloads and work requirements to accommodate the demands of the intensive, in-home services that MST entails. All this requires considerable commitment at all levels of a treatment agency—commitment that may be difficult to establish.

Cost/Savings

Aos et al. (1999) provide an independent cost–benefit analysis of MST, indicating that $13.45 in savings or benefits accrued for every dollar spent on MST.

Multidimensional Treatment Foster Care

Risk Factors Targeted

Multidimensional treatment foster care (MTFC) is designed for adolescents who have shown a pattern of repeated juvenile offending (Chamberlain, 1994) and targets various family and peer risk factors associated with the youth problem behaviors that are the focus of this book, including parental monitoring, providing consistent consequences for behavior, and reducing associations with deviant peers. The intervention involves placing the adolescent in the home of a foster parent who has been extensively trained in behavior management skills and who is continuously supported by intervention staff. Foster parents establish an indi vidualized plan designed to reinforce desired self-management, academic, and social behaviors and to limit the teen's contacts with deviant peers. Key features of the program include daily monitoring of the adolescent's behavior, with consistent consequences for even minor rule infractions. Once the adolescent's behavior is under control, he or she is—when possible—gradually returned to his or her home, and the biological parents receive the same type of intensive behavior management training and support from project staff as was provided to foster parents.

Evaluation

Chamberlain and colleagues evaluated early versions of this program in one quasi-experimental design and one randomized trial. Chamberlain (1990) showed that a very small sample ($N = 16$) of teens who received foster family care was significantly more likely to stay in and complete the treatment program and significantly less likely to be reincarcerated during and immediately after treatment than the 16 teens in the control group. Chamberlain and Reid (1991) found that, compared with 10 teens randomly assigned to traditional placements upon leaving the state mental hospital, 10 teens in the foster-parent group had lower rates of problems at the 3-month assessment and were placed outside the hospital significantly sooner than the control adolescents were.

Following these more limited evaluations, Chamberlain and Reid (1998) tested the program in a randomized controlled trial in which 85 boys ages 12–17 with criminal arrest and felony histories were randomly assigned to the program or to care provided by community-based group-care programs. The benefits of the program were substantial. Fewer boys in foster family care ran away from their placement and a greater proportion completed the program. They had fewer days in lockup or detention facilities and fewer days in the state training facility. Overall, they spent 60% fewer days incarcerated than boys in the alternative interventions. Moreover, these boys spent twice as much time living with their own parents or other relatives after the program was completed. Analysis of juvenile court records showed that boys in foster family care had fewer misdemeanor and felony arrests. In addition, they had fewer self-reported index crimes, felony assaults, and general delinquency. Eddy and Chamberlain (2000) provided evidence that the specific changes in the quality of adult care of the adolescent and the interdiction of associations with deviant peers were the effective ingredients leading to observed reductions in antisocial behavior.

Unpublished analyses of effects on substance use (Moore & Chamberlain, personal communication, November 2, 2000) indicated that, after 1 year in the program, young people who received foster family care reported lower levels of drug use and, after 2 years, less marijuana use (both of these differences approached significance, $p = .08$). By 24 months, those in foster family care reported significantly less smoking, suggesting possible benefits across a range of problem behaviors with a sample that was highly likely to have been involved with multiple problem behaviors before the intervention.

Although MTFC is a cost-effective alternative to incarceration for teens with serious criminal histories, it requires intensive training of dedicated foster parents. Supervision and staff support requirements are also extensive, and the problems these teens can pose in the community require committed, well-trained staff to manage the teens' behavior. These requirements may make this program difficult to implement with integrity and to sustain in community settings. Clearly, however, replication and demonstration projects would be extremely worthwhile, given that successfully intervening with this difficult population may deflect youth from trajectories as career criminals.

Cost/Savings

Aos et al. (1999) conducted an independent analysis of the cost-benefit of this program. They concluded that, compared with the usual community placement, MTFC could provide $22.58 in benefits and savings for each dollar spent on MTFC.

Pharmacotherapy for Treatment of Aggressive Behavior

For many decades, doctors have treated children and adolescents with medications for behavioral disorders. Although research has examined the effects of medication, those studies that met our criteria for rigorous clinical trials generally had small sample sizes and did not classify or describe the youth adequately. Many also used doses too low for children, who often need higher than adult doses to overcome rapid biotransformation by the liver. Thus, it is difficult to evaluate the efficacy of these medications for young people. This is particularly disconcerting given that many of these medications produce untoward side effects.

On the other hand, a greater number of clinical trials with randomized assignment have compared active medications to placebos for patients with severe medical disorders, such as schizophrenia, pervasive developmental disorder, anxiety disorder, mental retardation, autism, and, in some cases, aggressive behavior. Although many of these disorders are not consistently associated with delinquency and drug abuse, results of these studies may have important implications for treatment of these problems. The few well-controlled studies with youth we located suggest that some drugs may be useful in reducing childhood aggression and preventing its progression to more severe risk behavior.

There is some consensus that lithium is a relatively safe and effective short-term treatment for aggression in children with conduct disorder (CD), despite the need for further controlled studies, and although its use is associated with some adverse effects. Campbell and Cueva (1995) conducted a large critical overview of selected literature published over a 7-year period on the efficacy and safety of psychoactive agents in several childhood disorders involving aggressive behavior, including CD. They reviewed only reports of double-blind and placebo-controlled trials and open studies. They found supportive evidence for the utility of lithium in reducing aggression. One recently conducted double-blind randomized trial studying effects of lithium versus placebo with inpatient youth diagnosed with CD (average age = 12½) also found lithium to be statistically and clinically superior to placebo (Malone, Delaney, Luebbert, Cater, & Campbell, 2000).

Another family of medications often prescribed to children and adolescents includes the selective serotonin reuptake inhibitors (SSRIs). There was much hope for the utility of this class of drugs, given consistent evidence for low concentrations of the neurotransmitter serotonin and its metabolite in the central nervous system of aggressive animals and humans. Further, controlled clinical trials of SSRIs in depressed adults have suggested that aggressive behavior is less likely during treatment with these medications than with placebo. Unfortunately, no well-controlled studies of SSRIs have examined aggression in children (Constantino, Liberman, & Kincaid, 1997), although a few small clinical trials and case studies have shown some promise. Nevertheless, SSRI prescriptions for ADHD, aggression, and depression among young people have increased greatly in recent years, despite insufficient evidence for their safety and efficacy and a lack of clear guidelines for use (Rushton, Clark, & Freed, 2000).

Perhaps the most studied drug for youth is methylphenidate (MPH; trade name Ritalin), used in the treatment of ADHD (a frequent precursor of delinquency and drug abuse). Although not generally prescribed for CD, Ritalin may also be helpful in the treatment of aggression and noncompliance in children diagnosed with ADHD in addition to CD. Klorman et al. (1988) conducted two double-blind, placebo-controlled studies indicating that adolescents with ADHD who received MPH showed greater improvements in attention and compliance (according to parents and measures of cognitive function) than youth with ADHD who received placebo (Klorman et al., 1988).

These results seem to apply equally to aggressive and nonaggressive youth with ADHD: Barkley and colleagues found that aggressive and nonaggressive youth with ADHD respond in similar ways to MPH (Barkley, McMurray, Edelbrock, & Robbins, 1989). The exceptions were on measures of conduct, where the aggressive youth were rated as more extreme and subsequently showed greater degree of improvement during MPH treatment than did nonaggressive youth with ADHD (Barkley et al., 1989). Other studies have also shown MPH to reduce aggression in aggressive and oppositional youth with ADHD (Connor, Barkley, & Davis, 2000; Kaplan, Busner, Kupietz, Wassermann, & Segal, 1990).

Two other medications are, in some cases, administered to treat aggression in youth. Practitioners have used Valproate, an anticonvulsant, in the treatment of patients exhibiting aggressive and violent behaviors as far back as 1988. However, reports in the literature reflect uncontrolled studies, which is in marked contrast to the actual wide and established use of Valproate for the treatment of aggressive behaviors. Lindenmayer and Kotsaftis (2000) conducted an exhaustive search and discovered no double-blind, placebo-controlled study. However, a combination of the many case studies reported showed an overall response rate of 77.1%, suggesting a 50% reduction of aggressive behavior. The authors concluded that, although Valproate's general antiaggressive effect is promising, in the absence of controlled data, conclusions are presently limited.

Finally, some researchers used risperidone, an antipsychotic agent, in youths with CD and related aggression. Findling et al. (2000) examined the efficacy of risperidone in a 10-week, randomized, double-blind study. They randomly assigned 10 youths to receive placebo and 10 youths to receive risperidone. Risperidone was reportedly superior to placebo in ameliorating aggression on most measures without serious side effects. Because of the small sample size and the brief length of this study, further research is necessary to confirm these findings.

Juvenile Justice Interventions

Youth Diversion Programs

Several decades ago, labeling theorists suggested that first-time and nonserious offenders should not go to the juvenile courts but instead should receive counseling or mental health services. The belief was that counseling would prevent the adolescents from labeling themselves as delinquent, then behaving in ways that were consistent with their self-concept. According to a meta-analytic review of 44 studies of diversion interventions undertaken between 1967 and 1983, this overall movement did not appear to be effective in reducing recidivism (Gensheimer, Mayer, Gottschalk, & Davidson, 1986). However, teens were "diverted" to programs that differed quite widely in format and content, and often authors of these studies provided limited information on what comprised the intervention. Diversion to ineffective interventions is unlikely to produce positive benefits for youth.

A recent meta-analysis by Aos et al. (2001) came to somewhat different conclusions, indicating that diversion programs produce a modest crime-prevention benefit compared to regular juvenile court processing. One program that involves both diversion and the provision of a well-trained and carefully supervised mentor has produced considerably more impressive benefits. The Adolescent Diversion Project (Schillo, Monaghan, & Davidson, 1996) diverts youth from juvenile courts and assigns them to work with a college-student mentor, trained and supervised through participation in a university class on behavior change and mentoring. Treatment is behavioral in format and includes contracts with rewards for the youth. Aos et al. (2001) concluded that the program was able to reduce government costs $5,720 per youth and, with reduced victim costs, saved a total of $27,212 per youth.

This particular diversion program may have been more effective than previous programs of this type because it included the focus on specific goals and immediate consequences for behavior. This focus also characterized many of the programs that fared well in Lipsey and Wilson's (1998) meta-analysis. In any case, it would be a mistake to assume that any mentoring program would be effective in reducing recidivism or other adolescent problems. Furthermore, as we pointed out earlier, not all diversion programs are equal—the specifics of the diversion intervention matter.

Other Juvenile Justice Procedures

Aos et al. (2001) also reviewed other ways of handling delinquent teens within the juvenile justice system. They found that intensive probation and parole had modestly greater benefit compared with regular probation and parole caseloads. This may have occurred due to the increased contact (and monitoring) by the caseworker. Efforts to coordinate the services youth received were also associated with slightly better outcomes, as were various family treatment approaches evaluated. Although we should consider many of these findings tentative due to the absence of randomized controlled trials, they nonetheless suggest that organization structure as well as content of services may contribute to youth outcome.

Questionable Interventions

Unfortunately, some policies intended to reduce crime may be harmful (Aos et al., 2001). No one has evaluated some of these with randomized controlled trials, but the findings of other studies are so consistent that we mention them here. So-called "Scared Straight" interventions have a deleterious effect. These programs involve taking juvenile offenders to an adult prison to hear lectures by adult offenders about not pursuing a life of crime. On average, they increased offending by 13%, led to increased public expenditures of $6,572 (for added justice system involvement), and cost nearly $18,000 in additional crime victim costs. Not one of the eight studies Aos et al. (2001) reviewed indicated a meaningful positive effect on criminal behavior. We propose discontinuing such programs.

Boot camps are a cheaper alternative to prisons. Like army boot camps, they promote discipline, physical conditioning, and teamwork at the same time they are supposed to promote moral values. Officials first established them in Georgia and Oklahoma in 1983 and within a decade, 30 states had adopted them (Tonry & Lynch, 1996). Boot camps proliferated because they satisfied the public's competing desire to use intermediate sanctions and also to maintain the "punishing" quality of the intervention.

Aos et al. (2001) reported that, overall, boot camps significantly increased offending by 10% compared to sending juveniles to regular institutions. Of the four randomized controlled trial studies Aos and colleagues reviewed, none produced significant positive benefits and one led to significantly *more* criminal behavior in the boot camp group (compared to regular juvenile processing). Although initially cheaper than regular institutions, the total cost of boot camps—including the increased costs of additional criminal victims—is $3,587 per youth. Boot camps also involve bringing together groups of delinquent youth, a practice we view with caution, as described below. Based on these data, boot camps do not seem to be worthwhile investments.

Aos et al. (2001) also reported that a national evaluation of the Job Training Partnership Act indicated it increased offending. The act provides funds for training economically disadvantaged people. An evaluation of the program indicated that it increased offending by 10%, compared to offending by youth randomly assigned not to receive the program. The additional public-borne cost of the program is $4,562 per youth (for the program and the increased justice system costs). The total cost to society (including crime victim costs) is $12,082. Clearly, this program is harmful when implemented with youth.

Incarceration

Sampson and Laub (1997) reviewed evidence on how common juvenile justice practices may make it *more* likely that delinquent youth will commit additional crimes. In particular, they point to the formal stigmatization associated with arrest and conviction. A young person with a conviction may not be able to join a trade union or work in a trade that requires bonding (e.g., as a security guard or a hotel worker). Policies may bar them from gaining licensure for many occupations, including plumbing, electrical work, and nursing. This prevents disadvantaged young people from pursuing many lines of work that might keep them away from criminal activity.

In reanalyzing data from a long-term study of juvenile delinquency, researchers found that length of incarceration in both adolescence and young adulthood strongly related to difficulties with later job stability between ages 25 and 32 (Sampson & Laub, 1997). This was true even when they controlled for other variables that might affect job stability, including official arrest frequency, self-reported delinquency, sample attrition risk, and excessive drinking. Sampson and Laub (1997) reviewed additional studies that show that length of incarceration predicts poorer long-term employment, even when controlling for demographic and behavior variables related to employment. All these findings suggest that youth incarceration may have negative long-term consequences.

Sampson and Laub also noted that incarceration makes it less likely that young men will marry. Marriage and stable employment are both strong predictors of desistance from crime (Sampson & Laub, 1997). Thus, policies that promote incarceration—especially lengthy incarceration—may contribute to continued offending by reducing young men's employment and making family formation less likely. These policies also bring youth into contact with deviant peers, a process linked to negative outcomes (see later). Finally, Aos et al.'s (2001) meta-analysis showed no differences in crime reduction between incarceration and intensive probation; incarceration was much more costly to provide. Combined, these findings call into question recent moves toward mandatory minimum sentences for juvenile offenders, such as Measure 11 in Oregon that requires a 5-year minimum sentence for anyone over 15 convicted of one of 16 felonies (see website: *http:// www.open.org/~lwvor/M11JJ.htm*).

Why Do Some Practices Promote Delinquency?

Why are so many practices with delinquent youth associated with *worsening* rather than *lessening* antisocial behavior? Here we consider two explanations. The first draws on growing evidence that certain types of interactions among high-risk youth can contribute to the development of problem behaviors. The second examines how the types of negative consequences used in response to juvenile crime rarely have the characteristics required for punishment to be effective.

Congregating At-Risk Youth

Dishion (Dishion, McCord, & Poulin, 1999) became concerned about the issue of congregating at-risk youth when an intervention he thought would prevent problem behavior actually promoted it. He created a group program for middle school students (the Adolescent Transitions Program, described later) identified by their teachers as at risk. The program used state-of-the-art behavioral techniques to help these teens develop social and self-management skills. His experiment showed, however, that the youth assigned at random to the group program were more likely to take up smoking than those not assigned to this group. Moreover, the teens in the group program had significantly greater teacher-rated delinquency over the next 3 years than did the youth not in the group program (Dishion et al., 1999). The fact that this was a randomized controlled trial with a sizable sample contributed to concerns that this deterioration was due to something about the intervention.

As described in Chapter 4, one of the most robust findings about all the behavior problems targeted in this volume is that adolescents displaying these problems affiliate with each other. Dishion, Spracklen, Andrews, and Patterson (1996) showed one process by which teens promote problem behavior among their peers. They found that delinquent boys and their friends laughed and joked about deviant behavior much more than did nondelinquent boys. Furthermore, these patterns of laughing about deviance predicted deviant behavior 2 years later—even when initial deviant behavior was controlled. This led Dishion to worry that bringing at-risk young people into groups in an attempt to prevent deviant behavior may actually encourage the behavior the groups are trying to prevent.

Additional evidence suggests that this may be the case. In one famous study of delinquency—the Cambridge–Somerville Youth Study—researchers matched and randomly assigned boys to an intervention involving tutoring, medical treatment as needed, and mentoring (McCord,

1992). The boys in the control group received no special services. When followed in middle age, the treatment boys as a group had significantly poorer outcomes (on an index that included premature death, crime, and psychiatric illness) than did the control boys with whom they matched (Dishion et al., 1999). Further analyses showed that this was likely due to bad outcomes among members of the treatment group who had participated in summer camp twice or more. One possibility is that attending summer camp provided reinforcement for deviant behavior.

Similarly, O'Donnell (1996) reviewed a number of interventions for juvenile offenders that *increased* offending. All involved bringing at-risk or offending youth into contact with each other. Davidson, Redner, Amdur, and Mitchell (1990) reported a similar effect in their study of diversion programs for juvenile offenders.

Apparently, even well-designed interventions that adults provide with the best intentions can increase juvenile offending if these interventions cause at-risk youth to congregate. The story is not a simple one, however. Some of the approaches cited in this chapter showed beneficial effects of group treatment involving teens with problem behavior (e.g., Waldron et al., 2001). In addition, Dishion et al. (1999) found that treatment boys in the Cambridge–Somerville study who were involved in YMCA or Boy Scout groups did not show the same problems in adulthood associated with summer camp attendance. Thus, it is likely that bringing at-risk teens together only *under certain conditions* encourages problem behavior.

A clear and important question lies in identifying the conditions that lead to iatrogenic effects. Dishion et al. (1999) provided evidence that negative results occur when teens have the opportunity to reinforce each other's talk about deviant activities (e.g., bragging and snickering about rule violation and criminal behavior). These findings, in concert with their earlier work, suggest that settings in which these kinds of conversations go unmonitored and unchecked may be particularly risky.

Even though we do not fully understand the conditions under which bringing at-risk or problem teens together exacerbates their problems, we need to take a particularly close look whenever this occurs. For example, consider the growing practice of placing young people who are doing poorly academically in "alternative schools." According to Grunbaum et al. (1999), 280,000 students attended alternative schools in 1998—2% of the total high school population. These investigators administered the YRBS to a representative sample of these students to assess rates of problem behavior. Their findings indicated two things. First, these schools are disproportionately populated with minority students. Whites made up 42.7% of students, blacks were 20.8%, and Hispanics were 25.7%. Second, many of these students display serious behavior problems. Table 7.1 shows the rates of various problem behaviors compared with those for a nationally representative sample of regular high school students.

Table 7.1 shows clearly that a young person assigned to an alternative school will most assuredly attend a school with a higher proportion of multiproblem youth than he or she would otherwise encounter. High schools presumably also offer many opportunities for unsupervised conversations among teens. These data raise serious concerns about the effects of such placements for societal efforts to deter problem behavior.

The reasons for moving problem teens to alternative schools (and indeed for grouping them together in other settings) are not hard to surmise. Like Michael, these teens pose difficulties in the classroom because of their behavior problems and learning difficulties. Zero-tolerance policies, safe-schools legislation, and demand for more orderly schools have all contributed to the creation of alternative schools (Gregg, 1999). Yet the problems these create may exacerbate youths' difficulties.

In sum, growing evidence suggests that juvenile justice, treatment, and education interventions designed to reduce delinquency and other problem behaviors may at times actually increase these problems if they bring at-risk or delinquent youth together. Because these policies can actually make matters worse, it is important to discover why this occurs. Educators need to review and revise policies that create these arrangements. Furthermore, settings that involve troubled youth in groups should carefully assess whether they are producing the outcomes they intend or instead are having unintended negative effects.

TABLE 7.1. A Comparison of High School Youth Overall to Alternative High School Students on Selected Behavior Problems, United States, 1998 and 1999

	Alternative high school students[a]	Youth overall[b]
Current cigarette use	64.1%	16.8%
Lifetime use of cocaine	36.1%	9.5%
Carried a weapon	32.9%	17.3%
Driving after drinking	25.1%	13.1%
Had four or more sexual partners (lifetime)	50.4%	16.2%

[a]Data from the YRBS National Alternative High School Risk Behavior Survey, United States, 1998 (Grunbaum et al., 1999).
[b]Data from the YRBS, United States, 1999 (Kann et al., 2000).

Punishment Policies

Adults often respond to problem behaviors with punishment. It can start in the home with parents' harsh punitive efforts to control their children. Use of punishment continues in school settings as teachers and administrators rely heavily on detention, suspension, and criticism to deal with the behaviors they deem undesirable. We have built our juvenile justice system almost entirely on a punishment model instead of acknowledging youth who behave well. When young people violate the law and are caught, the system is highly likely to deliver punitive consequences. Indeed, in recent years, many states have moved toward greater use of punishment with juvenile offenders, including trying them in adult court and requiring mandatory minimum sentences for offenders as young as 15.

The bulk of these practices does not suppress problem behavior. Although swift, mild, and consistent negative consequences can decrease behavior, many punishment practices are too harsh, too inconsistent, and come too far after the fact to have much effect. In fact, many of these practices appear to increase the very behavior they try to reduce. As we described in Chapter 4, harsh and inconsistent discipline practices are a major contributor to the development of child and adolescent aggressive behavior (Reid & Patterson, 1991). Schools that make heavy use of such tactics are more likely to have high levels of disruptive behavior and vandalism than schools that use positive reinforcement for desired behavior (Mayer, 1972). In contrast, assisting schools in reducing the number of rules and the use of punishment to enforce them and increasing positive reinforcement for desired behavior can reduce disruptive behavior and vandalism (Mayer, 1999; Metzler et al., 2001).

Punishing young people through incarceration or even by requiring attendance at group programs involves bringing together young people with problems, which, as was just shown, can contribute to increased problem behavior. Prison sentences for adolescents increase the likelihood of criminal careers by removing the teens from the social and work settings that might lead them to marry and/or to get jobs—two factors that deter criminal behavior (Sampson, 1997). Here, existing policies are most clearly at variance with those policies that will promote desirable social behavior.

Interventions for Adolescent Substance Misuse

The literature on treatment of adolescent substance misuse and abuse is considerably less well developed than that addressing delinquency, possibly because illegal activities of teens provoke greater societal attention than does drug or alcohol use. Of course, many delinquent teens involved in the types of interventions for delinquency described previously also misuse drugs and alcohol. In fact, Henggeler et al. (1999) tested the effects of MST on drug misuse, and Waldron et al. (2001) adapted FFT for use specifically with drug-abusing teens.

Much of the customary treatment for alcohol and drug abuse among teens has been extrapolated from models used to treat adult addiction, such as 12-step programs (Brown et al., 1998). Unfortunately, few researchers have evaluated these programs using randomized controlled trials. Catalano, Hawkins, Wells, Miller, and Brewer (1991) reviewed the literature available at the time and succinctly concluded that "some treatment is better than no treatment . . . few comparisons of treatment method have consistently demonstrated the superiority of one method over another . . . post-treatment relapse rates are high" (p. 1086).

A burgeoning literature on treatment and indicated prevention has emerged since Catalano et al.'s (1991) review. Many interventions have focused on the family. Two of these—the Adolescent Transitions Program (ATP) and multidimensional family therapy (MDFT)—have shown replicated benefits in two or more randomized controlled trials. ATP targets high-risk teens. MDFT serves as both a selected (preventive) and indicated (treatment) intervention.

Adolescent Transitions Program

Risk Factors Targeted

ATP is an indicated prevention program delivered through middle schools to teens at risk for the development of drug misuse problems and delinquency. In studies of the program, staff invited families to participate if they had a middle school student who appeared to be at risk according to a risk factor screening that included emotional difficulties, problem behavior, stressful life events, academic difficulties, and alienation from parents. In one study, parents responded to advertising and phoned in for screening into the project (Dishion & Andrews, 1995). In another, teachers or family-service agency staff rated students (Irvine, Biglan, Smolkowski, Metzler, & Ary, 1999).

This program works with parents to incorporate and institute consequences for problem behavior, to limit access to problem situations, and to monitor the teen. Specifically, the intervention involves 12 90-minute sessions in which parents from 8–10 families are taught how to monitor and positively reinforce their children's behavior, set limits to prevent problem escalation, and problem solve with their children. The sessions provide videotaped models of parenting skills and many opportunities for role-play practice, discussion, and mutual support. Parents receive between-session assignments and each session begins with a discussion of the outcome of previous assignments. Up to three individual, in-home consultations are available to families as well.

Evaluation

Researchers evaluated the program in two randomized controlled trials. Dishion and Andrews (1995) randomized 158 families to one of four conditions. These were (1) a parent focus condition, in which parents received the ATP intervention; (2) a teen intervention, in which teens met together in groups designed to build their skills at setting and reaching prosocial goals; (3) a group that received both the family and teen intervention; and (4) a control group, in which families received videotapes and newsletters. These tapes and newsletters were the same as those used in the family-focused intervention, but in the control group, the families had no other contact with therapists or group leaders. Dishion and Andrews also assessed a quasi-experimental comparison group recruited via newspaper advertisements that was equivalent to the treated groups, received no intervention, but was not randomly assigned.

Parents and teens in the three treatment conditions showed less negative behavior in problem-solving discussions after the intervention, compared with the control conditions. The five conditions did not differ in mothers' reports of problem behaviors: All the groups showed marked decreases. Teacher reports of problem behaviors were marginally better immediately after treatment in the two parent conditions ($p = .06$) than in the other conditions.

By follow-up, this effect disappeared: The parent-focused groups did not differ from the controls in teacher ratings of problem behavior or in youth smoking. In fact, by follow-up another trend appeared: The two groups with the peer-focused intervention showed significantly worse teacher ratings of problem behavior and more smoking than did the other groups. This finding prompted concerns about treating high-risk teens in groups, as we discussed earlier.

Irvine et al. (1999) also evaluated the family-focused component of ATP with 303 families in eight small Oregon communities. The group leaders were nonprofessionals trained and supervised by three PhD-level clinical researchers. After random assignment, families either received the program immediately or waited 6 months to receive it. Program staff assessed all families at five time points. The program reduced coercive parental behavior toward their children and helped parents to improve their tracking and reinforcement of appropriate behavior, set expectations and define problems, remain calm in distressing situations, set limits, and solve problems. These improvements were not a result of parents avoiding their duties, because parents also reported being less lax in their discipline. The program also reduced parent-reported adolescent problem behavior. The effects of the program were even stronger for families that had attended four or more sessions.

One limitation of this evaluation is that the wait-list families entered the program after six months. Therefore, Irvine et al. could not assess whether the effects on the intervention group dissipated after a year in comparison to a control group, as they did in the Dishion and Andrews (1995) study. This is important because the control group in Dishion and Andrews study improved over time without the intervention. Although the intervention group continued to do well, the controls caught up by 1 year posttreatment. These effects are important to assess in estimating the potential of an intervention for long-term preventive effects.

A second problem in the Irvine et al. (1999) study is that it proved a challenge to get parents to attend: 26% percent of families did not attend a single session and only 46% attended seven or more sessions, despite the fact that, in an effort to establish rapport, each family received a home visit before the program.

In a more recent development, Dishion and colleagues (Dishion, Bullock, & Granic, 2002; Dishion, Kavanagh, Schneiger, Nelson, & Kaufman, 2002) embedded the ATP parenting program in a multitiered family intervention that began with a screening of middle school students to identify at-risk youngsters. They invited families to a Family Resource Center for a "checkup" of the family. Researchers assigned high-risk families at random to receive feedback about the results of the family checkup and invited them to receive further consultation and training.

Although 37% of the families did not participate in the family checkup, 30% of the families did so, and another 32% had some form of contact with the Family Resource Center. Young people whose families received assistance from the resource center had significantly less growth in involvement with deviant peers than those whose families did not get help from the resource center. Similarly, intervention youth had less increase in substance use over time.

Cost/Savings

To our knowledge, no studies have included economic evaluations of this program.

Multidimensional Family Therapy

Risk Factors Targeted

MDFT addresses several adolescent and family factors associated with adolescent drug use and antisocial behavior. Specifically, treatment attempts to build adolescents' social, emotional, and cognitive skills (e.g., develop better stress management skills and establish antidrug use attitudes); decrease teens' affiliation with deviant peers; and improve parent–child interactions and parenting behavior (Liddle, Henderson, Rowe, & Dakof, 2001). Therapists also work to improve families' interactions with extrafamilial agencies, such as schools and the juvenile justice system. Thus, key foci seem to involve responses to stress, drug-related attitudes, improving teen and parent skills, increasing appropriate consequences for drug use, and reducing opportunities for drug use. Therapists individualize the treatment depending on the youth's and the family's situation; treatment generally consists of 15–25 sessions over a 3–4 month period (Hogue, Liddle, Becker, & Johnson-Leckrone, 2002). Engaging and retaining families are early key foci of treatment.

Evaluation

Three studies have evaluated MDFT, two examining its utility in treating drug abuse and the third looking at its viability as a selective prevention intervention. In the first study, Liddle et al. (2001) recruited 182 families with a teen between the ages of 13 and 18 who reported using any illegal drug other than alcohol at least three times a week; 51% used more than two drugs and the remainder used marijuana and alcohol only. Researchers then randomly assigned families either to MDFT, a multifamily educational intervention (MEI), or to adolescent group therapy. MEI included groups of three or four families and focused on learning stress reduction strategies and on improving family organization, rules, problem solving, and communication. The adolescent group therapy condition emphasized building teens' social skills and providing peer support for drug refusal. Thus, this study provided a particularly stringent trial of MDFT because the alternative treatments also addressed risk factors associated with adolescent drug use.

As in other studies of adolescent drug abuse treatment, attrition was considerable. Sixteen percent who initially enrolled failed to attend any of the treatment sessions. An additional 30% of those who started MDFT dropped out, compared with 35% in the MEI condition and almost half (47%) of those assigned to adolescent group therapy.

Liddle et al. (2001) assessed families before treatment began, immediately after it ended, and at 6- and 12-month follow up. Unfortunately, measures were available only for those who completed treatment, which likely inflates treatment effects. Nonetheless, drug use declined significantly in all three treatments from pre- to post-, with MDFT producing the greatest changes. Parent reports of acting-out behavior also indicated significant improvements in all three groups, as did the adolescent's grade-point average, but the three treatments did not differ on these variables. All positive changes were sustained during the follow-up interval.

The second investigation of MDFT specifically targeted marijuana abusers, excluding teens who regularly abused other drugs or alcohol or who were sufficiently violent to pose a threat to others. Nonetheless, 53% met the diagnostic criteria for CD, and many reported risky sexual behaviors (e.g., 39% reported having multiple partners and 23% reported having had sex without protection in the last 90 days; Dennis et al., 2000); 73% were smokers (Dennis, 2002). Thus, participants were likely to have been predominantly multiproblem youth. In this ambitious large-scale study involving multiple sites in the eastern United States, Dennis et al. (2000) compared MDFT with two alternative treatments. The first was a five-session intervention with two sessions designed to increase the teen's motivation to change and three sessions devoted to refusal skills, gaining support for nondrug activities, and relapse prevention. The second was the adolescent community reinforcement approach, in which therapists worked with the adolescent or parent to teach the teen alternative skills for coping with problems and for changing the environmental reinforcers for continued substance use.

Written materials about the project provide analyses through a 6-month follow-up period (Dennis et al., 2000). All three groups reduced days of substance use, but outcomes did not differ for the three treatment groups.

In the final investigation of MDFT, Hogue et al. (2002) screened African American adolescents ages 11–14 who enrolled in a community youth-enrichment program in a disadvantaged inner city neighborhood. Hogue and colleagues invited adolescents who self-reported serious risk factors for drug use or antisocial behavior to participate, matched on demographic factors and randomly assigned to either MDFT or a no-treatment control condition. About 57% of those offered MDFT agreed to participate. Pre–post comparisons indicated that MDFT reduced reports of peer antisocial behavior and improved reports of teens' self-concept and school bonding. The groups did not differ on measures of school antisocial behavior, externalizing behavior problems, drug use, or drug-use attitudes. Few teens in the project reported having used alcohol (6%), marijuana (2%), or tobacco (13%) before the study, however. Rates of parent-reported behavior problems were also in the normal range. Unfortunately, no follow-up data are available yet for this sample. Given the relatively low rates of problem behavior, these data would be particularly important to assess whether MDFT prevented future problems.

In sum, MDFT shows some promise for reducing adolescent drug abuse, but so do a number of comparative alternative treatments. Its effectiveness as a prevention intervention is less clear, but the jury is still out until researchers can collect longer-term follow-up data. In addition, MDFT—like MST and FFT—is quite individualized and may accordingly be particularly dependent on therapist judgment.

Cost/Savings

To our knowledge, no one has conducted formal cost/benefit or cost/effectiveness assessments of MDFT, but Dennis et al. (2000) reported an average per-subject cost for treatment of $1,471 in one site and $2,762 in another.

Other Treatments for Adolescent Substance Abuse

Well-controlled evaluations of treatments for adolescent substance abuse are on the rise, but few replications of promising treatment have appeared. In addition, many interventions with promising posttest results have not yet gathered or analyzed their follow-up data (e.g., Dennis et al., 2000).

Those studies using random assignment that have produced preliminary findings often compare different viable treatments rather than comparing a single intervention with no treatment (considered to be unethical in these cases because of the severe problems associated with substance abuse) or treatment as usual. Many of these comparisons have shown reductions in drug use with various types of treatment (e.g., Dennis et al., 2000; Liddle, Dakof, & Henderson, 2002; Waldron et al., 2001).

In one of the most comprehensive studies of this sort, Dennis et al. (2000) actually conducted two different studies. We just described one of these, which compared a brief intervention with two more intensive approaches. In the second part of their study, they randomly assigned teens to one of three interventions. These were (1) the brief motivational/cognitive therapy treatment, (2) the same treatment plus more intensive skill building for the adolescent, or (3) the previous two interventions plus additional support for families and case management services. Of particular note, they provided these interventions in community sites, making results more likely to generalize to other sites using the interventions. Importantly, recruitment and retention rates in this study were excellent: About 85% of families invited to participate agreed to so, about two-thirds of the teens and their families completed the treatments to which they had been assigned, and virtually all families enrolled in the study initially completed follow-up assessments. Although Dennis and colleagues have not completely analyzed the data from this massive undertaking, initial results indicate that the treatments produced similar results on most measures of drug use and compared favorably to results described in earlier studies examining outcomes of adolescent drug treatment. At the same time, only about one-third of the teens living in the community (i.e., not incarcerated or in residential treatment) a year after the study reported no cannabis use and no substance-related problems. Thus, these interventions provide promising starts but require improvements to help more drug-abusing youth become drug-free.

Family interventions such as FFT, MST, and MDFT provide particularly promising avenues to develop further for drug-abusing teens (Ozechowski & Liddle, 2000). In addition, and in order to extend the reach of interventions to this important population, researchers must clearly specify and evaluate procedures associated with recent improvements in systematically recruiting and retaining families in drug abuse treatment (e.g., Dennis et al., 2000).

In addition, teens who are serious drug abusers face physiological symptoms of addiction and withdrawal due to their drug use. A number of medications have been useful in treating adult substance abuse (O'Brien, 1997), but few have evaluated these drugs for use with teens (Weinberg, Rahdert, Colliver, & Glantz, 1998). Some evidence suggests that naltrexone, a drug used to reduce craving and risk of relapse with adult alcoholics, may be safe to use with adolescents. Initial data from small samples of alcohol-using teens have been promising (Chabune, Leboye, & Mouren-Simeoni, 2000). Clearly, however, this area warrants further exploration.

Treatments for Risky Sexual Behavior

Most interventions to reduce risky sexual behavior combine indicated and selected approaches by offering intervention to groups of teens who are likely to have already been involved in behavior that risks HIV and other STDs or pregnancy. Investigators have examined the effects of interventions delivered to (1) homeless and runaway youth in shelters, a group at high risk for HIV and other STDs; (2) youth attending public health, family planning, and STD clinics; (3) substance-abusing youth in residential treatment; (4) youth in juvenile detention centers; and (5) gay and bisexual male adolescents (see Kirby, 2001; Rotheram-Borus et al., 2000 for reviews).

Most youth attend groups in which they learn about safe-sex practices and receive skill training for dealing with high-risk sexual situations
(Rotheram-Borus et al., 2000). Although several programs have proven
successful at reducing teens' reports of risky sexual behavior in randomized controlled trials with high-risk populations, to our knowledge
researchers have replicated only one, Becoming a Responsible Teen
(B.A.R.T.), in randomized controlled trials.

Becoming a Responsible Teen

Risk Factors Targeted

St. Lawrence and colleagues adapted a program that had been successful
in altering high-risk behavior in adult gay men (Kelly, St. Lawrence,
Hood, & Brasfield, 1989) to use with substance-dependent youth in a
residential facility (St. Lawrence, Jefferson, Alleyne, & Brasfield, 1995)
and with African American youth attending a public health services center (St. Lawrence, Brasfield, et al., 1995). The intervention (B.A.R.T.)
consisted of either six (St. Lawrence, Jefferson, et al., 1995) or eight (St.
Lawrence, Brasfield, et al., 1995) group sessions.

The intervention focused primarily on building youths' skills in sexual situations. One session involved learning technical skills for using
condoms. Youths practiced assertion and partner communication skills
(three sessions), along with anticipating and developing strategies for
risky situations the teens had encountered in the past (one session).
Teens also spent one session learning information about HIV-AIDS in
didactive and interactive activities.

Evaluation

St. Lawrence, Jefferson, et al. (1995) randomly assigned 34 adolescent
males and females in residential treatment for substance misuse to either B.A.R.T. or the single educational session included in the B.A.R.T.
curriculum. Although the evaluation was limited by the small sample
and the fact that treatment and control groups differed at baseline, the
results were impressive—particularly so because these were multiproblem teens. Despite the low statistical power afforded by the small
sample, the groups differed significantly in reports of extremely high-
risk sexual behaviors, including exchanging sex for money or drugs
and engaging in casual sex. Six of the control participants received
treatment for a sexually transmitted disease in the 2 months after the
intervention, compared with only one of the B.A.R.T. participants.
Teens were still in the residential program at postassessment, however,

so whether these results would maintain once they left the residential setting is an open question.

In a second evaluation, St. Lawrence, Brasfield, et al. (1995) randomly assigned 246 African American male and female adolescent patients at a public health center to either B.A.R.T. or the same control condition used in the study just described. They assessed outcomes immediately after the intervention, then again at 6- and 12-month follow-up. The sample showed some indication of sexual risk behavior: 8.6% had been treated for an STD in the 2 months prior to the program, 13.1% had children, about 39% had been sexually active in the 8 weeks before the program, and the sample reported an average of 1.8 sexual partners in the previous year.

The B.A.R.T. intervention produced substantially greater improvements in role-played skills for handling potentially problematic situations than the one-session education control condition. In addition, teens who received B.A.R.T. reported less unprotected sex of various sorts and more condom use than the control teens. Gains were particularly evident for boys, who had higher rates of sexual behavior before the intervention than girls did. Girls' reports of condom use 1 year after B.A.R.T. indicated that they maintained their treatment gains, whereas boys' use had declined and no longer differed from condom use by the control boys.

St. Lawrence, Brasfield, et al. (1995) also examined rates of intercourse for those who had and had not been sexually active before treatment, showing significant differences between both subsamples at 1-year follow-up. Among those who were sexually active before the intervention, 43% of the controls compared to only 27% of the B.A.R.T. group were still sexually active. Among those who were abstinent at the beginning of the program, 31% of the controls had become sexually active, compared to only 12% of the B.A.R.T. teens. These findings are particularly important because they show that HIV–risk reduction programs that focus explicitly on sexual situations and condom use do not increase sexual intercourse frequency. Kirby (2001) conducted an extensive review of literature on prevention of pregnancy and came to the same conclusion.

Another important implication of St. Lawrence, Brasfield, et al. (1995) is that some programs that explicitly discuss alternative approaches to avoiding sexual risk in addition to abstinence may in fact promote abstinence. This contrasts with abstinence-only programs, which—although few in number and methodologically limited—have not been particularly effective at reducing intercourse frequency (Kirby, 2001). Of course, it should also be noted that HIV and pregnancy prevention approaches generally are more likely to show significant effects on use of condoms than on frequency of intercourse or initiation of sexual activity (Kirby, 2001).

Cost/Savings

To our knowledge, no studies have evaluated this program in terms of its economic impact. If reductions in reports of risky behavior translate into lower rates of HIV infection, pregnancy, and STDs, however, the economic benefits could be substantial.

Other Interventions for Risky Sexual Behavior

A number of other evaluations have studied interventions for teens at risk for HIV/STDs. Rotheram-Borus et al. (2000) reviewed programs for preventing HIV. Of the nine studies they reviewed that provided interventions to high-risk teens (excluding the St. Lawrence studies described previously), five showed positive effects on condom use and four showed no effects. Rotheram-Borus et al. (2000) suggested that the more successful programs used group mixed-gender formats with multiple sessions, emphasized behaviors rather than just attitudes or knowledge, and had adult leaders.

Studies reviewed by Rotheram-Borus et al. (2000) were multi-session interventions conducted in various community settings. Another venue for reaching sexually active teenagers is a medical clinic, when teens come in for appointments. Kirby (2001) reviewed six studies of brief interventions delivered during clinic appointments in medical settings, four of which were randomized controlled trials. The most consistently effective of these in producing increased use of contraception and condoms were brief interventions with a 10–20-minute educational component (e.g., slide-tape presentation) related to HIV/STD prevention, followed by a personalized conversation about contraception or demonstration and role play of condom use. These interventions clearly warrant greater empirical scrutiny because they are brief, likely to be cost-effective, and able to reach many adolescents through health care delivery systems. It is not clear, however, how many of the teens who participated in these studies were engaging in risky sexual behavior prior to the intervention; thus specific effects on multi-problem youth need to be established.

Research on treatment of risky sexual behavior among teens, like that on smoking cessation and drug abuse treatment, is less developed than studies seeking to reduce antisocial behavior. Perhaps this is because interventions to reduce HIV risk behaviors among teens are politically controversial: Some maintain that to talk about sexual activity is to condone it, and others fear that risk prevention programs will lead to more, rather than less, sexual behavior. As Rotheram-Borus (2000) points out, the range of interventions targeting adolescents has been limited, with virtually no programs developed with widespread implementation in mind. In addition, most programs focus on skill building in individual adolescents and relatively few focus on other mechanisms that may be involved in risky sexual behavior. Almost no interventions have addressed family and peer factors related to sexual risk taking, except as they relate to communication with romantic partners. Finally, as mentioned in Chapter 6, policy-related interventions for preventing HIV/STD/pregnancy have been underexplored, perhaps because of political controversies associated with universal approaches to reducing risky adolescent sexual behavior.

Another issue that future research needs to address involves measurement. Virtually all studies assessing the effects of HIV and pregnancy risk prevention/reduction have used self-reports of sexual behavior to measure their effects. Some researchers have voiced concerns, however, that a variety of biasing factors may influence these reports, particularly after treatment (Malow, Gustan, Ziskind, McMahon, & St. Lawrence, 1998), and suggest that researchers take stronger measures to verify the accuracy of the information that teens report. Beside providing improved ways of measuring risky sexual behavior, studies that examine actual pregnancy, HIV infection, and STD rates will be important as this field moves forward. These studies will be difficult to do, however, because not all risky behavior results in these outcomes; because these outcomes are relatively rare, even in high-risk populations; and because adolescents are not continuously sexually active. All these factors mean that research will require long-term follow-up of large samples to have enough statistical power to detect significant effects.

TOBACCO USE CESSATION FOR ADOLESCENTS

Perhaps because about one in three adolescent smokers will eventually die of a smoking-related illness, investigators have developed smoking cessation programs for adolescents. Like adults, the majority of adolescent smokers say that they want to quit (Lantz et al., 2000). However, most adolescents are not familiar with the concept of a smoking-cessation program and are disinclined to seek professional assistance (Lantz et al., 2000). Most adult smokers also would prefer to quit on their own (Personal Improvement Computer Systems, 2001).

Advice from health care professionals to stop smoking has proven to significantly increase the proportion of adult smokers who quit (Hollis, Lichtenstein, Vogt, Stevens, & Biglan, 1993). However, whether physician advice to quit will work among adolescents is less clear. In addition, it currently appears that many fewer adolescent than adult smokers receive such advice from health care providers (Lantz et al., 2000).

Sussman, Lichtman, Ritta, and Pallonen (1999) reviewed 17 evaluations of tobacco cessation programs for adolescents. Of the 17 studies, only 3 employed group design experiments. There was also considerable heterogeneity in intervention methods and in the theories on which researchers based the interventions, making it even more difficult to draw clear inferences about what, if anything, works. One consistency across studies was the use of clinics, with 12 of the studies providing clinic-based interventions in school settings and 2 providing them outside schools. The mean number of sessions across studies was 6.3 (range 1 to 20). Participants ranged from 12 to 22 years old. Among the 12 studies that reported a quit rate, the mean quit rate at posttest was 20.7% (0.0 to 36%). It dropped to 13% at follow-up. Data from six studies suggested that adolescents who did not quit reduced their rates of use.

The Sussman et al. (1999) review does not include a well-controlled randomized trial that investigators conducted at Kaiser-Permanente in Portland, Oregon (Vogt, Lichtenstein, Ary, & Biglan, 1989). Despite a series of contacts with a nurse and phone follow-ups, the intervention did not significantly improve cessation among treated adolescents compared to a control condition that provided health information unrelated to smoking.

In sum, in spite of the fact that smoking-cessation programs for adults have clear benefit (Biglan, 2001), there is still insufficient evidence that any existing program helps adolescents quit smoking. Adolescents may be less experienced than adults in coping with unpleasant feelings that accompany quitting the use of tobacco. Alternatively, teens may hide their tobacco use from parents and others who could serve as sources of support for quitting. Regardless of the reasons, researchers must develop and test new approaches to adolescent smoking cessation via randomized controlled trials. In addition, because smoking among teens is illegal and teens often hide their smoking from adults, it will be important to develop and evaluate effective methods of reaching teen smokers to encourage their participation in these interventions.

SUMMARY AND RECOMMENDATIONS

Several comprehensive interventions that target family interactions, peer-group involvement, and problems in school have been shown to reduce antisocial behavior. These include FFT, MST, and foster family treatment. Interventionists have used FFT and MST with teens referred for drug-abuse problems, with some success. These treatments specifically

POLICY RECOMMENDATIONS

• Adoption of evidence-based practices for treating problem adolescents will reduce their numbers. Many of the interventions with proven effects for treating individual children and families require considerable clinical skill to implement. This in turn requires appropriately sized caseloads, appropriate training, and appropriate supervision to ensure continued treatment fidelity.

• Practices that bring at-risk and behavior problem teens together into groups should be carefully examined for negative effects, particularly when interactions among youth are unsupervised and are likely to revolve around deviant behavior.

• Professions that implement interventions for multiproblem youth should develop "best practice" guidelines based on the best available scientific evidence. These guidelines should be widely disseminated and updated routinely as new knowledge accumulates. They should be taught routinely as part of professional education programs.

target empirically based risk factors strongly associated with delinquent behavior. Some researchers have evaluated medications, but not with the large samples and scientific rigor necessary for clear conclusions.

Meta-analysis has identified some juvenile justice interventions that have shown modest positive effect, but others may be harmful. Boot camps for juveniles, shock incarceration, and "scared straight" programs, for example, have produced negative effects.

Equally worrisome are findings from randomized controlled trials that occasionally a group of at-risk teens treated together shows significantly worse behavior than control teens. A sufficient number of these findings have emerged so that they cannot be considered flukes. These findings raise serious concerns about customary aggregation of high-risk or problem youth in school and jail settings. Greater attention to these settings and to studying the processes that promote unintended negative effects is imperative.

Compared with the delinquency area, we know far less about treatment of adolescent substance misuse, risky sexual behavior, and smoking cessation. Investigators in these areas have instead examined preventive strategies (see Chapter 6), although adolescent drug-abuse treatment research has improved markedly in quantity and quality in the last several years. Promising treatments exist for teen risky sexual behavior and for drug abuse, but to our knowledge, none of these programs is in wide-

RESEARCH RECOMMENDATIONS

- Although several interventions have had significant effects in randomized controlled trials, many teens either do not respond to treatment or relapse. Researchers should systematically study treatment responders so that interventions can continue to improve their effectiveness.

- Study methods for recruiting and retaining teens and families in interventions.

- Identify and study the effectiveness of methods to promote the adoption of evidence-based treatments in clinical and medical settings.

- Replicate the effects of treatments shown to be effective in community settings in preparation for wide-scale dissemination.

- Develop new treatments with dissemination efforts in mind.

- Identify methods for promoting and assessing treatment fidelity in community settings.

- Research on treating individual behavior problems (e.g., drug abuse) should include measures of related behavior problems to assess generality of effect.

- Identify under what specific conditions, and for whom, treatment of at-risk youth produces unanticipated negative effects. Peer processes are particularly suspect, warranting close empirical scrutiny.

spread use and few have developed materials and technology needed for widespread dissemination. We should replicate the most promising of them.

Unlike prevention programs, treatment programs for problem behavior tend to be highly focused on the target problem, despite the fact that teens with serious problems in one area are likely to display other problems as well. Imagine if Michael were to receive treatment for his behavior problems: He would need to meet regularly with his parole officer, and receive MST for antisocial behavior and drug misuse. If that did not work for his drug misuse, his mother would need to participate in MST. Michael would also need to go to classes to reduce risky sexual behavior and sign up for a stop-smoking program. What are the odds that an unmotivated teen and a busy, stressed, economically disadvantaged single parent would follow through on all of these treatment plans?

This proliferation of services for specific problems may or may not be required. Future studies should evaluate whether treatment programs that focus on a single problem also affect related problems. These studies should also examine whether co-occurring problems impede progress of treatments that target only one of several correlated difficulties. Ultimately we need to identify interventions that efficiently alter the most important risk factors for diverse problem behaviors and see if they are the most economical way to reduce diverse problems. For example, interventions such as MST that focus on changing the peer, family, and school environments appear to alter the conditions that contribute to a wide range of problems.

It is equally as essential, however, that we attempt to better understand which interventions work for which adolescents. There likely will not be any one intervention, even for multiple problem behaviors, that will affect all youth in the same way; individual differences must be taken into account. This is not surprising, given the fact that there may be many different pathways leading to the development of the kinds of problems Michael displays.

One impediment to implementing evidence-based interventions for adolescents with serious behavior problems lies in the many disciplines and organizations that are involved in dealing with these youth. Professionals in education, psychiatry, psychology, social work, juvenile justice, family planning, and family medical practice can all be involved. For a community to affect the prevalence of serious youth behavior problems at a community level, it is necessary for all individuals to use "best practices" in their field. At times, this will mean discontinuing existing practices that may be harmful. The current structure of many service provision organizations in contemporary U.S. communities may mean converting one professional at a time—a nearly impossible task.

One alternative to this laborious process is to provide incentives that promote improved practices and that will encourage professionals to evaluate their work and to adopt evidence-based practices. In Chapter 9, we discuss this issue in more detail.

Finally, it may go without saying that potentially effective interventions for multiproblem youth often run aground on the shoals of political objections. This is particularly the case with interventions for risky sexual behavior, but it can also be the case with drug abuse and smoking cessation. With juvenile crime, societal desires to "get tough on crime" may inadvertently lead to policies that satisfy these desires at the expense of effective crime reduction. Media efforts could educate the public about the importance of evaluating different sorts of intervention, then basing decisions on documented outcomes rather than anticipated outcomes to shift the tide toward greater attention to evidence that an intervention does or does not work. After all, do we ultimately want to expend enormous societal costs and efforts based only on ideology or on anecdotes about single dramatic outcomes? Would we rather spend the same capital and effort on approaches that have been shown to work for many children like Michael? We will explore these issues again in Chapter 9.

8

Comprehensive Community
and Statewide Interventions

The previous chapters examined the effects of specific interventions and policies evaluated in isolation from each other. However, it is possible that these interventions could be combined into comprehensive interventions and could affect the rates of problems in entire populations of communities or states. In this chapter, we describe six community interventions that combined a number of programs and policies and were evaluated in experimental or quasi-experimental ways. We also describe some recent statewide efforts that—although not evaluated through experimental designs—indicate the potential for affecting the populations of entire states.

Although comprehensive community interventions have the potential to prevent the entire range of youth problems, the well-evaluated ones have thus far focused only on the prevention of substance use. One focused on reducing tobacco use, four on reducing alcohol use and alcohol-related problems, and one on all forms of substance use. Given the interrelationships among youth problems, the many influences they have in common, and the many programs and policies that can affect those problems, the next generation of community interventions will need to use comprehensive approaches to preventing the entire range of youth problems.

COMMUNITY INTERVENTIONS

Project SixTeen

Intervention

Project SixTeen tested a community intervention to prevent adolescent tobacco use. It had five components: (1) a classroom curriculum designed to prevent tobacco use, (2) media advocacy for preventing tobacco use, (3) youth antitobacco activities, (4) family communications about tobacco use, and (5) reduction of illegal sales of tobacco to young people. The school-based program was Project PATH (Biglan, James, LaChance, Zoref, & Joffe, 1988), which contained the chief components of interactive programs described in Chapter 7.

Evaluation

Researchers evaluated the effects of the intervention by assigning eight communities at random to receive the entire intervention and eight others to receive only the classroom curriculum. Biglan, Ary, Duncan, Black, and Smolkowski (2000) assessed effects among seventh and ninth graders through five annual surveys of the prevalence of self-reported smoking and smokeless tobacco (ST) use in the month before assessment. They also assessed antisocial behavior and other substance use.

Compared with communities that received only the school-based program, the community intervention led to significantly lower prevalence of cigarette use 1 and 5 years after the program began. The effect after 4 years approached significance. The community intervention also led to a lower prevalence of ST among ninth-grade boys at Time 2, with ST use decreasing in intervention communities but not in control communities. Despite the fact that the program did not specifically target alcohol or marijuana use, there were significant effects on the slope of alcohol use among ninth graders. This means that over the 4 years, alcohol use was not increasing as rapidly in intervention communities as in school-based-only communities. Moreover, there was a significant effect on the quadratic slope of marijuana for all students. Over the 4 years, marijuana use was curving upward in school-based communities but curving downward in intervention communities. Consistent with the gateway hypothesis (Kandel, 2002), preventing tobacco use may have contributed to preventing the use of other substances.

Project Northland

Intervention

This two-phase intervention targeted alcohol use among early adolescents (Perry et al., 1993, 1996, 1998, 2000). In the first phase, Project Northland targeted students in grades 6 through 8. The program relied principally on persuasion, norm setting, and reducing opportunities to drink. It was designed to improve parent–child communication about alcohol use, enhance students' reasons for not using alcohol, strengthen students' beliefs that they were capable of resisting alcohol, reduce peer influences on drinking, improve alcohol use norms, and reduce students' ease of access to alcohol. The strategies used included parental involvement and education, social–behavioral curricula delivered in the schools, peer leadership opportunities, and communitywide task force activities. In the second phase, when students were in grades 11 and 12, Project Northland attempted to implement local policies requiring RBS for on- and off-premise alcohol establishments. Researchers implemented a gold-card system with local merchants to give discounts to students who pledged to remain alcohol and drug free (Veblen-Mortenson et al., 1999), thereby adding incentives for promises to abstain and additional measures to limit teens' access to alcohol.

Evaluation

Investigators randomly assigned 24 school districts to intervention or control conditions. They assessed alcohol use and other behaviors at the end of grades 6–12. The first phase of the intervention led to substantial reductions in alcohol use. At the end of the eighth grade, intervention students reported significantly less alcohol use in the past week and in the past month and reduced peer influence on behavior, compared to students in control communities (Perry et al., 1996). Students receiving the program also had better attitudes and normative beliefs regarding alcohol use than did those in comparison communities. Those who did not use alcohol at the beginning of the project reported significantly less alcohol, marijuana, and cigarette use at the end of eighth grade than did teens in the control school districts, but teens already involved in early substance use did not benefit similarly. This raises questions about the extent to which those teens likely to develop multiple problems would benefit from this intervention.

By the 10th grade, the effects of the program on alcohol use had decayed (Perry et al., 1998). Intervening again with the second phase seemed to counteract this decay: At the end of the 12th grade, the increase in alcohol use and binge drinking was again significantly less in the intervention schools than in the control schools (Perry et al., 2002). In addition, there was a significant reduction in commercial access to alcohol.

Communities Mobilizing for Change on Alcohol

Intervention

Communities Mobilizing for Change on Alcohol (CMCA) focused on using the media and changing policies affecting adolescent alcohol use rather than on efforts to change adolescents' motivation to use alcohol (Wagenaar, Murray, Gehan, et al., 2000; Wagenaar, Murray, Wolfson, & Forster, 1994). A primary goal involved changing community policies regarding access to alcohol by those under 21, thus limiting youths' opportunities to drink. Through numerous contacts with groups and organizations that might affect policies, practices, and norms for minors' access to alcohol, researchers created a strategy team in each community to lead efforts to bring about change (Wagenaar et al., 1999). This team used media advocacy to increase media coverage of alcohol issues in the community. The strategy teams also implemented various activities to reduce youth access to alcohol. These activities included efforts designed to stop alcohol merchants from selling to young people, increased enforcement of laws regarding underage sales, changes in community events to make alcohol less readily available to young people, prevention of underage drinking parties at hotels, information provided to parents, and alternative sentencing for youth who violated drinking laws. The specific activities varied across communities.

Evaluation

Scientists evaluated CMCA in a randomized trial in which they assigned 15 Minnesota and Wisconsin communities to receive or not receive the program. The CMCA communities had lower levels of alcohol sales to minors in their retail outlets and had marginally lower sales to minors at bars and restaurants. Phone surveys of 18- to 20-year-olds indicated that those in the CMCA communities were less likely to try to buy alcohol and less likely to provide alcohol to others. The proportion of 18- to 20-year-olds who reported drinking in the past 30 days was marginally lower in intervention than in control communities. However, there was no effect on the prevalence of heavy drinking in this age group and there were no significant effects on the drinking behavior of 12th graders (who were surveyed in school). Arrests of 18- to 20-year-olds for driving under the influence of alcohol declined significantly more in CMCA communities than in control communities (Wagenaar, Murray, Gehan, et al., 2000). The difference for 15- to 17-year-olds approached significance.

Saving Lives Project

Intervention

Hingson and colleagues designed the *Saving Lives Project* to reduce alcohol-impaired driving and related problems such as speeding (Hingson, McGovern, et al., 1996). They conducted the work in six Massachusetts communities. In each community, a full-time city employee organized a task force of representatives from city departments to work on the project. The task force designed the specific activities for its community. These activities included media campaigns, business information programs, speeding and drunk driving awareness days, speed-watch telephone hotlines, police training, high school peer-led education, *Students against Drunk Driving* chapters, and college prevention programs.

Evaluation

Researchers evaluated these interventions through a quasi-experimental design in which five comparison communities served as controls. Although the control communities were slightly more affluent than the experimental sites, they had similar demographic characteristics, rates of traffic citations, and fatal crashes. Outcomes measured included fatal and injury crashes, seat belt use, auto speed, traffic citations, and telephone surveys of self-reported drinking and driving. Over the 5 years of the program, *Saving Lives* cities experienced a decline in all fatal car crashes and in alcohol-related fatal crashes when compared to the rest of Massachusetts. Compared to the 5 years before the intervention, the *Saving Lives* cities had a 42% reduction in fatal auto crashes, a 47% reduction in the number of fatally injured drivers who were positive for alcohol, and an 8% decline in 16- to 25-year-old crash injuries. In addition, there was a decline in self-reported driving after drinking among youth and about a 50% reduction in observed speeding. The greatest fatal and injury crash reductions occurred in the 15- to 25-year-old age group.

Community Trials Project

Intervention

This project tested a five-component community intervention to reduce alcohol-related harm among people of all ages (Holder et al., 1997). It sought to reduce the primary sources of harm related to alcohol: drunken-driving injuries and fatalities; injuries and deaths related to violence; and drowning, burns, and falls.

The Community Trials Project had five intervention components. One was a *Media and Mobilization* component to develop community organization and support for the goals and strategies of the project and to use local news to increase public support of environmental strategies. The second was an RBS component to reduce service to intoxicated patrons at bars and restaurants. The third was a *Sales to Youth* component to reduce underage access. The last two components were a *Drinking and Driving* component to increase local enforcement of DUI laws and an *Access* component to reduce the availability of alcohol. That component focused principally on reducing opportunities for youth to obtain alcohol and on the consequences received for one type of alcohol misuse—driving while intoxicated.

Evaluation

Project staff evaluated the effects of the program by comparing three communities that received the intervention with matched comparison communities. The communities selected had a population of over 100,000 and were not bedroom communities. Their alcohol problem indicators were about equal to the state average. Each community was racially diverse, with 40% or more minority group members.

Each of the intervention components affected its target in the communities in which it took place. Of particular interest for our purposes is the fact that the *Sales to Youth* component produced a significant reduction in alcohol sales to minors. Overall, off-premise outlets in experimental communities were half as likely to sell alcohol to minors as those outlets in the comparison sites. This was the joint result of special training of clerks and managers to conduct age ID checks, the development of effective off-premise outlet policies, and, especially, the threat of enforcement of laws against sales to minors (Grube, 1997). Moreover, the *Drinking and Driving* component increased enforcement of drinking and driving laws and a significantly reduced alcohol-involved traffic crashes (Voas, Holder, & Gruenewald, 1997).

Comparing experimental and control communities, the intervention produced significant reductions in nighttime injury crashes (10% lower in experimental than in comparison communities) and in crashes in which the police found the driver to "have been drinking" (6%). Assault injuries observed in emergency departments were 43% lower in the intervention communities than in the comparison communities, and assaults requiring hospitalization were 2% lower. Reports of driving after "having had too much to drink" were 49% lower and self-reports of driving when "over the legal limit" were 51% lower. Although the drinking population increased slightly in the experimental sites over the course of the study, there was a significant reduction in problematic alcohol use: Average drinks per occasion declined by 6% and the variance in drinking patterns (an indirect measure of heavy drinking) declined 21% (Holder et al., 2000). Unfortunately, researchers did not specifically evaluate alcohol use by young people.

Midwestern Prevention Program

Intervention

Researchers designed the Midwestern Prevention Program (MPP) to prevent any type of substance use. They evaluated MPP in Kansas City, Missouri, and Indianapolis, Indiana. The program had five components: (1) classroom curriculum, (2) parent–child activities, (3) a school task force working on school policies and parent–child activities, (4) media promotion of prevention policies and norms, and (5) the creation of community action committees to promote drug prevention in community organizations such as churches and work places. The classroom curriculum targeted students in grade 6 (for those entering middle school) or 7 (for those entering junior high school).

Evaluation

Pentz and colleagues evaluated MPP in Kansas City using a quasi-experimental design in which they randomly assigned some schools to MPP and some to delayed-intervention conditions, while other schools were assigned based on scheduling. Later they added the Indianapolis site, where they randomly assigned school clusters to conditions. Both MPP and comparison youth were exposed to the media campaigns and to the school and community policy initiatives. Thus, comparison of treatment and control conditions evaluated only the additive effects of the school and parenting aspects of the program.

Apparently, the school and parent–child activities were beneficial. Pentz, Dwyer, et al. (1989) found that in Kansas City, intervention youth had a significantly lower increase in cigarette, alcohol, and marijuana use in the prior week at 1-year follow-up. Program effects on smoking persisted at 2-year follow-up in the Kansas City sample and affected the prevalence of heavy and light smoking equally (Pentz, McKinnon, et al., 1989). In 9th and 10th grades, expired carbon monoxide measures of smoking were also lower in MPP than in the comparison groups (Pentz,

Dwyer, et al., 1989). Results after 3½ years in the Indianapolis study, which randomly assigned students to conditions, showed significantly less tobacco and marijuana (but not alcohol) use in MPP than in comparison schools. Post hoc analyses of the Indiana schools indicated that results found in private and parochial—not public—schools were largely responsible for the positive intervention effects in Indianapolis (Pentz et al., 1994).

Of particular interest are two studies examining the effects of MPP in high-risk samples of youth. Johnson et al. (1990) reported on only those students in the Kansas City sample who received MPP or delayed intervention (by random assignment). They examined whether the effectiveness of the MPP school/parent components differed as a function of risk factors assessed at baseline, which included gender and grade of the youth; whether the youth reported tobacco, alcohol, or marijuana use during the pretest; and student reports of friends' or parents' use of alcohol, tobacco, or marijuana. Although risk was highly associated with substance use, the intervention was equally effective with high- and low-risk youth. The results indicated that the program was more effective for seventh- than for sixth-grade students.

Using a different approach, Chou et al. (1998) examined data collected from the Indianapolis participants who reported any drug or alcohol use during the month before baseline. Researchers looked at data obtained up to 3½ years after baseline. In particularly stringent analyses,[1] they examined the percentage of participants whose reports of substance use during the past month declined from one assessment to the next. They found that across all follow-ups, MPP produced significant declines in cigarette, alcohol, and marijuana use. Additional analyses for each follow-up point, however, showed limited effects for baseline marijuana users and effects that diminished over time for early alcohol and cigarette users.

Pentz, Trebow, Hansen, and MacKinnon (1990) examined whether the degree of implementation of the program affected outcome. It did. Teachers reported providing between 3 and 10 of the 10 scheduled classes (mean = 8.8); no teacher reported deviating more than slightly from the curriculum. Amount of exposure to the curriculum reported by teachers was significantly associated with lower rates of virtually all alcohol, tobacco, and marijuana use variables assessed 18 months after baseline.

---

[1]The authors extrapolated missing data by substituting the level of substance use reported on average at the next follow-up assessment and used a very conservative alpha level.

STATEWIDE CAMPAIGNS

As described in Chapter 6, states have implemented many policy inter-ventions. Because states regulate alcohol use, the minimum drinking age is a statewide policy substantially evaluated at the individual state level. Even before the federal requirement for a minimum drinking age of 21, many states already had such an age for most or all beverages.

Statewide efforts to affect other youth problem behaviors are also emerging. These efforts are important because of their potential to affect large numbers of communities and youth. Since 1989, five states have implemented campaigns to reduce tobacco use. These states are Califor-nia, Massachusetts, Arizona, Oregon, and Florida. In the first four of these states, efforts began with an increase in the tax on tobacco prod-ucts, which provided some funds for antitobacco activities. In Florida, the program began after money became available from a settlement of the state's lawsuit against the tobacco companies. Each state targeted adolescents and all but Florida targeted adults as well. All the states included mass media and support of school-based programs as compo-nents of the campaign. Four of the states provided money to local lead agencies to support local efforts to reduce tobacco use.

Wakefield and Chaloupka (2000) reviewed the evidence regarding the effects of these efforts. They concluded that the combination of pro-gram efforts and increased tobacco taxes reduced cigarette consumption more than taxes alone would have done. They reported effects for adolescents as well as adults. They reported reductions in smoking in California and Massachusetts. Since that time, the Florida Health Department has reported that the prevalence of middle school smoking had declined from 18.5 to 8.6%, a 54% decline. Among high school stu-dents, current smoking declined 24%, from 27.4 to 20.9%. In Oregon, the Oregon Health Division reported that smoking among eighth grad-ers fell from 22% in 1996 to 13% in 2000, a reduction of 41%. Smoking among 11th grade students fell from 28% in 1996 to 22% in 2000, a reduction of 21%. At least in the tobacco area, these efforts stand as models of what comprehensive statewide programs can achieve.

THE POTENTIAL OF COMMUNITY INTERVENTIONS

The evidence reviewed in this chapter shows that it is possible to reduce the prevalence of substance use in entire communities. Media, commu-nity organizing, enactment and enforcement of relevant ordinances, and programs directed at youth and their parents all can contribute to reduc-ing tobacco, alcohol, or other drug use as well as many of the problems

EXPERIMENTAL EVALUATION OF COMMUNITY INTERVENTIONS

Throughout this volume, we have emphasized the importance of randomized controlled trials in evaluating interventions. Community interventions are particularly difficult to evaluate in this way, however. Random assignment works to control alternative explanations of treatment effects only when large numbers of units are employed. When researchers randomly place large numbers of cases into different conditions, individual differences of the cases balance out across the different conditions because of the randomization process. However, gathering large numbers of communities for random assignment is not feasible either politically or economically. In addition, when only a few communities are available, random assignment will necessarily equalize communities assigned to each condition.

We do not need randomized controlled trials to evaluate community interventions, however. An alternative strategy is the multiple baseline design in which scientists repeatedly measure relevant outcomes in several communities and implement the intervention one community at a time (Biglan, Ary, & Wagenaar, 2000). Evidence that the intervention was effective comes from two sources: (1) the outcome changes noticeably in each community only after it receives the intervention, and (2) the outcome fails to change in the communities that have not yet received the intervention. These designs require fewer communities than randomized trials do and permit each community to receive the intervention.

Such a design provides a less expensive way to evaluate the effects of an intervention. Perhaps more important, these designs are better suited to learning about functional relationships between community processes and their context. In randomized controlled trials, it is generally assumed that one knows what the relevant independent variables are and the study is conducted to see if the effects of the independent variables are generalizable across communities.

that result from alcohol use. At the same time, these studies indicate that it is feasible to evaluate community interventions in a controlled fashion.

However, the evidence reviewed in the other parts of this book suggests that existing community interventions are more limited in scope than they could be. Given that substance use is related to other risky behaviors and that all these behaviors share many common influences, we should be developing and evaluating comprehensive community interventions that attempt to prevent multiple problem behaviors by altering influences throughout the lifespan.

Antisocial behavior is especially important to address in comprehensive interventions. As we have seen, antisocial behavior in childhood typically precedes, and contributes to, the development of substance abuse and high-risk sexual behavior. As we showed in Chapter 5, numerous efficacious interventions target influences on the development of antisocial behavior. The time has come to develop and evaluate comprehensive community interventions that include components focused on antisocial behavior.

It is also important to evaluate comprehensive community interventions for preventing risky sexual behavior. We are unaware of any experimental evaluations that evaluate multifaceted community-based approaches to preventing this problem. Although diverse views in communities about how to deal with adolescent sexual behavior will make communitywide approaches based on consensus difficult to develop, this problem does not obviate the need to prevent pregnancy, HIV infection, and STDs among youth. In addition, community efforts to reduce other problem behaviors should assess the effects of those problems on risky sexual behavior, because—given its relationship to other problems—preventing those problems may prevent risky sexual behavior.

One example of a comprehensive intervention with the potential to prevent aggressive behavior and all its sequelae is the "Triple-P: Positive Parenting Program" tiered approach in Australia (Sanders, 1999; Sanders, Markie-Dadds, et al., 2000). Triple-P targets parents of children from birth through age 12, with the goal of improving parents' knowledge, skills, and confidence about childrearing and preventing child behavior problems and enhancing child development. Triple-P uses media campaigns, primary care interventions of differing intensities, more intensive parenting interventions for children with greater risk of developing behavior problems, and school-based intervention opportunities. Thus, researchers can deliver the basic content of the intervention in various venues, increasing not only its flexibility but also parents' access to the program. Importantly, Sanders and colleagues have made considerable efforts to train medical and mental health professionals to deliver Triple-P interventions to enhance the reach of the intervention, because so many children visit pediatricians or other physicians on a regular basis. Although no one has evaluated the multilevel approach of Triple-P in whole communities, evaluation has shown that many of its components contribute to reductions in problem behavior (Sanders, 1999). Approaches such as this have considerable potential for reducing the incidence and prevalence of aggressive behavior in childhood because they target multiple settings in which parents are likely to raise concerns about child behavior and provide a wide variety of prevention and treatment interventions. These interventions nonetheless share common core content, goals, and emphases based on research findings about important components of effective parenting.

The multilevel approach of Triple-P also highlights the need for partnerships across the different organizations that have the potential to affect the lives of children and teenagers. The interventions described in this chapter either combined school-based universal prevention programs with media and policy interventions or implemented media and public policy changes alone. Notably lacking were community efforts that included components directed toward children already identified as demonstrating one or more of the behavior problems that concern us here. Instead, communities tended to consider those children to be the responsibility of the clinical treatment, special education, or juvenile justice system. Yet, as we saw in Chapter 2, these children potentially can have a huge effect on community prevalence rates of various serious behavior problems. Including the portions of the service sectors that come in contact with at-risk children in community interventions would be an important step in creating comprehensive community attempts to reduce smoking, risky sexual behavior, serious antisocial behavior, and alcohol and drug misuse.

Comprehensive community interventions might address components directed at each of the influences presented in Table 4.2 (see Chapter 4). Most interventions examined in this chapter used persuasion, changing group norms, building teens' skills at resisting persuasion to use substances, limiting opportunities for problem behavior, and providing consequences for problems (e.g., improved enforcement of drunk driving laws).

Interventions could focus on multiple phases of the lifespan in the interest of reducing problem incidence and prevalence—both concurrently and in years to come. For example, communitywide intervention focused on the prenatal and postnatal period might include programs for reducing smoking during pregnancy. It could also provide effective nurse-visitation and preschool programs to assist caregivers when children are infants and toddlers. There could be screening for children with aggressive behavior problems when they enter school (Walker, Severson, Todis, & Block-Pedego, 1990); behavior management, effective instruction, and social skills components in school; and behavioral parenting skills training for parents. A comprehensive approach might also include policy components that require such programs to be available, as well as the provision of after-school programs for latchkey children. Media might routinely offer programming that models and teaches good parenting in entertaining ways (cf. Sanders, Montgomery, & Brechman-Toussaint, 2000). An intervention focused on middle school years might include components to improve schoolwide behavior management or parenting programs for parents of at-risk youth (e.g., Dishion & Andrews, 1995). It might include policies to reduce access to tobacco and alcohol, youth activities to discourage substance use (e.g., Biglan, Ary, Yudelson, Duncan, & Hood, 1996), school-based substance use prevention programs, and evidence-based mental health for children and teenagers. It might also include review and modification of juvenile justice policies that bring at-risk youth into contact with each other.

Policy interventions could also borrow what has worked in reducing tobacco and drug use and extend these lessons to policies that could affect risky sexual and antisocial behavior. A key focus of the community interventions for tobacco or alcohol use has been to discourage the use of the substance or the harms associated with its use. We found no similar lines of research for antisocial or risky sexual behavior.

Particularly with antisocial behavior, there is no shortage of policies designed to affect it. There are laws against each type of behavior and a very active criminal justice system. However, as indicated previously, many of these policies are ineffectual in preventing future problems and some may be counterproductive or harmful. We recommend instead the development and testing of policies to reduce the formation of deviant peer groups and the opportunities for engagement in antisocial behavior, as well as those that would alter school, family, and community influences on antisocial behavior. We could apply the same general principles to risky sexual behavior.

Policy strategies are important components in comprehensive community interventions. The policy strategies should, as the tobacco and alcohol policies already do, focus on altering the environment to decrease youth problems and to provide incentives to youth, families, and community organizations for such reductions. Policies can be used to alter the community in a way that discourages undesired behaviors, for example, by identifying and modifying community settings in which deviant peer groups can gather, particularly when unsupervised. The effectiveness of such policy strategies that go beyond those already tested are unknown, but the intent to create a comprehensive community prevention intervention will require a mix of evidence-based program components and tested, or at least potentially effective, policy strategies.

Evaluation of these broad-scale community interventions should be comprehensive, long term, and geared toward both assessing immediate and longer-term effects and moving to the next generation of effective prevention and intervention efforts. Researchers should use measures with demonstrated reliability and validity. These should include surveys, archival and direct observation measures of adolescent problem behaviors, related health outcomes (e.g., sexually transmitted diseases, pregnancy rates, smoking rates, binge drinking, and drinking and driving crash rates), and the environment for adolescents (e.g., access to tobacco and alcohol, parental monitoring).

A final word of caution: Some of the weaker findings we have reported come from comprehensive interventions in which community groups each selected different strategies to implement. This probably

RECOMMENDATIONS FOR RESEARCH

- There should be a coordinated effort on the part of National Institute of Health institutes and foundations to fund the experimental evaluation of comprehensive community interventions targeting the entire range of youth problems.

- Research should examine comprehensive interventions that combine universal, selective, and targeted interventions and that include media and policy components.

- These interventions should address risk and protective factors across the lifespan.

- Evaluations of comprehensive community interventions should determine whether they prevent the development of multiple problem behaviors.

- There should be experimental evaluations of comprehensive community interventions targeting antisocial behavior.

- There should be cost–benefit analyses of effects of comprehensive interventions.

- Comprehensive community approaches are ill-suited to testing combinations of interventions with no prior record of effectiveness. Even if such interventions are successful, it is impossible to identify their effective components. A better approach is to test comprehensive approaches that combine interventions that have each been shown—individually—to produce benefits.

resulted from different groups choosing interventions of differing effectiveness. On the one hand, it is important for communities to be able to review and choose the strategies that meet their needs and are acceptable to the public. On the other hand, it is important not to equate *choice* with *effectiveness*. Some interventions that sound wonderful do not work (e.g., DARE). It is important to select strategies based on evidence that they are likely to have an impact on youth behavior, not on how good they sound in the absence of evidence. Ineffective interventions waste time and money. More important, they involve youth such as Michael without altering their destiny or improving their lives.

RECOMMENDATIONS FOR PRACTICE

- State and national funding agencies dealing with the various problem behaviors should cooperate to develop a system for supporting states and communities to implement, with fidelity, empirically supported practices that have been shown to affect one or more youth problem behaviors.

- Communities should systematically review whether they are using evidence-based strategies to reduce serious adolescent behavior problems.
  — They should review family-focused interventions and school, neighborhood, and community practices, including policies regarding tobacco and alcohol.
  — They should review whether they have policies or programs that have unintended negative effects, such as juvenile justice policies that cause at-risk youth to congregate.

- State and national funding agencies should support the development of systems in states and communities to monitor the entire range of youth problems.

9

Integrating Science and Practice to Enhance the Well-Being of Children and Adolescents

Michael's girlfriend, Barbara, gives birth to a baby boy. Tommy is a healthy, full-term infant, due to Barbara's enrollment in a program for pregnant teens, where she learned to quit smoking and drinking and was able to improve her nutrition.

When Tommy is 3, Barbara attends college part-time and works part-time. She ends her relationship with Michael, who moves away and seldom sends child support. Because of her low income, Barbara qualifies for Head Start and enrolls Tommy in a program close to home. Head Start includes parent training, which helps Barbara to handle Tommy in better ways. Due to Barbara's consistent discipline, the frequent tantrums Tommy had as a toddler occur only rarely by the time he is 4 years old.

When Tommy starts school, he knows his letters and cooperates well with others. In the second grade, he has trouble learning to read but his school provides tutoring, and by grade 3, he is reading at grade level. Although he has a tendency to be disruptive because he loves attention, his first-grade teacher provides appropriate consequences and soon this tendency is under control. He gets along well with others, and is a funny, engaging child. Still, parenting is a challenge for Barbara as she finishes her bachelor's degree and works full-time.

As Tommy grows up, he and his mother have a good relationship—even though they sometimes bicker a little over rules. Barbara cannot afford to move out of her neighborhood, which worries her as Tommy begins middle school. Nevertheless, she always knows where he is and who is with him. She tries to steer him away from bad influences. Eventually, some of Tommy's friends begin to experiment with tobacco and alcohol. However, Tommy is involved in a smoking and substance-abuse prevention program at school, and although some of it seems "kind of lame," most of it really makes sense to him. His teacher invites him to train as a peer facilitator and Tommy may do it—he has seen ads about helping other kids stay off drugs and alcohol. He does not want to grow up like his father.

Imagine what communities could be like in, say, 2020 if they took full advantage of the information contained in the previous chapters. Community members would share a vision of what young people need in order to develop successfully. They would inform this vision with evidence about the most common problems that threaten successful development and what could help to prevent those problems. They would examine every decision about community life—from planning to ordinances—in terms of their implications for the well-being of young people. Members of community organizations would routinely answer questions about how their efforts contributed to young people's success. Community members would be encouraged and empowered to build communities in which the well-being of young people was among their highest priorities.

These communities would nurture and celebrate their children. They would recognize and reward desirable behavior, not only on the part of young people, but also from every community member. When problems occurred, adults would intervene quickly—without abuse—and effectively to nip children's difficulties in the bud. All children would have access to services and practices shown to be effective in preventing the emergence of problems and in promoting well-being. Conflicts would be resolved through active listening, mutual dialogue, and compromise. In short, such communities would use the nurturing practices of effective families and schools throughout community life and would strengthen them with effective policies and regulations that are fairly enforced.

These communities would have sophisticated systems for measuring how their children were doing. Community members would be able to obtain data on the prevalence of child and adolescent problems through archival records, surveys, and data on the risk and protective factors that influence adolescent development. The data would enable community members to tell whether particular problems were getting worse or better. Evidence of increases in particular problem behaviors or the conditions that contribute to them would prompt the communities to take needed action.

These communities would be committed to using cost-effective policies and programs. Their members would understand the value of choosing programs and policies that showed evidence of having worked elsewhere. However, they would temper that understanding with the realization that whatever the origins of a practice, a community must continue to evaluate how it is working and make sure that effective practices are implemented with fidelity.

Behavioral scientists would play an important role in these communities. They would not make decisions about a community's policies, programs, or means of implementation. Instead, scientists would provide information the community needed to make good decisions, and they would help the community evaluate how well it was achieving its goals for young people.

Because of the practices that evolved in the community, it would become a better place to grow up. Fewer families would live in poverty. Child and spousal abuse would become rare because of programs and policies to prevent unhealthy pregnancies and to help newly forming families get off to a harmonious and healthy start. From early childhood through high school, young people would be taught effectively and acquire a lifelong love of learning. Young people who were having psychological or behavioral problems would receive assistance in overcoming these threats to their successful development. They would receive assistance based on best practice guidelines derived from the best available scientific evidence on effective interventions. Tobacco, alcohol, and illicit drugs would not be accessible to young people and advertising and entertainment media would not glorify or promote their use. Because the conditions for successful development would be so improved, the prevalence of young people with problems of antisocial behavior, substance use, and high-risk sexual behavior would be far less than they had been 20 years previously. There would also be a decrease in other problems not discussed in as much detail in this volume, such as academic failure and depression. As a result, young people would live more productive and satisfying lives: The sons and daughters of Michael and the many youth like him would find new destinies, as did Tommy.

This vision of child-friendly communities is far from fictional. Most of the just imagined practices are reality in some communities, though no community has adopted all of them. For example:

- Vermont has experienced striking reductions in a wide variety of social indicators, including child abuse, high school dropouts, children without health insurance, teen births, mothers without prenatal care, and property crime (Hogan, 1999). The state's progress came about through a process of creating community partnerships among local stakeholders; setting specific goals for indicators of youth, family, and community well-being; devising a system for assessing those indicators; and carefully evaluating changes in them.

- The Work Group on Health Promotion and Community Development at the University of Kansas (University of Kansas, 2003) assists communities throughout the world in developing measurable goals for youth and community well-being using approaches that ensure input from all sectors of the community and facilitate the development of a consensus among community members about the steps to be taken.
- The Social Development Research Group (SDRG) at the University of Washington is helping communities throughout the nation to assess and modify risk and protective factors and to adopt research-based strategies for affecting them (Brewer et al., 1995; Hawkins, 1999). A growing number of organizations are identifying, supporting, and promoting the adoption of empirically supported practices. We presented a partial list in Chapter 5.
- Communities in Kansas and Missouri have begun formally to adopt a policy that requires lawmakers to evaluate any regulation or ordinance in terms of its effects on young people (Stephen Fawcett, personal communication, February, 1999).

It may be possible to accelerate evolution toward more effective childrearing practices in communities by describing the specific goals and activities that are essential to achieving the vision we just described. Thus, in this chapter, we sketch a vision of communities optimally organized to prevent the development of problems—especially multiple behavior problems—and to support successful development. We also describe what steps might be needed to get us there. We have organized the discussion in terms of sets of practices needed at the community level. Moreover, because communities are more likely to evolve in the hoped-for direction if they have effective support from state and national organizations, we describe important state and national practices as well.

We developed the vision articulated in this chapter based on collaboration with a group of 26 scientists and practitioners.[1] They provided

---

[1]Those who participated include Lynda Anderson, Judith Auerbach, Cathy Backinger, Jim Caccamo, Virginia Cain, Richard Catalano, Patti Chamberlain, Lucy Davidson, Dennis Embry, Stephen Fawcett, Connie Ferrara, Brian Flay, Con Hogan, Jan Howard, David MacKinnon, Carol Metzler, Pat Mrazek, David Olds, Dennis Prager, David Racine, Heather Ringeisen, Liz Robertson, Mark Rosenberg, Sonja Schoenwald, Richard Spoth, and Alex Wagenaar. We are grateful for their assistance and participation, but we and not they are responsible for the material presented here. This note does not infer their personal or organizational endorsement.

reactions to several iterations of documents that described what optimal communities might be like and what research and infrastructure development might facilitate the evolution of communities toward more effective childrearing. Many participated in meetings that involved brainstorming and discussion.

DEVELOPING COLLABORATIVE PARTNERSHIPS WITH A SHARED VISION

The foundation for a community's optimization of its childrearing practices could be the development of collaborative partnerships, with a shared vision of what childrearing in the community should resemble (Fawcett, Francisco, Paine-Andrews, & Schultz, 2000). The vision would specify the outcomes that the community desires for its children; the optimal conditions to ensure their successful development; and the practices, programs, and policies that seem likely to ensure optimal conditions. Those who articulate the vision would be part of a collaborative partnership of community groups and organizations from multiple sectors of the community who agreed to come together for the common purpose of improving outcomes for young people (Roussos & Fawcett, 2000).

Creating partnerships around such a vision can mobilize significantly more community change than would occur in its absence (Roussos & Fawcett, 2000). Communities that lack a shared vision will tend to have organizations working at cross-purposes, with different priorities and different analyses of what the community needs to affect its youth. Sectors of the community that could make a difference for young people will not take part or may even resist because no one has worked with them to articulate how they could contribute. The community will miss opportunities to prevent problems by failing to address key risk or protective factors that a comprehensive vision would identify. Its organizations will not be accountable for their contribution to affecting wellbeing in the entire population of young people because a population-based perspective will not be salient. In essence, the process of creating a partnership with a shared vision creates social capital (Sampson et al., 1997); it organizes and mobilizes groups and organizations so that they are better able to affect youth development.

An effective vision specifies population-based goals for the community. That is, desired outcomes should be stated in terms of the incidence or prevalence of problems or successes, such as the number of teen pregnancies, proportion of high school students who smoke, number of children with aggressive behavior problems, number of students who go on to college, and so on.

THE VALUE OF A SHARED VISION: A CASE STUDY OF TOBACCO USE

Efforts to reduce tobacco use in the United States have been more successful than those targeting problems like delinquency (Biglan & Taylor, 2000). One reason may be that the tobacco control community has been organized and mobilized by a well-worked-out view of the tobacco problem that is scientifically accurate, yet readily understood and communicated to lay people. This analysis:

- Articulated the cost of tobacco use in ways that were scientifically accurate, yet persuasive (e.g., "It's like two Boeing 747's crash every day of the year, killing everyone on board. That's how many people smoking kills.").

- Clarified the major factors that contribute to tobacco use.

- Identified the things that were needed to reduce tobacco use.

As scientists and public health advocates have worked in concert, numerous changes in public policy occurred and contributed to substantial reductions in tobacco use in the United States. Because a scientifically accurate, yet easily understood, vision of the tobacco problem came to be widely shared, we have been able to bring about changes in tobacco use that no one could have imagined 20 years ago.

Population-based goals are important. They are particularly important for organizations that have typically focused on helping individual young people. They require looking beyond one's work with individuals to examining whether the organization is contributing to the overall well-being of young people in the community. Furthermore, looking at population goals makes the need for partnerships crystal-clear. No single intervention or policy we have reviewed here is likely to affect all youth. Many, such as the treatment strategies described in Chapter 8, are unlikely to make even a dent in incidence and prevalence rates on their own. Yet, if all adults with the potential to implement effective policies and practices did their share and worked together, they could affect entire populations. But everyone—policymakers, juvenile justice professionals, therapists, teachers, school administrators, medical professionals, shopkeepers who sell tobacco and alcohol, clergy, parents, day-care providers—must do his or her share to make this happen.

The Process of Developing These Partnerships

Roussos and Fawcett (2000) reviewed studies of collaborative partnerships as a strategy for improving community well-being. They define a collaborative partnership as "an alliance among people and organizations from multiple sectors, such as schools and businesses, working together to achieve a common purpose" (p. 369). They note that such partnerships may arise from a social planning strategy in which experts take the lead or from grass-roots efforts in which persons with a particular concern take the initiative. What appears to be essential for a successful partnership is engagement of all the people and organizations that could affect or benefit from the success of the effort.

Fawcett et al. (2000) have described a process of active listening in which those attempting to form a collaborative partnership seek input from diverse members of the community. Community leaders can identify the concerns of the community through systematic surveys of relevant sectors of the community and in public forums. Thus, a small group of community leaders can conduct listening activities and make presentations that will lead to a diverse and growing number of community members giving explicit support to improving childrearing in their community. These processes make it more likely that plans for community change that are developed will reflect the views and have the support of those who might be affected by them.

Roussos and Fawcett (2000) conclude from their review of the literature that leadership is needed to create collaborative partnerships and keep them functioning. Unfortunately, there is little empirical guidance as to how a community can identify, train, or support effective leaders. Roussos and Fawcett suggest that good leaders will need to be able to frame and communicate the vision and mission of the partnership to diverse sectors of the community. They will need to be able to facilitate meetings and network and negotiate with many types of people.

One model of collaborative partnerships that has been widely applied in drug abuse prevention is that of Communities That Care (Hawkins, 1999; Hawkins & Catalano, 1992). In that model, leaders of key sectors of the community (business, education, religion, law enforcement, health care, and government) get assistance—typically from a technical assistant from the state alcohol and drug office—in forming a task force to work on reducing youth drug use in the community. The community task force receives training on the major risk and protective factors for drug abuse and then receives more assistance in assessing the level of those factors in their community. The Communities that Care group (a for-profit arm based on the research of Hawkins and Catalano) obtains survey data from adolescents, combines it with archival data, and provides a profile of the community's strengths and weaknesses. The task force sets goals outlining which risk and protective factors they want to change and—with the assistance of a state-level person or

SDRG—identifies, implements, and evaluates empirically based interventions likely to affect those factors.

One device for gathering support for a vision is the creation of a proclamation (Biglan et al., 1995). In this strategy, the community asks organizations and individuals to lend their names to a brief statement of what the community seeks to do to improve the well-being of children and adolescents. A proclamation takes advantage of well-established social and psychological principles of social influence. It elicits a social commitment from the signatories and provides visible evidence that others in the community support the initiative. Signing the proclamation is a small step that begins a process of eliciting larger commitments. The process of gathering support for it provides a concrete and specific method of building the partnership and produces an early success for those organizing the effort.

The process of achieving a shared vision may be as important as actually achieving the vision. When diverse groups consider what they want for children, public discussion focuses on the question. This process sensitizes community members to the needs of young people and gathers support and commitment from them, because they feel that the developed program is consonant with their desires. Innovations are likely to emerge as community members discuss how they would like their community to be.

The vision may focus initially on only a few outcomes. A community can do a limited number of things at one time. For example, a community might choose to focus on lowering the rates of delinquency. Establishing a shared vision of what the community would be with less delinquency will create a goal that forms the basis for problem solving. If a subsequent initiative results in observable reductions in delinquency, it will reinforce the efforts of those who have contributed to the outcome. Once it meets one goal, the community can add new goals so that the vision specifies an increasing number of ways the community can optimize conditions for youth.

The Role of Behavioral Scientists

A sizable literature examines the role of behavioral scientists in working with communities (e.g., Fawcett, Francisco, Paine-Andrews, & Schultz, 2000; Kelly, 1988). Major issues raised repeatedly involve a need to empower disadvantaged groups in communities (Rappaport, 1987) and to avoid having researchers impose their goals or strategies (Kelly, 1988).

In our view, it is not the role of behavioral scientists to decide what communities should do about childrearing. Rather, their role is to provide technical expertise to help a community use democratic and participatory methods to achieve a consensus about what that community should do. First, behavioral scientists have a duty to provide clear and accurate evidence about the epidemiology, cost, etiology, prevention, and treatment of youth problems, as well as the conditions shown by evidence to optimize successful youth development and intervention. Second, they can assist in gathering, analyzing, and interpreting local data that facilitate decision making. The nature of these data would be based on input from community members about goals and practices they plan to implement. Data would include information on problems and well-being of children and adolescents and the conditions in the community that promote or detract from youth development. Finally, behavioral scientists could design and implement systems to evaluate programs and policies put in place.

The Role of State and National Groups in Fostering Community Visions

Our collaborative group on community practices identified several things that state or national organizations could do to foster the development of a shared vision of effective childrearing in local communities. First, state- and national-level organizations could develop a shared vision of what they need to do to prevent problems in the development of children and adolescents. That vision would articulate:

- The most common and costly problems of childhood and adolescence and interconnections among those problems.
- Based on the best science available, the most important factors influencing both healthy and problem development.
- What is known about effective policies, strategies, and programs to prevent child and adolescent problems, based on methodologically sound evaluations and preferably involving replication and randomized controlled trials whenever feasible.
- The costs that effective prevention of child and adolescent problems would avoid; if the analysis could break down those costs for each state and Congressional District, it would be even better.

This analysis may look a lot like the material presented in this book. That similarity is no accident.

Second, a consortium of national- and state-level organizations could conduct a media campaign to communicate its shared vision of the requirements for maximizing successful youth development. Such a social marketing campaign could build a national consensus about what is

> NEEDED RESEARCH
>
> • Experimentally evaluate methods for forming partnerships and establishing a shared vision.
>
> • Identify processes that are most effective in achieving consensus about community goals and the community's methods of pursuing those goals.
>
> • Evaluate consensus-building methods in terms of (1) the proportion of individuals and organizations in the community that subscribe to the vision, (2) the degree to which the achievement of consensus leads to the community implementing new efforts to affect youth, and (3) observed changes in the incidence or prevalence of youth problems.

needed that would influence efforts in every community. This is precisely what is happening in the tobacco and alcohol control fields.

Third, the techniques for helping communities arrive at a shared vision of what they want their childrearing to be could be more widely disseminated by state and national organizations. To some extent, this is already happening.

Fourth, the Surgeon General could issue an annual report on the well-being of children and adolescents. This would take advantage of the Surgeon General's "bully pulpit" and could focus the nation on a small number of well-defined measures of child and adolescent problems needing assistance. To the extent that the Surgeon General derives the report from widely assessed indicators of youth problems and well-being, it would influence increasing numbers of communities to obtain those measures.

ONGOING ASSESSMENT OF CHILD AND ADOLESCENT PROBLEMS AND WELL-BEING

Measurement of child and adolescent problems and well-being is essential to a community's efforts to improve outcomes for youth. Thanks to the growing use of survey and archival data, it will soon be possible for every community to have reasonably accurate estimates of the incidence and prevalence of youth problem and successful behavior as well as estimates of the conditions that influence youth development. As their use becomes more widespread, these assessment systems will play an increasing role in guiding prevention efforts. Accurate estimates of the

FEATURES OF A SHARED COMMUNITY VISION

- Articulates a clear and compelling account of what communities need to prevent youth problems and to ensure successful development.

- Organizes epidemiological, etiological, and intervention facts to motivate public support for needed programs and policies.

- Bases decisions about programs and policies regarding children on significant participation from all community members, including the disadvantaged, minorities, and youth.

- Community leaders routinely convene local organizations, practitioners, and providers to clarify their roles in implementing support of youth development.

- Thanks to ongoing advocacy, the vision routinely and effectively enters public discussions about civic life.

- Advocacy ensures that data about youth well-being play a prominent role in public discussion and thus guide decision making.

- Programs and policies exist in order to achieve desired effects on the *population* of young people.

- Every organization and community member is routinely asked "What can you do to contribute to the well-being of children and adolescents in your area?"

- Community members celebrate positive results.

proportion of young people engaging in various prosocial and problem behaviors can let the community know if it is achieving its goals. Over time, the widespread use of such systems will contribute to the selection of more effective practices, as high levels of problems (or risk factors) prompt communities to modify their practices and evidence of improvements leads them to maintain effective practices.

The practice of monitoring youth problem behavior and well-being is becoming more widespread. Many states have set up systems for assessing the educational progress of their students in an effort to hold schools accountable. The assessment of tobacco, alcohol, and other drug use and of antisocial behavior in nationally representative samples of adolescents is now routine. The CDC has created a system for obtaining representative state-level data on numerous health and behavioral problems (CDC, 2002a), and an increasing number of states and school districts use such assessments to evaluate the health and well-being of adolescents. We expect that the use of such assessments will continue to spread, systems for integrating data from survey and archival sources will be refined, and the data will increasingly guide the efforts of communities to ensure child and youth well-being.

We envision development of the following:

- Communities routinely assess behavioral, psychological, and academic skills of young people to evaluate whether community efforts are preventing problems and promoting successful development.
- Communities routinely assess risk and protective factors affecting child and adolescent development at all levels, from the individual and family to the neighborhood and community.
- Communities assess in particular the behavior problems and risk and protective factors that characterize multiproblem youth.
- The assessment system provides rapid feedback and allows decision makers to create summaries, examine trends, and aggregate data from the school, neighborhood, or town up to state and national levels.
- Communities routinely review their progress and make decisions about needed changes in policies and programs, as suggested by the data.

Communities might evolve toward a comprehensive assessment system in stages. Initially, they might establish a basic minimum set of youth indicators that every state and community agree to monitor. Once the system is up and working, communities might add indicators of risk and protective factors at all levels (e.g., school, neighborhood, and community). Ultimately, the system would integrate various sorts of data from youth, families, teachers, and others working with youth and would weave the use of the data into community life so that it guided decision making.

Respecting Individual Rights

The establishment of such an assessment system requires the cooperation of community members. An extensive assessment system has the potential, however, to raise suspicion and mistrust unless it is established in a way that respects the rights of the individual. Community members will cooperate in data collection only if they believe that responding to the system is in their interest and that assessors will protect their privacy. Collection of data about young people and their families has the potential for abuse. Only if investigators build strict privacy protections into the system will community members be willing to participate.

We suggest several safeguards. Many of these protections are a routine part of most research, approved by boards charged with protecting the rights of research participants, and should be part of community monitoring as well. The first involves informed consent. Before any assessment of children, parents should understand the nature of the assessment and have the opportunity to refuse to have their child assessed. Even if the parents allow assessment of their child, the child should be able to refuse to participate or to decline to answer individual questions. There should be no penalty for refusal to participate. Some might argue that letting students refuse to participate will harm the accuracy of estimates. That may be, but coercing them to participate will lead to resistance and noncooperation that could harm the estimates just as much and could result in the termination of assessment entirely.

A second safeguard involves data privacy. If the primary purpose of the survey system is to estimate the prevalence of behaviors in the youth population, assessors can collect the survey data anonymously. This will increase people's privacy and may increase their willingness to participate. In addition, researchers should use the data to assess only groups, not individuals, and should ensure families of this control. Program staff should consult lawyers about areas of assessment that might require notification of law enforcement or social services agencies, and youth and their parents should know about the limits of confidentiality before completing any assessments. These issues would be important to address whenever organizations survey youth about illegal activities.

The assessment system should be one in which all community organizations working with young people participate. These organizations would contribute data to it and would use the data from these assessments to guide their work. They would probably need technical assistance and additional resources to collect and analyze valid data about their respondents. Over time, however, their collection and analysis of data would help the groups shape more effective programs.

A National Assessment System

Perhaps the most important thing that needs to happen at the national level is the design of a national assessment system that states and local communities could use. We could call this system *Vital Signs*. Such a system would define the aspects of adolescent functioning that current epidemiological evidence suggests are important to track. The system could include both problems and positive aspects of youth development. It would include the measurement of risk and protective factors, including those involving schools, family members, or communities. It would reflect a consensus within the public health community about the most important aspects of child and adolescent functioning that need assessing.

From the perspective espoused in this book, this system should include some way of assessing the difficulties that characterize multiproblem youth.

The *Vital Signs* system could be quite flexible. It could have modules allowing states and communities to choose the subsets of domains they wanted to measure but still collect the data in the same way. Thus, communities at the local, state, and national levels could examine the incidence and prevalence rates and directly compare the data, so that a community could compare its progress to that of another community.

Communities could specify a sampling design that provided accurate estimates at the state and national levels but allowed disaggregation down to the community level. This specification would allow communities to examine the relative importance of different outcomes and risk and protective factors, identify those on which it most needs to concentrate (Catalano, Berglund, Ryan, Lonczak, & Hawkins, 1999), and make comparisons to larger social units.

As consensus emerges about the aspects of adolescent functioning that are most important to monitor, it becomes possible to develop officially recognized indices of adolescent problem behavior and well-being. Obvious candidate indices include the rate of teenage childbearing; new cases of HIV and STDs among teens; the proportion of young people who drop out of or complete high school; the rates of index crimes committed by juveniles; the rates of arrests for these crimes; and the rates of tobacco, alcohol, and other drug use and abuse. Estimates of the national rates of these events can already be derived from the many national surveys of adolescents and archival records on crime and school dropout, but inconsistencies in how these measures are defined and recorded may make aggregation and comparison across states and communities difficult. As assessment systems develop and become more refined and more consistent in states and local communities, the accuracy of these estimates will improve. Eventually, an appropriate goal would be to have indices that are accurate for local communities and that can be aggregated at the county, state, and national levels.

An important first step in constructing a national data collection system might involve bringing together to design the system the organizations that have developed national- or state-level assessments systems of child or adolescent well-being. One example of this kind of system is the Kids Count annual report cards issued by the Annie E. Casey Foundation for the nation and each state. The report cards grade states on how they take care of their young people, using available measures of child and adolescent well-being. The report cards draw attention to the general issue of child and youth well-being and pinpoint areas in which states need to improve. They have become an essential tool in advocating for the welfare of young people.

Federal and state governments could strengthen efforts such as Kids Count if they adopted or adapted the system to provide officially recognized indices of adolescent problems and well-being. At the federal level, the Surgeon General's Office could create official indices of adolescent functioning for the nation, and state governments could use the information the Office obtained. In addition to adding prestige to these indices, formal government recognition of them would lay the foundation for policy development. For example, in Chapter 6, we described how the federal Synar amendment required states to systematically measure and reduce the level of illegal sales of tobacco to young people. As measures of other aspects of well-being become widely accepted, policies requiring efforts to improve them will become possible.

In developing such data-driven policymaking to improve the well-being of children and adolescents, the nation would be doing nothing more than it did to manage the economy. Figure 9.1 shows annual changes in the gross domestic product (GDP) from 1946 to 1996. Daniel Patrick Moynihan (1996) used this chart to illustrate how our management of the economy had improved. Notice that in about 1947 the variability in GDP went down considerably and that the measure currently seldom goes below zero. As increasingly more accurate economic indicators became available, it became possible to adjust more precisely the economic policy in light of the numbers and to avoid large inflationary or deflationary moves. The Employment Act of 1946, which made it official government policy to attempt to moderate both inflation and deflation, advanced improvement in economic management.

Improving the development of children and adolescents may prove more complex and difficult to achieve. But it will surely be advanced by formal adoption of a set of indicators of child and youth well-being that tells us precisely how well communities, states, and the nation are raising our children—indicators that can lead to changes in policies, based on scientific knowledge of how those changes are likely to affect *Vital Signs* indicators.

Technical Assistance to States and Local Communities

Some states and most communities will require technical assistance to implement assessment systems. Indeed, the development of such systems will require training people who are skilled in survey and sampling design, in the collection of data, and in analysis and interpretation of those data. We believe that ultimately every community will have an expert who supervises the collection, reduction, and analysis of the data and

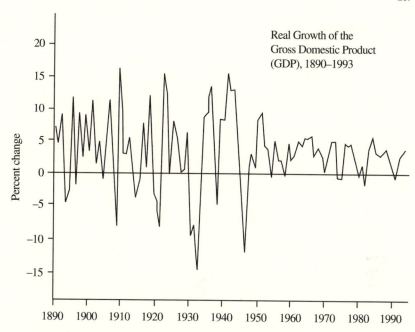

FIGURE 9.1. From Moynihan (1996). Copyright 1996 by Harvard University Press. Reprinted by permission. Data provided by the U.S. Department of Commerce, Bureau of Economic Analysis. Chart prepared by the Joint Economic Committee.

assists community leaders in interpretation of those data. Initially, a national entity could provide training and consultation to states on the design and implementation of state-level systems. This national entity should assist state offices in developing their own capacity to provide technical assistance to communities in the use of the data. Universities should be encouraged to develop training programs for those who will manage such data systems.

Even before a national assessment system is developed, states and communities need help using existing assessment.systems. For example, the YRBS of the CDC (2002b) provides data on a wide variety of risk behaviors from representative samples of schools in each state. We have cited numerous studies based on the YRBS data in this volume and used the YRBS data to produce some of the estimates in Chapter 2. The survey is available for additional schools who would like data on how their students are doing, provided resources are available to pay for the assessment. We suspect that state agencies could make schools and communities more aware of the value of the existing data. Organizations at the national level could provide states with assistance in promoting the use of such assessment systems in communities and individual schools. Communities would also need help in getting the data reduced, analyzed, and interpreted. It is likely that a state-level office in each state or a national level entity could provide individual schools and communities with summaries of data collected from systems such as the YRBS. Ultimately, user-friendly websites will be available that allow those with access to the data to produce a variety of summaries and breakdowns, as needed by the community or school.

Needed Research

Several lines of research could contribute to the development of community-level assessment systems. First, cross-sectional reliability and validity studies, comparing different measurement instruments, are needed to clarify the degree to which different measures of the same construct (e.g., a youth behavior or a risk factor) are comparable. Ultimately, such research would contribute to the establishment of standard items for all assessments.

Second, we need to develop and test systems for integrating epidemiological and etiological evidence with community input to create an assessment system with high credibility that is useful to all parties. This research could develop ways of quickly and efficiently reducing assessment data and making it effectively available to all decision makers. It could examine how and to what extent organizations in the community make use of data and what variables influence use of data.

Third, we need research on the degree to which assessment systems influence decision making about priorities, policies, and programs. Investigators could experimentally evaluate strategies for helping communities and their organizations to use data in decision making in order to identify the most effective methods of bringing data to bear on decision making.

EMPIRICALLY SUPPORTED INTERVENTIONS ACROSS THE LIFESPAN AND ACROSS MULTIPLE LEVELS OF INFLUENCE

Perhaps the single most important thing communities can do to prevent adolescent problem behavior and promote successful development is to implement effective policies and programs. The preceding chapters document numerous opportunities to foster successful development from the prenatal period through adolescence. For virtually every identified influence on development—from family circumstances to biological influences to the media—there are evidence-based strategies that can potentially prevent problem development. Communities should carefully examine each possible influence and make sure that their programs and policies minimize risk factors and maximize protective factors. Adopting an empirically supported intervention will not guarantee a beneficial outcome, but its chances of success are better than those for unevaluated interventions.

Optimally, communities would:

- Choose programs and policies affecting young people based on evidence for their effectiveness and cost-effectiveness, their fit with identified needs of the local populations, and the organization's role in the community.
- Consider all possible interventions for all age levels from childhood through adolescence.
- Examine universal, selective, and indicated interventions targeting biology, individuals, families, schools, peers, and neighborhoods.
- Employ all possible methods of intervention and involve individuals in medical, clinical, educational, policy, and media fields.
- Provide sufficient training, administrative support, and monitoring of fidelity of implementation to ensure success of their programs.
- Have effective and valid systems in place to identify and refer people who would benefit from selected and indicated interventions.
- Implement universal interventions based on data about which risk factors in the specific community need attention and on evidence of the previous effectiveness of the intervention.
- Evaluate any untried intervention particularly carefully and in a controlled fashion to gauge its effectiveness.
- Use data to identify harmful or useless practices and eliminate or improve them.
- Provide rewards to organizations for contributing to positive outcomes, adopting empirically supported practices, and evaluating the effects of those practices.

Actions to Increase Communities' Capacity to Implement Effective Programs and Policies

Developing Consensus Standards Regarding "Best Practices"

Numerous organizations have compiled lists of programs and policies that empirical evidence shows to be valuable. We summarized these in

Chapter 6. Although these efforts reflect the growing recognition that evidence-based interventions can improve outcomes for young people, the diversity of standards that organizations have used may undermine efforts to promote the most effective programs. Some lists include programs shown to produce only pre–post changes for a single sample. This encourages organizations to continue the use of inadequately evaluated programs. If prevention scientists spoke with one voice about standards for selecting programs and policies, it would better promote the use of those standards and increase the use of the best supported practices. These should include *both* standards for adequate evaluation of programs and policies *and* information about degree and type of behavior change required for a program to call itself "effective." Many evaluative efforts have focused principally on the former, at the expense of the latter (Foster, Biglan, & Katz, 2001).

In Chapters 5–7, we discussed the criteria we used to choose programs and policies that we reviewed individually and that might be worthy of disseminating. For interventions targeting individual children and families, these included (1) evidence that they affected child or adolescent behavior more than a comparison or control condition did, (2) evaluation using a randomized controlled trial, and (3) use of reliable and valid measures. In Chapter 7, we required that effects be replicated. For policy evaluations, we did not require a randomized controlled trial but instead required replication of effects using alternative methods of studying the issue and effective control for potential alternative explanations (see Chapters 5–7 for elaboration).

Others might argue for a different set of standards, of course— particularly in areas in which randomized trials are rare or extremely difficult to conduct. One way of illuminating and possibly resolving these discrepancies is to begin an organized discussion that brings together different organizations that have been identifying best practices, so that some consensus about standards could be developed. If we can do that, decision making will be easier for those who must select programs and policies and it will increase the demand for programs and policies that meet the highest standard.

Social Marketing to Increase Public Demand for Empirically Supported Interventions

It will do little good to articulate what works if that information is not effectively communicated to decision makers. Foundations and scientific and governmental organizations are increasingly seeking effective ways to communicate this information. It would strengthen those efforts if these organizations collaborated in funded advocacy campaigns to let state and community leaders know about programs and policies shown to have some effect. Briefings and workshops could inform policymakers and journalists about the most supported interventions and educate them about standards to use in evaluating emerging research. Organizations could enhance their media coverage of "best practices" programs and policies through press releases, op-ed pieces, and cultivation of contacts with journalists.

The public should learn about these practices. Information about best practices is likely to increase public demand for these services. This, in turn, will require a greater supply of these sorts of programs, policies, and interventions. Media coverage of the latest developments in child and adolescent treatment and prevention research could raise awareness of state-of-the-science developments, just as the media cover research on the latest cancer drug and longitudinal studies of the relationship between nutritional practices and health outcomes.

Policies to Foster the Adoption of Effective Practices

The ultimate goal of all who have contact with children should be the implementation of effective practices that prevent problems and encourage healthy development. We argue that practices shown to be of benefit through high-quality experimental evaluations are good bets to be effective. However, we also acknowledge that those evaluations do not guarantee success. An empirically supported practice might fail because its implementation may lack the necessary care or resources. It may be ineffective due to differences between the original population involved in the research and the population in which it is adopted. Thus, no one can assume effectiveness, even for the best supported practices.

In addition, even our best interventions are not 100% effective, and communities will want to improve on these. They may also wish to try something innovative. How will they know if the improvement or innovation is effective? That is one reason that the development of assessment systems in each community is so important. Communities will need continuing evidence of whether they are having the effects they desire.

This analysis suggests two different types of policies that might foster effectiveness in communities. One type would set up contingencies favoring the implementation of empirically supported programs and policies. An example would be requiring that organizations receive funding only for programs with a high level of empirical support. Such policies would make the most sense in areas in which there is strong and consistent evidence about the efficacy of programs.

The second type of policy would not specify what practices communities or organizations needed to adopt but would require that whatever is adopted must bring about a change in a targeted indicator of well-being in order to continue. The Synar amendment, described in Chapter 6, is an example of such a policy. Federal policy could require states to focus on specific aspects of adolescent well-being and put resources into improving them. State policy could require the same of counties and communities.

For example, a policy could require a state or local community to measure and report the rate of alcohol-related car crashes involving teenagers each year and to take steps to reduce them. In Chapter 6, we reviewed several things that states and communities can do to achieve such reductions. At the federal level, such a policy could require—as the Synar amendment did—that states lose some of their block grant funds for substance abuse treatment if they do not lower the rate of alcohol-involved crashes of young people. This type of policy would require that an assessment system be in place. Over time, it could foster the selection of many effective practices, as communities discard or modify those that were not associated with improvement in the indicator or retain and expand those that were associated with improvements.

Developing the Capacity of Researchers to Disseminate Empirically Supported Practices

Researchers who developed most of the programs described in Chapters 5–7 have limited capacity to support dissemination. Researchers generally do not receive training in how to disseminate programs in user-friendly ways to communities and research provides almost no data-based guidance about how best to do it. Instead, researchers learn to disseminate their work via highly technical scientific papers in peer-reviewed journals, supplemented with the occasional technical book. Moreover, there are few incentives for dissemination to the public. Scientists' pay, promotion, and further funding for research are contingent on their conducting and publishing more research—not by assisting organizations in adopting previously tested programs.

Several things must change to alter this state of affairs. First, we need mechanisms to increase funding for training and consultation in how to implement empirically supported programs. A good model is the Blueprints project at the Center for the Study and Prevention of Violence (*http://www.colorado.edu/cspv/blueprints/*), which has identified 11 programs indicated by experimental evidence to be effective for reducing delinquency and violence. Through a mechanism that funds the developers of these programs, the project provides training and technical assistance for implementation of these 11 programs. Table 9.1 provides information about other organizations actively assisting communities and organizations in the implementation of research-based practices.

Second, we need to develop a cadre of implementation specialists trained to assist communities in implementing empirically based practices (James & Biglan, 2000). These individuals should be skilled at implementing the interventions they were disseminating as well as training and consulting in organizations that are adopting those interventions. Moreover, if we are correct that ongoing evaluation of implemented programs will become more common, specialists of this sort will have to be skilled in helping organizations set up systematic evaluations. Graduate programs in community and clinical psychology and those in prevention science and public health would seem to be the logical places to train these specialists.

Third, we need a better science of dissemination. As noted previously, limited research has examined "best practices" for disseminating "best practices" in ways that increase the likelihood that the practices being disseminated will be adopted and implemented well. We discuss this topic in more detail in the next section.

Research Needed to Implement Effective Interventions

Two research initiatives could foster the implementation of effective programs and policies in communities. The first is the development of better partnerships between communities and those conducting research on the prevention and reduction of adolescent problem behaviors. The second is a new line of research that would experimentally evaluate strategies for getting empirically supported interventions adopted, well implemented, and evaluated.

Developing True Partnerships between Researchers and Communities

The recent development of the Clinical Trials Network (CTN) by the National Institute on Drug Abuse (NIDA; *http://www.nida.nih.gov/ CTN/index.htm*) provides a model for how research on reducing the prevalence of adolescent problem behaviors might proceed. The CTN consists of "nodes" around the country that link research organizations with up to 10 clinical facilities. They evaluate the effectiveness of research-based treatments when implemented in treatment settings. In doing these studies, researchers have to deal with challenges involved in training and maintaining fidelity of implementation in the settings where the treatments must ultimately be provided. This requires that the researchers devise and evaluate effective methods of implementing inter-

TABLE 9.1. Organizations Assisting in the Implementation of Research-Based Practices

Organization/agency	Mission	Contact information
Collaborative for Academic, Social, and Emotional Learning (CASEL)	Establish social and emotional learning (SEL) as an integral part of education from pre-high school. International network of researchers/practitioners in SEL, prevention, positive youth development, character education, and school reform.	CASEL, University of Illinois, Chicago, Department of Psychology (m/c 285), 1007 West Harrison, Chicago, IL 60607-7137; phone: 312-413-9406; e-mail: *casel@uic.edu;* website: *http://www.casel.org*
Center for Substance Abuse Prevention (CSAP)	Decrease substance use/abuse by bringing effective prevention to every community. Provide leadership in policy/program development; help to prevent the onset of illegal drug use, underage alcohol and tobacco use; and reduce negative consequences of using substances.	Ruth Sanchez-Way, Director; phone: 301-443-0365; website: *http://www.samhsa.gov/centers/ csap/csap.html* Office of Communications at SAMHSA; phone: 301-443-8956; e-mail: *info@samhsa.gov*
Community Tool Box at the University of Kansas	Promote community health and development by connecting people, ideas, and resources.	4082 Dole Human Development Center, 1000 Sunnyside Avenue, University of Kansas, Lawrence, KS 66045; phone: 785-864-0533; fax: 785-864-5281; website: *http://ctb.lsi.ukans.edu/* e-mail: *Toolbox@ky.edu.*
National Center for Improving the Tools of Educators, University of Oregon (NCITE)	Advance the quality and effectiveness of educational technology, media, and materials (TMM) for those with disabilities and create a marketplace demand for TMM.	Douglas Carnine, Director; Edward Kame'enui, Associate Director; NCITE, 805 Lincoln, Eugene, OR 97401; e-mail: *ncite@darkwing.uoregon.edu;* website: *http:// idea.uoregon.edu/~ncite/*

Social Development Research Group, University of Washington	Nationally known, interdisciplinary team united to understand and promote healthy behaviors, positive social development among children, adolescents, and young adults.	9725 Third Avenue NE, Suite 401, Seattle, WA 98115; phone: 206-685-1997; fax: 206-543-4507; e-mail: *sdrg@u.washington.edu*; website: *http://depts.washington.edu/sdrg/*
Society for Prevention Research (SPR)	A scientific, multidisciplinary forum for prevention science. They invite investigators from underrepresented research specialties to join SPR.	1300 I Street NW, # 250 West, Washington, DC 20005; phone: 202-216-9670; fax: 202-216-9671; website: *http://www.preventionresearch.org/*
National Institute of Health (Small Business Innovation Research and Small Business Technology Transfer)	Steward of medical and behavioral research for the United States. Science in pursuit of fundamental knowledge about the nature and behavior of living systems and its application to extend healthy life and reduce illness and disability.	Website: *http://grants.nih.gov/grants/funding/sbir.htm#sbir*

ventions in these settings. Such information is essential to any further dissemination of these interventions. Moreover, if an intervention is found to be effective in these settings, one can have considerable confidence that its effects can be replicated in similar treatment facilities—an assumption that is less tenable for treatments evaluated in research settings, where patients can be extensively screened and there are greater resources for ensuring fidelity of implementation.

The next generation of studies on the prevention of adolescent problem behaviors might follow such a model. Research organizations might establish partnerships with sets of communities so that they could develop collaborative studies in which they assist the community in establishing specific goals, help to create a system for measuring youth problems and implementing one or more interventions, and experimentally evaluate the effects of interventions. Such an arrangement would force researchers to learn how to assist communities in setting goals and assessing problems or well-being. Indeed, experimental evaluations of such strategies for assisting communities could constitute a first round of studies.

Such collaborations would also force researchers to deal with all the obstacles to effective implementation in community settings. That would lead to refinements in interventions and implementation strategies for these interventions that would make it easier to disseminate them with effectiveness. Ideally researchers should clearly describe these strategies as they evolve, a practice that would be made much more likely if federal and local funds were available to evaluate dissemination strategies. As an additional benefit, we could have greater confidence in the disseminability of interventions that had an effect in these "real world" settings.

Ideally, such a network would be set up through a cooperative arrangement among multiple federal agencies and foundations. As this book documents, the next generation of prevention studies needs to target the prevention of a range of adolescent problems and be particularly sensitive to multiproblem youth. Thus, the outcome of this research would be relevant to the missions of several National Institutes of Health, including NIDA, National Institute of Mental Health, National Institute of Child Health and Human Development, National Institute on Alcoholism and Alcohol Abuse, and National Cancer Institute. It would also be relevant to the mission of the CDC.

Experimental Evaluations of Dissemination Strategies

Identifying effective strategies for assisting communities in adopting empirically based practices will require experimental evaluations of those strategies (Biglan, Mrazek, Carnine, & Flay, 2003; James & Biglan, 2002). In these studies, the primary dependent variable will be the implementation of the program or policy. For example, if the program were a classroom management procedure, the study would evaluate whether the dissemination strategy led teachers to implement the procedure as intended by its developers.

The use of experimental procedures to evaluate dissemination strategies has lagged behind the use of experimentation to develop interventions. It is admittedly costly to evaluate dissemination strategies: One may need to evaluate implementation with large numbers of teachers, schools, or even communities. However, we cannot repeal the logic of experimental design just because it is costly. If we want to find reliable ways of getting schools, treatment facilities, community organizations, or whole communities to implement empirically supported programs or policies, the best course will be to experimentally evaluate well-defined dissemination strategies.

The experiments need not be randomized trials. This is true especially in the initial development of knowledge about what may influence organizations to implement an intervention with fidelity. The most efficient designs may involve interrupted time-series experiments in which repeated measures of the targeted practice are obtained in a small number of organizations and the strategy for fostering implementation is introduced in one organization at a time (Biglan, Ary, & Wagenaar, 2000). We described this multiple baseline design in Chapter 8.

THE INNOVATING AND EVALUATING SOCIETY

If we take seriously the notion that a program or policy that has worked well in one setting may not work in another, then we cannot settle for the static implementation of empirically supported practices in new communities. Communities differ in many known and unknown ways; thus we cannot be sure that a practice that worked in one will work in another. Moreover, we cannot be sure that a practice that proved useful when initially implemented will continue to be effective, or that good practices cannot be made even better. Finally, no one would assume that useful innovations come only from the research community. Thus, the effective community of the future will be one that knows how to innovate, but also knows how to evaluate whether its practices are contributing to the well-being of young people. We might characterize that community as follows:

- Policymakers and the public understand and strongly support the value of experimental evaluations of programs and policies.
- The community encourages innovations to enhance the successful development of its young people, but it always evaluates the

impact of those innovations, ideally by comparing them with data from current best practices.

- The community regularly evaluates the costs and benefits of its programs and policies to determine their impact on child and adolescent well-being.
- Evaluation tools exist and the community knows about them. Decision makers in the community have access to them and know how to use them.
- The community follows a cycle of self-improvement. Feedback about evaluations of programs and policies serves to support and refine innovations.

We could evolve improved childrearing practices more rapidly if the previously listed practices were common in states and communities. Imagine that communities experimentally evaluated every new program or policy intended to affect children or adolescents and based decisions on these data. Practices that had a detectable impact would tend to continue; others would adopt them. Those that did not make an impact would wither. Experimental evaluation of programs and policies is no less than what is required of every prescription drug. Why should we not demand that our educational, mental health, and criminal justice systems use all available tools to select more effective policies and programs?

Evolution toward an experimenting society is already well under way. We have been able to identify and document a wealth of programs and policies thanks to the increasing use of and attention to experimental evaluations. As the value of experimental evidence becomes more widely understood and accepted, it will further increase demand and support for experimental evaluations. We look forward to the day when no policymaker will be able to propose a new program or policy without hearing many voices from many constituencies raised to ask, "Are there any data on how well this works? How will you evaluate whether or not it is working here?"

It may seem that using experimental procedures to evaluate programs and policies is too complicated and expensive for wide use. However, many practices once known to only a few are now widespread because of the benefit of these procedures. Examples include quality-control techniques in manufacturing and the use of cell phones and computers. Given the benefit of precise methods for discerning the effects of different interventions or practices on human beings, why should they not become more common?

The increased use of experimental evaluations is one example of the integration of science and practice needed if scientific knowledge is to be of practical benefit. Increasingly, practice will occur in the context of organized efforts to evaluate its effects. Thus, science will inform practice, not simply through the export of knowledge from research to practice settings but through the integration of scientific methods into the management of practice settings. In turn, practice concerns will influence science by speaking to the generalizability of findings and illuminating concerns for scientists to address. This is already happening as scientists begin to study issues such as how communities can encourage participants to enroll in potentially beneficial prevention programs.

Finally, we need to promote the practice of continuous quality improvement among all organizations that affect human health or behavior. The well-functioning community of the future will be one in which organizations that affect human well-being will routinely experimentally evaluate the effects of their programs and policies and modify them in light of what they learn. This will require that those who manage such organizations receive training in measurement and experimental evaluation, and that scientists continue to develop practical, user-friendly, and scientifically sound methods for evaluating programs and policies in communities.

Supporting the Development of Innovation and Evaluation in Communities

The collaborative group (see page 225) that assisted in examining how to translate science into practice identified four things that would support the evolution of the practices identified in this chapter. First, we need to develop a network of practitioners, policymakers, and scientists who are committed to fostering increased use of experimental methods of evaluation in states and communities. The network would share information about efforts to encourage such evaluation and could support each other in assisting states and communities in implementing evaluations.

Second, scientific organizations and those who fund research and practices relevant to youth well-being should advocate for experimental evaluations. We need to inform legislators and other decision makers about the value of experimental designs and the rudiments of appropriate designs. We need to increase journalists' understanding of experimental evaluations. Ultimately, we need to push for making funding contingent on organizations experimentally evaluating their policies and programs. This advocacy effort would go hand-in-hand with advocacy for empirically supported practices. The message is straightforward: Here are some things that might work in your state or community and here are some ways to be sure they are working.

Third, researchers need mechanisms for funding to assist communities in evaluating the effects of programs and policies. Previously, we called for the development of a network of researcher–community collaborations. This is one way to assist communities in developing their capacity to evaluate what they do.

Fourth, we need to train more people to help communities with these tasks (James & Biglan, 2002). As the number of people trained in prevention science and community psychology grows, the ability to evaluate will be increasingly available to communities. It might seem that we should wait until there is a demand for such people. However, creating a cadre of trained people can foster the development of a practice. For example, Japanese auto companies' advances in quality-control techniques have been attributed to the availability on the shop floor of trained engineers; the skills contributed to the development of the practice, rather than the need for the practice creating the demand for the skill (Halberstam, 1987).

Considerable knowledge exists to guide how we think about the problems of youth, and we now know that many approaches to prevention and intervention can prevent difficulties in children such as Michael. We must develop collaborative partnerships with a shared vision, facilitate ongoing assessment of child and adolescent problems and well-being, encourage empirically supported interventions across the lifespan and across multiple levels of influence, and support an innovative and evaluating society. With concerted efforts by those involved in childrearing, communities can implement "best practice" policies and practices that have the potential to turn many potential Michaels into Tommys. Further, communities can help accelerate our progress in improving the lives of youth by contributing to the knowledge base via systematic evaluations of established as well as innovative efforts. This information will in turn help coalitions of community members and scientists develop and test the next generation of effective practices.

NEEDED RESEARCH

- Conduct experimental evaluations of campaigns to get policymakers to implement valid evaluations of policies and programs.

- Identify circumstances in which experimental designs other than randomized controlled trials can enable improved evaluations. We noted the value of interrupted time-series experiments earlier. Research to assess the optimal situations in which to use such designs would be valuable.

References

Aarons, S. J., Jenkins, R. R., Raine, T. R., El Khorazaty, M. N., Woodward, K. M., Williams, R. L., et al. (2000). Postponing sexual intercourse among urban junior high school students—a randomized controlled evaluation. *Journal of Adolescent Health, 27*(4), 236–247.

Acierno, R., Kilpatrick, D. G., Resnick, H., Saunders, B., De Arellano, M., & Best, C. (2000). Assault, PTSD, family substance use, and depression as risk factors for cigarette use in youth: Findings from the National Survey of Adolescents. *Journal of Traumatic Stress, 13*(3), 381–396.

Adams, E. K., & Melvin, C. L. (1998). Costs of maternal conditions attributable to smoking during pregnancy. *American Journal of Preventive Medicine, 15*, 212–219.

Ainsworth, M. S., Blehar, M. C., Waters, E., & Wall, S. (1978). *Patterns of attachment: A psychological study of the strange situation.* Hillsdale, NJ: Erlbaum.

Alan Guttmacher Institute. (1999). Facts in brief: Teen sex and pregnancy. Retrieved March 28, 2003, from *http://www.agi-usa.org/pubs/fb_teen_sex. html.*

Alexander, J. F., Barton, C., Gordon, D., Grotpeter, J., Hansson, K., Harrison, R., et al. (1998). *Blueprints for violence prevention, book three: Functional family therapy.* Boulder, CO: Center for the Study and Prevention of Violence.

Alexander, J. F., Barton, C., Schiavo, R. S., & Parsons, B. V. (1976). Behavioral intervention with families of delinquents: Therapist characteristics and outcome. *Journal of Consulting and Clinical Psychology, 44*(4), 656–664.

Alexander, J. F., & Parsons, B. V. (1973). Short-term behavioral intervention with delinquent families: Impact on family process and recidivism. *Journal of Abnormal Psychology, 3*, 219–225.

American Psychiatric Association (1987). *Diagnostic and statistical manual of mental disorders* (3rd ed., rev.). Washington, DC: Author.

American Psychiatric Association (1994). *Diagnostic and statistical manual of mental disorders* (4th ed.). Washington, DC: Author.

Anisman, H., & Merali, Z. (1999). Understanding stress: Characteristics and caveats. *Alcohol Research and Health, 23,* 241–249.

Aos, S., Phipps, P., Barnoski, R., & Lieb, R. (1999). *The comparative costs and benefits of programs to reduce crime: a review of national research findings with implications for Washington state.* Olympia: Washington State Institute for Public Policy.

Aos, S., Phipps, P., Barnoski, R., & Lieb, R. (2001). *The comparative costs and benefits of programs to reduce crime (Updated).* Olympia: Washington State Institute for Public Policy.

Armbruster, P., & Fallon, T. (1994). Clinical, sociodemographic, and systems risk factors for attrition in a children's mental health clinic. *American Journal of Orthopsychiatry, 64*(4), 577–585.

Arnett, J. J. (1999). Adolescent storm and stress, reconsidered. *American Psychologist, 54,* 317–326.

Arthur, W. B. (1981). The economics of risks to life. *American Economic Review, 71,* 54–64.

Ary, D. V., Duncan, T. E., Biglan, A., Metzler, C. W., Noell, J. W., & Smolkowski, K. (1999). Development of adolescent problem behavior. *Journal of Abnormal Child Psychology, 27*(2), 141–150.

Ary, D. V., Duncan, T. E., Duncan, S. C., & Hops, H. (1999). Adolescent problem behavior: The influence of parents and peers. *Behaviour Research and Therapy, 37*(3), 217–230.

Aseltine, R. H., Jr, Gore, S., & Colten, M. E. (1998). The co-occurrence of depression and substance abuse in late adolescence. *Development and Psychopathology, 10,* 549–570.

Atkinson, D. R., & Gim, R. H. (1989). Asian-American cultural identity and attitudes toward mental health services. *Journal of Counseling Psychology, 36*(2), 209–212.

Baker, T. K., Johnson, M. B., Voas, R. B., & Lange, J. E. (2000). Reduce youthful binge drinking: Call an election in Mexico. *Journal of Safety Research, 31*(2), 61–69.

Baltes, P. B., Reese, H. W., & Lipsitt, L. P. (1980). Life-span developmental psychology. *Annual Review of Psychology, 31,* 65–110.

Barber, B. K. (1996). Parental psychological control: Revisiting a neglected construct. *Child Development, 67*(6), 3296–3319.

Barber, J. G., & Grichting, W. L. (1990). Australia's media campaign against drug abuse. *International Journal of the Addictions, 25*(6), 693–708.

Barkley, R. A., McMurray, M. B., Edelbrock, C. S., & Robbins, K. (1989). The response of aggressive and nonaggressive ADHD children to two doses of methylphenidate. *Journal of the American Academy of Child and Adolescent Psychiatry, 28*(6), 873–881.

Barnett, W. S. (1995). Long-term effects of early childhood programs on cognitive and school outcomes. *The future of children: Long-term outcomes of early childhood programs, 5*(3), 25–50.

Barnett, W. S. (2000). Economics of early childhood intervention. In J. P. Shonkoff

& S. J. Meisel (Eds.), *Handbook of early childhood intervention* (2nd ed., pp. 589–610). Cambridge, UK: Cambridge University Press.

Barone, C., Weissberg, R. P., Kasprow, W. J., Voyce, C. K., Arthur, M. W., & Shriver, T. P. (1995). Involvement in multiple problem behaviors of young urban adolescents. *Journal of Primary Prevention, 15*(3), 261–283.

Barrera, M., Jr., Biglan, A., Ary, D. V., & Li, F. (2001). Replication of a problem behavior model with American Indian, Hispanic, and Caucasian youth. *Journal of Early Adolescence, 21,* 133–157.

Barrish, H. H., Saunders, M., & Wold, M. M. (1969). Good behavior game: Effects of individual contingencies for group consequences on disruptive behavior in a classroom. *Journal of Applied Behavior Analysis, 2,* 119–124.

Barton, C., Alexander, J. F., Waldron, H., Turner, C. W., & Warburton, J. (1985). Generalizing treatment effects of functional family therapy: Three replications. *American Journal of Family Therapy, 13*(3), 16–26.

Bates, J. E., Pettit, G. S., Dodge, K. A., & Ridge, B. (1998). Interaction of temperamental resistance to control and restrictive parenting in the development of externalizing behavior. *Developmental Psychology, 34*(5), 982–995.

Bauman, K. E., Brown, J. D., Bryan, E. S., Fisher, L. A., Padgett, C. A., & Sweeney, J. M. (1988). Three mass media campaigns to prevent adolescent cigarette smoking. *Preventive Medicine, 17,* 510–530.

Bauman, K. E., LaPrelle, J., Brown, J. D., Koch, G. G., & Padgett, C. A. (1991). The influence of three mass media campaigns on variables related to adolescent cigarette smoking: results of a field experiment. *American Journal of Public Health, 81*(5), 597–604.

Bergman, L. R., & Magnusson, D. (1991). Stability and change in patterns of extrinsic adjustment problems. In D. Magnusson (Ed.), *Problems and methods in longitudinal research: Stability and change* (pp. 323–346). Cambridge, MA: Cambridge University Press.

Biener, L., & Siegel, M. (2000). Tobacco marketing and adolescent smoking: More support for a causal inference. *American Journal of Public Health, 90*(3), 407–411.

Biglan, A. (1995). *Changing cultural practices: A contextualist framework for intervention research.* Reno, NV: Context Press.

Biglan, A. (2001). *Expert report in the case of United States of America vs. Philip Morris, Incorporated et al.,* Civil Action No. 99-CV-2496 (GK).

Biglan, A. (2003a). Selection by consequences: One unifying principle for a transdisciplinary science of prevention. *Prevention Science, 4*(4), 213–232.

Biglan, A. (2003b). The generic features of effective childrearing. In A. Biglan, M. C. Wang, & H. J. Walberg (Eds.), *Preventing youth problems* (pp. 221–246). New York: Kluwer Academic.

Biglan, A., Ary, D. V., Duncan, T. E., Black, C., & Smolkowski, K. (2000). A randomized control trial of a community intervention to prevent adolescent tobacco use. *Tobacco Control, 9,* 24–32.

Biglan, A., Ary, D. V., Koehn, V., Levings, D., Smith, S., Wright, Z., et al. (1996). Mobilizing positive reinforcement in communities to reduce youth access to tobacco. *American Journal of Community Psychology, 24*(5), 625–638.

Biglan, A., Ary, D. V., & Wagenaar, A. C. (2000). The value of interrupted time-series experiments for community intervention research. *Prevention Research, 1,* 31–49.

Biglan, A., Ary, D., Yudelson, H., Duncan, T. E., & Hood, D. (1996). Experimental evaluation of a modular approach to mobilizing anti-tobacco influences of peers and parents. *American Journal of Community Psychology, 24,* 311–339.

Biglan, A., Flay, B., & Foster, S. (2003). The prevention of drug abuse. In A. Biglan, M. C. Wang, & H. J. Walberg (Eds.), *Preventing youth problems* (pp. 87–111). New York: Kluwer Academic.

Biglan, A., Henderson, J., Humphreys, D., Yasui, M., Whisman, R., Black, C., et al. (1995). Mobilising positive reinforcement to reduce youth access to tobacco. *Tobacco Control, 4,* 42–48.

Biglan, A., James, L. E., LaChance, P., Zoref, L., & Joffe, J. (1988). Videotaped materials in a school-based smoking prevention program. *Preventive Medicine, 17,* 559–584.

Biglan, A., Metzler, C. W., Wirt, R., Ary, D., Noell, J., Ochs, L., et al. (1990). Social and behavioral factors associated with high-risk sexual behavior among adolescents. *Journal of Behavioral Medicine, 13*(3), 245–261.

Biglan, A., Mrazek, P., Carnine, D. W., & Flay, B. R. (2003). The integration of research and practice in the prevention of youth problem behaviors. *American Psychologist, 58*(6–7), 433–440.

Biglan, A., & Smolkowski, K. (2002). Intervention effects on adolescent drug use and critical influences on the development of problem behavior. In D. B. Kandel (Ed.), *Stages and pathways of drug involvement: Examining the gateway hypothesis* (pp. 158–183). New York: Cambridge University Press.

Biglan, A., & Taylor, T. K. (2000). Why have we been more successful in reducing tobacco use than violent crime? *American Journal of Community Psychology, 28*(3), 269–302.

Blum, R. W., Beuhring, T., Shew, M. L., Bearinger, L. H., Sieving, R. E., & Resnick, M. D. (2000). The effects of race/ethnicity, income, and family structure on adolescent risk behaviors. *American Journal of Public Health, 90*(12), 1879–1884.

Bogenschneider, M., & Stone, M. (1997). Delivering parent education to low and high-risk parents of adolescents via age-paced newsletters. *Family Relations, 46,* 123–134.

Botvin, G.J. (1996). Substance abuse prevention through life skills training. In R. D. Peters & R. J. McMahon (Eds.), *Preventing childhood disorders, substance abuse, and delinquency* (pp. 215–240). Thousand Oaks, CA: Sage.

Botvin, G. J., Baker, E., Dusenbury, L., Botvin, E. M., & Diaz, T. (1995). Long-term follow-up results of a randomized drug abuse prevention trial in a white middle-class population. *Journal of the American Medical Association, 273,* 1106–1112.

Botvin, G. J., Baker, E., Dusenbury, L., Botvin, E. M., & Filazzola, A. D. (1993). *Preventing adolescent drug abuse through a multi-modal cognitive-behavioral approach: Results of a six-year study.* Ithaca, NY: Cornell University Medical College, Institute for Prevention Research.

Botvin, G. J., Baker, E., Dusenbury, L., Tortu, S., & Botvin, E. M. (1990). Preventing adolescent drug abuse through a multi-modal cognitive-behavioral approach: Results of a 3-year study. *Journal of Consulting and Clinical Psychology, 58*(4), 437–446.

Botvin, G. J., Baker, E., Filazzola, A. D., & Botvin, E. M. (1990). A cognitive-behavioral approach to substance abuse prevention: One-year follow-up. *Addictive Behaviors, 15*(1), 47–63.

Botvin, G. J., Baker, E., Renick, N. L., Filazzola, A. D., & Botvin, E. M. (1984). A cognitive-behavioral approach to substance abuse prevention. *Addictive Behaviors, 9,* 137–147.

Botvin, G. J., Batson, H. W., Witts-Vitale, S., Bess, V., Baker, E., & Dusenbury, L. (1989). A psychosocial approach to smoking prevention for urban black youth. *Public Health Reports, 104,* 573–582.

Botvin, G. J., Dusenbury, L., Baker, E., James-Ortiz, S., & Kerner, J. (1989). A skills training approach to smoking prevention among Hispanic youth. *Journal of Behavioral Medicine, 12*(3), 279–296.

Botvin, G. J., Dusenbury, L., Baker, E., James-Ortiz, S., Botvin, E. M., & Kerner, J. (1992). Smoking prevention among urban minority youth: Assessing effects on outcome and mediating variables. *Health Psychology, 11*(5), 290–299.

Botvin, G. J., Griffin, K. W., Diaz, T., Scheier, L. M., Williams, C., & Epstein, J. A. (2000). Preventing illicit drug use in adolescents: Long-term follow-up data from a randomized control trial of a school population. *Addictive Behaviors, 25,* 769–774.

Botvin, G. J., Renick, N. L., & Baker, E. (1983). The effects of scheduling format and booster sessions on a broad-spectrum psychosocial approach to smoking prevention. *Journal of Behavioral Medicine, 6*(4), 359–379.

Brennan, P. A., Grekin, E. R., & Mednick, S. A. (1999). Maternal smoking during pregnancy and adult male criminal outcomes. *Archives of General Psychiatry, 56*(3), 215–219.

Brennan, P. A., Grekin, E. R., Mortensen, E. L., & Mednick, S. A. (2002). Maternal smoking during pregnancy and offspring criminal arrest and hospitalization for substance abuse: A test of gender specific relationships. *American Journal of Psychiatry, 159,* 48–54.

Brestan, E. V., & Eyberg, S. M. (1998). Effective psychosocial treatments of conduct-disordered children and adolescents: 29 years, 82 studies, and 5,272 kids. *Journal of Consulting and Clinical Psychology, 27,* 180–189.

Brewer, D. D., Hawkins, J. D., Catalano, R. F., & Neckerman, H. J. (1995). Preventing serious, violent, and chronic juvenile offending: A review of evaluations of selected strategies in childhood, adolescence, and the community. In J. C. Howell, B. Krisberg, J. D. Hawkins, & J. J. Wilson (Eds.), *A sourcebook: Serious, violent, and chronic juvenile offenders* (pp. 61–141). Thousand Oaks, CA: Sage.

Briggs, X. S. (1997). Moving up versus moving out: Neighborhood effects in housing mobility programs. *Housing Policy Debate, 8,* 195–234.

Brody, G. H., & Forehand, R. (1993). Prospective associations among family form, family process, and adolescents' alcohol and drug use. *Behaviour Research and Therapy, 31,* 587–593.

Brondino, M. J., Henggeler, S. W., Rowland, M. D., Pickrel, S. G., Cunningham, P.

B., & Schoenwald, S. K. (1997). Multisystemic therapy and the ethnic minority client: Culturally responsive and clinically effective. In D. K. Wilson, J. R. Rodrigue, & W. C. Taylor (Eds.), *Health-promoting and health-compromising behaviors among minority adolescents* (pp. 229–250). Washington, DC: American Psychological Association.

Bronfenbrenner, U. (1979). Contexts of child rearing: Problems and prospects. *American Psychologist, 34*(10), 844–850.

Brook, J. S., Cohen, P., Whiteman, M., & Gordon, A. S. (1992). Psychosocial risk factors in the transition from moderate to heavy use or abuse of drugs. In M. D. Glantz & R. W. Pickens (Eds.), *Vulnerability to drug abuse* (pp. 359–388). Washington, DC: American Psychological Association.

Brook, J. S., Whiteman, M., & Gordon, A. S. (1982). Qualitative and quantitative aspects of adolescent drug use: Interplay of personality, family, and peer correlates. *Psychological Reports, 51*(3, Pt 2), 1151–1163.

Brooks-Gunn, J., Duncan, G. J., Klebanov, P. K., & Sealand, N. (1993). Do neighborhoods influence child and adolescent development? *American Journal of Sociology, 99*(2), 353–395.

Brown, B. (1999). Optimizing expression of the common human genome for child development. *Current Directions in Psychological Science, 8*(2), 37–41.

Brown, S. A., Gleghorn, A., Schuckit, M. A., Myers, M. G., & Mott, M. A. (1996). Conduct disorder among adolescent alcohol and drug abusers. *Journal of Studies on Alcohol, 57*(3), 314–324.

Brown, S. A., Myers, M. G., Lippke, L., Tapert, S. F., Stewart, D. G., & Vik, P. W. (1998). Psychometric evaluation of the customary drinking and drug use record (CDDR): A measure of adolescent alcohol and drug involvement. *Journal of Studies in Alcohol, 59*, 427–438.

Cadoret, R. J., Cain, C. A., & Grove, W. M. (1980). Development of alcoholism in adoptees raised apart from alcoholic biologic relatives. *Archives of General Psychiatry, 37*(5), 561–563.

Cadoret, R. J., Troughton, E., O'Gorman. T. W., & Heywood, E. (1986). An adoption study of genetic and environmental factors in drug abuse. *Archives of General Psychiatry, 43*(12), 1131–1136.

Cameron, M., Cavallo, A., & Sullivan, G. (1992). *Evaluation of the random breath testing initiative in Victoria 1989–1991. Multivariate time series approach.* Report No. 38. Victoria, Australia: Monash University.

Cameron, M., Diamantopoulou, K., Mullan, N., Dyte, D., & Gantzer, S. (1997). *Evaluation of the country random breath testing and publicity program in Victoria, 1993–1994.* Report No. 126. Victoria, Australia: Monash University.

Campbell, F. A., Ramey, C. T., Pungello, E., Sparling, J., & Miller-Johnson, S. (2002). Early childhood education: Young adult outcomes from the Abecedarian Project. *Applied Developmental Science, 6*(1), 42–57.

Campbell, M., & Cueva, J. E. (1995). Psychopharmacology in child and adolescent psychiatry: A review of the past seven years: I. *Journal of the American Academy of Child and Adolescent Psychiatry, 34*(9), 1124–1132.

Caspi, A., Begg, D., Dickson, N., Harrington, H., Langley, J., Moffitt, T. E., et al.

(1997). Personality differences predict health-risk behaviors in young adulthood: Evidence from a longitudinal study. *Journal of Personality and Social Psychology, 73*(5), 1052–1063.

Caspi, A., Lynam, D., Moffitt, T. E., & Silva, P. A. (1993). Unraveling girls' delinquency: Biological, dispositional, and contextual contributions to adolescent misbehavior. *Developmental Psychology, 29*(1), 19–30.

Casswell, S., & Zhang, J. F. (1998). Impact of liking for advertising and brand allegiance on drinking and alcohol-related aggression: A longitudinal study. *Addiction, 93*(8), 1209–1217.

Casteel, C., & Peek-Asa, C. (2000). Crime prevention through environmental design (CPTED) in reducing robberies. *American Journal of Preventive Medicine, 18*(4), 99–115.

Catalano, R. F., Berglund, M. L., Ryan, J. A. M., Lonczak, H. S., & Hawkins, J. D. (1999). *Positive youth development in the United States: Research findings on evaluations of the Positive Youth Development Program.* Report to the U.S. Department of Health and Human Services, Office of the Assistant Secretary for Planning and Evaluation and NICHD. Retrieved January 15, 2003, from *http://aspe.hhs.gov/hsp/PositiveYouthDev99/index.htm.*

Catalano, R. F., & Hawkins, J. D. (1995). *Risk focused prevention: Using the Social Development Strategy.* Seattle, WA: Developmental Research and Programs.

Catalano, R. F., Hawkins, J. D., Wells, E. A., Miller, J., & Brewer, D. (1991). Evaluation of the effectiveness of adolescent drug abuse treatment, assessment of risks for relapse, and promising approaches for relapse prevention. *International Journal of the Addictions, 25*(9A & 10A), 1085–1140.

Caulkins, J., Crawford, G., & Reuter, P. (1993). Simulation of adaptive response: A model of drug interdiction. *Mathematical and Computer Modelling, 17*(2), 37–52.

Center for Human Resource Research. (2001). *National Longitudinal Surveys 1997.* Prepared for the U.S. Department of Labor, Bureau of Labor Statistics. Columbus: Ohio State University.

Center for the Study and Prevention of Violence. (2003). *The Blueprints Project* [On-line]. Available: *http://www.colorado/edu/research/scpv/blueprints.*

Centers for Disease Control and Prevention, Division of Adult and Community Health, National Center for Chronic Disease Prevention and Health Promotion. (2002). *Behavioral Risk Factor Surveillance System online prevalence data, 1995–2000.* Retrieved March 4, 2003, from *http://www.cdc.gov/brfss/index.htm.*

Centers for Disease Control and Prevention. (1989). *Reducing the health consequences of smoking: 25 years of progress. A report of the Surgeon General* (DHSS Publication No. CDC 89-8411). Washington, DC: U.S. Department of Health and Human Services.

Centers for Disease Control and Prevention. (1996). Youth risk behavior surveillance, 1995. *Morbidity and Mortality Weekly Report, 45*(20), 413–418.

Centers for Disease Control and Prevention. (1998). *HIV/AIDS Surveillance Report, 10*(1).

Centers for Disease Control and Prevention. (2000a). *HIV/AIDS Surveillance Report, 12*(1).

Centers for Disease Control and Prevention. (2000b). Youth risk behavior surveillance: United States, 1999. *Morbidity and Mortality Weekly Report, 49*(SS05), 1–96.

Centers for Disease Control and Prevention. (2002a). *Vital Statistics of the United States, 1998*. Retrieved April 12, 2002 from *http://www.cdc.gov/nchs/products/pubs/pubd/vsus/vsus.htm.*

Centers for Disease Control and Prevention. (2002b). Youth Risk Behavior Surveillance—United States, 2001. (2002). *Morbidity and Mortality Weekly Report, 51*(SS04), 1–64.

Chabune, N., Leboye, M., & Mouren-Simeoni, M. C. (2000). Opiate antagonists in children and adolescents. *European Child and Adolescent Psychiatry, 9,* 44–50.

Chaiken, J. M., & Chaiken, M. R. (1990). Drugs and predatory crime. In M. Tonry & J. Q. Wilson (Eds.), *Drugs and crime* (pp. 203–239). Chicago: University of Chicago Press.

Chaloupka, F. J., & Grossman, M. (1996). *Price, tobacco control policies and youth smoking.* NBER Working Paper 5740.

Chaloupka, F. J., Grossman, M., & Tauras, J. A. (1997). Public policy and youth smokeless tobacco use. *Southern Economic Journal, 64*(2), 503–516.

Chaloupka, F. J., & Laixuthai, A. (1997). Do youths substitute alcohol and marijuana? Some econometric evidence. *Eastern Economic Journal, 23*(3), 253–276.

Chaloupka, F. J., & Pacula, R. L. (2000). Economics and anti-health behavior: The economic analysis of substance use and abuse. In W. K. Bickel & R. E. Vuchinich (Eds.), *Economics and anti-health behavior: The economic analysis of substance use and abuse* (pp. 89–111). Mahwah, NJ: Erlbaum.

Chaloupka, F. J., Saffer, H., & Grossman, M. (1993). Alcohol control policies and motor vehicle fatalities. *Journal of Legal Studies, 22*(1), 161–186.

Chaloupka, F. J., & Wechsler, H. (1997). Price, tobacco-control policies, and smoking among young adults. *Journal of Health Economics, 16,* 359–373.

Chamberlain, P. (1990). Comparative evaluation of specialized foster care for seriously delinquent youths: A first step. *Community Alternatives: International Journal of Family Care, 2*(2), 21–36.

Chamberlain, P. (1994). *Family connections: Treatment foster care for adolescents with delinquency.* Eugene, OR: Castalia.

Chamberlain, P., & Reid, J. B. (1991). Using a specialized foster-care community treatment model for children and adolescents leaving the state mental hospital. *Journal of Community Psychology, 19*(3), 266–276.

Chamberlain, P., & Reid, J. B. (1998). Comparison of two community alternative to incarceration for chronic juvenile offenders. *Journal of Consulting and Clinical Psychology, 66*(4), 624–633.

Chambless, D. L, Sanderson, W. C., Shoham, V., Johnson, S. B., Pope, K. S., Crits-Christoph, P., et al. (1996). An update on empirically validated therapies. *The Clinical Psychologist, 49*(2), 5–18.

Chambless, D. L., Baker, M. J., Baucom, D. H., Beutler, L. E., Calhoun, K. S., Crits-Christoph, P., et al. (1998). Update on empirically validated therapies: II. *The Clinical Psychologist, 51,* 3–16.

Chambless, D. L., & Hollon, S. (1998). Defining empirically supported therapies. *Journal of Consulting and Clinical Psychology, 66*(1), 7–18.

Chessare, J. B., Pascoe, M., & Baugh, E. F. (1986). Smoking during pregnancy and child maltreatment: Is there an association? *International Journal of Biosocial Research, 8,* 37–42.

Chilcoat, H. D., & Breslau, N. (1999). Pathways from ADHD to early drug use. *Journal of the American Academy of Child and Adolescent Psychiatry, 38*(11), 1347–1354.

Chou, C., Montgomery, S., Pentz, M. A., Rohrback, L. A., Johnson, A., Flay, B. R., et al. (1998). Effects of a community-based prevention program on decreasing drug use in high-risk adolescents. *American Journal of Public Health, 88,* 944–948.

Chung, P. J., Garfield, C. F., Rathouz, P. J., Lauderdale, D. S., Best, D., & Lantos, J. (2002). Youth targeting by tobacco manufacturers since the Master Settlement Agreement. *Health Affairs, 21*(2), 254–263.

Clarke, S. H., & Campbell, F. A. (1998). Can intervention early prevent crime later? The Abecedarian Project compared with other programs. *Early Childhood Research Quarterly, 13*(2), 319–343.

Cloninger, C. R., & Gottesman, I. I. (1987). Genetic and environmental factors in antisocial behavior disorders. In S. A. Mednick, T. E. Moffitt, & S. A. Stack (Eds.), *The causes of crime: New biological approaches* (pp. 92–109). New York: Cambridge University Press.

Coate, D., & Grossman, M. (1988). Effects of alcoholic beverage prices and legal drinking ages on youth alcohol use. *Journal of Law and Economics, 31*(1), 145–171.

Cohen, M. (1998). The monetary value of saving a high-risk youth. *Journal of Quantitative Criminology, 14,* 5–33.

Cohen, M. A. (1988). Pain, suffering, and jury awards: A study of the cost of crime to victims. *Law and Society Review, 22,* 537–555.

Colon, I. (1982). The influence of state monopoly of alcohol distribution and the frequency of package stores on single motor vehicle fatalities. *American Journal of Drug and Alcohol Abuse, 9*(3), 325–331.

Comstock, G., & Paik, H. (1991). *Television and the American child.* San Diego: Academic Press.

Conduct Problems Prevention Research Group. (1999a). Initial impact of the fast track prevention trial for conduct problems: I. The high-risk sample. *Journal of Consulting and Clinical Psychology, 67*(5), 631–647.

Conduct Problems Prevention Research Group. (1999b). Initial impact of the Fast Track prevention trial for conduct problems: II. Classroom effects. *Journal of Consulting and Clinical Psychology, 67*(5), 648–657.

Conduct Problems Prevention Research Group. (2002). Evaluation of the first 3 years of the Fast Track prevention trial with children at high risk for adolescent conduct problems. *Journal of Abnormal Child Psychology, 30*(1), 19–35.

Connolly, G. M., Casswell, S., Zhang, J. F., & Silva, P. A. (1994). Alcohol in the mass media and drinking by adolescents: A longitudinal study. *Addiction, 89*(10), 1255–1263.

Connor, D. F., Barkley, R. A., & Davis, H. T. (2000). A pilot study of methylpheni-date, clonidine, or the combination in ADHD comorbid with aggressive oppositional defiant or conduct disorder. *Clinical Pediatrics (Philadelphia)*, *39*(1), 15–25.

Constantino, J. N., Liberman, M., & Kincaid, M. (1997). Effects of serotonin reuptake inhibitors on aggressive behavior in psychiatrically hospitalized ad-olescents: Results of an open trial. *Journal of Child and Adolescent Psycho-pharmacology*, *7*(1), 31–44

Cook, P. J. (1981). The effect of liquor taxes on drinking, cirrhosis, and auto acci-dents. In M. H. Moore & D. R. Gerstein (Eds.), *Alcohol and public policy: Beyond the shadow of prohibition* (pp. 255–285). Washington, DC: National Academy Press.

Cook, P. J., & Tauchen, G. (1982). The effect of liquor taxes on heavy drinking. *Bell Journal of Economics*, *13*, 379–390.

Cox, D., Cox, A. D., & Moschis, G. P. (1990). When consumer behavior goes bad: An investigation of adolescent shoplifting. *Journal of Consumer Research*, *17*, 149–159.

Coyle, K., Kirby, D., Marin, B., Gomez, C., & Gregorich, S. (2000). *Effect of Draw the Line/Respect the Line on sexual behavior in middle schools.* Unpublished briefing paper.

Crick, N. R., & Dodge, K. A. (1994). A review and reformulation of social infor-mation-processing mechanisms in children's social adjustment. *Psychological Bulletin*, *115*(1), 74–101.

Crockett, S. J., Mullis, R., Perry, C. L., & Luepker, R. V. (1989). Parent educa-tion in youth-directed nutrition interventions. *Preventive Medicine*, *18*, 475–491.

Cromwell, J., Bartosch, W. J., Fiore, M. C., Hasselblad, V., & Baker, T. (1997). Cost-effectiveness of the clinical practice recommendations in the AHCPR guideline for smoking cessation. *Journal of the American Medical Associa-tion*, *278*, 1759–1766.

Cummings, K., Hyland, M., Saunders-Martin, A., & Perla, J. (1997). *What retail-ers are doing to prevent tobacco sales to minors.* Unpublished manuscript.

Cummings, K. M., Sciandra, R., Pechacek, T. F., Orlandi, M., & Lynn, W. R. (1992). Where teenagers get their cigarettes: A survey of the purchasing hab-its of 13–16 year olds in 12 US communities. *Tobacco Control*, *1*, 264–267.

Davidson, W. S., II, Redner, R., Amdur, R. L., & Mitchell, C. M. (1990). *Alterna-tive treatments for troubled youth: The case of diversion from the justice sys-tem.* New York: Plenum Press.

Dawson, G., Ashman, S. B., & Carver, L. J. (2000). The role of early experience in shaping behavioral and brain development and its implications for social pol-icy. *Development and Psychopathology*, *12*(4), 695–712.

DeCicca, P., Kenkel, D., & Mathios, A. (2000). Racial differences in the determi-nants of smoking onset. *Journal of Risk and Uncertainty*, *21*(2/3).

DeCicca, P., Kenkel, D., & Mathios, A. (2002). Putting out the fires: Will higher taxes reduce the onset of youth smoking? *Journal of Political Economy*, *110*(1), 144–169.

Deckel, A. W., & Hesselbrock, V. (1996). Behavioral and cognitive measurements predict scores on the MAST: A 3-year prospective study. *Alcoholism: Clinical and Experimental Research, 20*(7), 1173–1178.

Dee, T. S. (1999). State alcohol policies, teen drinking and traffic fatalities. *Journal of Public Economics, 72*(2), 289–315.

De Kloet, E. R., Korte, S. M., Rots, N. Y., & Kruk, M. R. (1996). Stress hormones, genotype, and brain organization: Implications for aggression. In C. F. Ferris & T. Grisso (Eds.), *Understanding aggressive behavior in children* (pp. 179–191). New York: New York Academy of Sciences.

Dembo, R., Williams, L., Wothke, W., Schmeidler, J., Getreu, A., Berry, E., et al. (1992). The generality of deviance: Replication of a structural model among high-risk youths. *Journal of Research in Crime and Delinquency, 29*(2), 200–216.

Dennis, M. L (2002, May). (Invited Commentary). Treatment research on adolescent drug and alcohol abuse: Despite progress, many challenges remain. *Connection, A Newsletter Linking the Users and Producers of Drug Abuse Services Research, 1–2*(7). Retrieved October 15, 2002, from *http://www.academyhealth.org.*

Dennis, M. L., Babor, T. F., Diamond, G., Donaldson, J., Godley, S. H., Titus, J. C., et al. (2000). *Cooperative agreement for a multisite study of the effectiveness of treatment for cannabis (marijuana)-dependent youth.* Rockville, MD: Center for Substance Abuse Treatment. Retrieved March 7, 2003, from *http://www.chestnut.org/LI/cyt/findings/.*

Derzon, J. H., & Lipsey, M. W. (2002). A meta-analysis of the effectiveness of mass-communication for changing substance-use knowledge, attitudes, and behavior. In W. D. Crano & M. Burgoon (Eds.), *Mass media and drug prevention: Classic and contemporary theories and research* (pp. 231–258). Mahwah, NJ: Erlbaum.

DeWolff, M., & van IJzendoorn, M. H. (1997). Sensitivity and attachment: A meta-analysis on parental antecedents of infant attachment. *Child Development, 68*(4), 571–591.

DiFranza, J. R. (2000). World's best practice in tobacco control: Reducing youth access to tobacco. *Tobacco Control, 9,* 235–236.

DiFranza, J. R., Savageau, J. A., & Aisquith, B. F. (1996). Youth access to tobacco: The effects of age, gender, vending machine locks, and "it's the law" programs. *American Journal of Public Health, 86*(2), 221–224.

DiFranza, J. R., & Tye, J. B. (1990). Who profits from tobacco sales to children? *Journal of the American Medical Association, 263*(20), 2784–2787.

DiNardo, J. (1993). Law enforcement, the price of cocaine and cocaine use. *Mathematical and Computer Modelling, 17*(2), 53–64.

Dishion, T. J., & Andrews, D. W. (1995). Preventing escalation in problem behaviors with high-risk young adolescents: Immediate and 1-year outcomes. *Journal of Consulting and Clinical Psychology, 63,* 538–548.

Dishion, T. J., Bullock, B. M., & Granic, I. (2002). Pragmatism in modeling peer influence: Dynamics, outcomes, and change processes. In D. Cicchetti & S. Hinshaw (Eds.), How prevention intervention studies in the field of developmental psychopathology can inform development theories and models [Special Issue]. *Development and Psychopathology, 14*(4), 969–981.

Dishion, T. J., Capaldi, D., Spracklen, K. M., & Li, F. (1995). Peer ecology of male adolescent drug use. *Development and Psychopathology, 7*(4), 803–824.

Dishion, T. J., French, D., & Patterson, G. R. (1995). The development and ecology of antisocial behavior. In D. Cicchetti & D. Cohen (Eds.), *Manual of developmental psychopathology: Vol. 2. Risk, disorder, and adaptation* (pp. 421–471). New York: Wiley.

Dishion, T. J., Kavanagh, K., Schneiger, A., Nelson, S., & Kaufman, N. (2002). Preventing early adolescent substance use: A family-centered strategy for the public middle-school ecology. In R. L. Spoth, K. Kavanagh, & T. J. Dishion (Eds.), Universal family-centered prevention strategies: Current findings and critical issues for public health impact [Special Issue]. *Prevention Science, 3,* 191–201.

Dishion, T. J., McCord, J., & Poulin, F. (1999). When interventions harm: Peer groups and problem behavior. *American Psychologist, 54*(9), 755–764.

Dishion, T. J., Spracklen, K. M., Andrews, D. W., & Patterson, G. R. (1996). Deviancy training in male adolescents friendships. *Behavior Therapy, 27*(3), 373–390.

Disney, E. R., Elkins, I. J., McGue, M., & Iacono, W. G. (1999). Effects of ADHD, conduct disorder, and gender of substance use and abuse in adolescence. *American Journal of Psychiatry, 156*(10), 1515–1521.

Dolan, L. J., Kellam, S. G., Brown, C. H., Werthamer-Larsson, L., Rebok, G. W., Mayer, L. S., et al. (1993). The short-term impact of two classroom based preventive intervention trials on aggressive and shy behaviors and poor achievement. *Journal of Applied Developmental Psychology, 14,* 317–345.

Donovan, J. E., & Jessor, R. (1985). Structure of problem behavior in adolescence and young adulthood. *Journal of Consulting and Clinical Psychology, 53*(6), 890–904.

Donovan, J. E., Jessor, R., & Costa, F.M. (1988). Syndrome of problem behavior in adolescence: A replication. *Journal of Consulting and Clinical Psychology, 56*(5), 762–765.

Dresser, J., & Gliksman, L. (1998). Comparing statewide alcohol-server training systems. *Pharmacology, Biochemistry, and Behavior, 61,* 150.

Drotar, D., Stein, R. E. K., & Perrin, E. C. (1995). Methodological issues in using the Child Behavior Checklist and its related instruments in clinical child psychology research. *Journal of Clinical Child Psychology, 24*(2), 184–192.

Drummond, A. E., Sullivan, G., & Cavallo, A. (1992). *An evaluation of the random breath testing initiative in Victoria 1989–1990: Quasi-experimental time series approach.* Victoria, Australia: Monash University Accident Research Centre.

Drummond, D. C. (2000). UK government announces first major relaxation in the alcohol licensing laws for nearly a century: Drinking in the UK goes 24/7. *Addiction, 95*(7), 997–998.

Duffy, M. (1995). Advertising in demand systems for alcoholic drinks and tobacco: A comparative study. *Journal of Policy Modeling, 17,* 557–577.

Duncan, S. C., Duncan, T. E., Biglan, A., & Ary, D. (1998). Contributions of the social context to the development of adolescent substance use: A multivariate latent growth modeling approach. *Drug and Alcohol Dependence, 50*(1), 57–71.

Eccles, J. S., & Midgley, C. (1990). Changes in academic motivation and self-perception during early adolescence. In R. Montemayor, G. R. Adams, & T. P. Gullota (Eds.), *From childhood to adolescence: A transitional period?* (pp. 134–55). Thousand Oaks, CA: Sage.

Eddy, J. M., & Chamberlain, P. (2000). Family management and deviant peer association as mediators of the impact of treatment condition on youth antisocial behavior. *Journal of Consulting and Clinical Psychology, 68*(5), 857–863.

Eddy, J. M., Reid, J. B., & Fetrow, R. A. (2000). An elementary school-based prevention program targeting modifiable antecedents of youth delinquency and violence: Linking the Interests of Families and Teachers (LIFT). *Journal of Emotional and Behavioral Disorders, 8*(3), 165–186.

Eiden, R. D., & Leonard, K. E. (1996). Paternal alcohol use and the mother-infant relationship. *Development and Psychopathology, 8*(2), 307–323.

Eiden, R. D., Peterson, M., & Coleman, T. (1999). Maternal cocaine use and the care-giving environment during early childhood. *Psychology of Addictive Behaviors, 13*(4), 293–302.

Eisen, M., Zellman, G. L., & McAlister, A. L. (1990). Evaluating the impact of a theory-based sexuality and contraceptive education program. *Family Planning Perspectives, 22*(6), 261–271.

Elder, G. H., & Caspi, A. (1988). Economic stress in lives: Developmental perspectives. *Journal of Social Issues, 44*(4), 25–45.

Elder, J. P., Perry, C. L., Stone, E. J., Johnson, C. C., Yang, M., Edmundson, E. W., et al. (1996). Tobacco use measurement, prediction, and intervention in elementary schools in four states: The CATCH study. *Preventive Medicine: An International Devoted to Practice and Theory, 25*(4), 486–494.

Ellickson, P., Saner, H., & McGuigan, K. A. (1997). Profiles of violent youth: Substance use and other concurrent problems. *American Journal of Public Health, 87*(6), 985–991.

Elliott, D. S., Huizinga, D., & Menard, S. (1989). *Multiple problem youth: Delinquency, substance use, and mental health problems.* New York: Springer-Verlag.

Ellis, B. J., McFadyen-Ketchum, S., Dodge, K. A., Pettit, G. S., & Bates, J. E. (1999). Quality of early family relationships and individual differences in the timing of pubertal maturation in girls: A longitudinal test of an evolutionary model. *Journal of Personality and Social Psychology, 77*(2), 387–401.

Embry, D. D. (2000). *The PAX Acts Game Solution: Applying replicated research and current evaluation from the Good Behavior Game for achievement and prevention in schools.* A Special presentation to the National Crime Prevention Council. Tucson, AZ: PAXIS Institute.

Emshoff, J., & Moeti, R. (1986). *Preventive intervention with children of alcoholics.* Paper presented at the meeting of the Southeastern Psychological Association, Orlando, FL.

Ennett, S. T., Tobler, N. S., Ringwalt, C. L., & Flewelling, R. L. (1994). How effective is drug abuse resistance education? A meta-analysis of Project DARE outcome evaluations. *American Journal of Public Health, 84*(9), 1394–1401.

Ensminger, M. E. (1990). Sexual activity and problem behaviors among Black, urban adolescents. *Child Development, 61*(6), 2032–2046.

Evans, W. N., & Farrelly, M. C. (1997). *The compensating behavior of smokers: Taxes, tar, and nicotine.* College Park: University of Maryland, Department of Economics.

Evans, W. N., & Huang, L. X. (1998). *Cigarette taxes and teen smoking: New evidence from panels of repeated cross-sections,* Working paper. College Park: Department of Economics, University of Maryland.

Expert Panel on Safe, Disciplined, and Drug-Free Schools. (1999). *Guidelines for submitting safe, disciplined, and drug-free schools programs for designation as promising or exemplary.* Washington, DC: U.S. Department of Education.

Fagan, J., Weis, J. G., & Cheng, Y-T. (1990). Delinquency and substance use among inner-city students. *Journal of Drug Issues, 20*(3), 351–402.

Farrell, A. D., Danish, S. J., & Howard, C. W. (1992). Relationship between drug use and other problem behaviors in urban adolescents. *Journal of Consulting and Clinical Psychology, 60*(5), 705–712.

Faulkner, A. H., & Cranston, K. (1998). Correlates of same-sex sexual behavior in a random sample of Massachusetts high school students. *American Journal of Public Health, 88,* 262–266.

Fawcett, S. B., Francisco, V. T., Paine-Andrews, A., & Schultz, J. A. (2000). A dialogue. A model memorandum of collaboration: A proposal. *Public Health Reports, 115,* 174–179.

Feighery, E. C., Altman, D. G., & Shaffer, G. (1991). The effects of combining education and enforcement to reduce tobacco sales to minors: A study of four Northern California communities. *Journal of the American Medical Association, 266,* 3168–3171.

Ferdinand, R. F., & Verhulst, F. C. (1994). The prediction of poor outcome in young adults: Comparison of the Young Adult Self-Report, the General Health Questionnaire, and the Symptom Checklist. *Acta Psychiatrica Scandinavica, 89*(6), 405–410.

Ferguson, S. A., Fields, M., & Voas, R. B. (2000). *Enforcement of zero tolerance laws in the United States.* Paper presented to the 15th International Conference on Alcohol, Drugs, and Traffic Safety, Stockholm, Sweden.

Fergusson, D. M. (1999). Prenatal smoking and antisocial behavior. *Archives of General Psychiatry, 56*(3), 223–224.

Fergusson, D. M., Horwood, L. J., & Lynskey, M. T. (1994a). The childhoods of multiple problem adolescents: A 15-year longitudinal study. *Journal of Child Psychology and Psychiatry and Allied Disciplines, 35*(6), 1123–1140.

Fergusson, D. M., Horwood, L. J., & Lynskey, M. T. (1994b). The comorbidities of adolescent problem behaviors: A latent class model. *Journal of Abnormal Child Psychology, 22*(3), 339–354.

Fergusson, D. M., Woodward, L. J., & Horwood, L. J. (1998). Maternal smoking during pregnancy and psychiatric adjustment in late adolescence. *Archives of General Psychiatry, 55*(8), 721–727.

Fichtenberg, C. M., & Glantz, S. A. (2002). Youth access interventions do not affect youth smoking. *Pediatrics, 109,* 1088–1092.

Fick, A. C., & Thomas, S. M. (1995). Growing up in a violent environment: Relationship to health-related beliefs and behaviors. *Youth and Society, 27*(2), 136–147.

Findling, R. L., McNamara, N. K., Branicky, L. A., Schluchter, M. D., Lemon, E., & Blumer, J. L. (2000). A double blind pilot study of risperidone in the treatment of conduct disorder. *Journal of the American Academy of Child and Adolescent Psychiatry, 39*(4), 509–516.

Fisher, A., Chestnut, L. G., & Violette, D. M (1989). The value of reducing risks of death: A note on new evidence. *Journal of Policy Analysis and Management, 8*(1), 88–100.

Flay, B. R., & Allred, C. G. (2003). Long-term effects of the Positive Action Program: A comprehensive, positive youth development program. *American Journal of Health Behavior, 27*(Suppl. 1), 56–521

Flay, B. R., Allred, C. G., & Ordway, N. (2001). Effects of the Positive Action program on achievement and discipline: Two matched-control comparisons. *Prevention Science, 2*(2), 71–89.

Flay, B. R., Brannon, B. R., Johnson, C. A., Hansen, W. B., Ulene, A. L., Whitney-Saltiel, D. A., et al. (1988). The television school and family smoking prevention and cessation project. *Preventive Medicine, 17,* 585–607.

Flynn, B. S., Worden, J. K., Secker-Walker, R. H., Pirie, P. L., Badger, G. J., Carpenter, J. H., et al. (1994). Mass media and school interventions for cigarette smoking prevention: Effects two years after completion. *American Journal of Public Health, 84,* 1148–1150.

Flynn, B. S., Worden, J. K., Secker-Walker, R. H., Pirie, P. L., Badger, G. J., & Carpenter, J. H. (1997). Long-term responses of higher and lower risk youths to smoking prevention interventions. *Preventive Medicine, 26*(3), 389–394.

Flynn K. (1999, February 14). Shooting in the Bronx: The investigation: Four officers not obliged to explain the shooting. *The New York Times,* p. A38.

Forehand, R., & Long, N. (1988). Outpatient treatment of the acting out child: Procedures, long-term follow-up data, and clinical problems. *Advances in Behaviour Research and Therapy, 10*(3), 129–177.

Forehand, R. L., & McMahon, R. J. (1981). *Helping the noncompliant child: A clinician's guide to parent training.* New York: Guilford Press.

Forster, J. L., Hourigan, M., & McGovern, P. G. (1992). Availability of cigarettes to underage youth in three communities. *Preventive Medicine, 21*(3), 320–328.

Forster, J. L., Hourigan, M. E., & Kelder S. (1992). Locking devices on cigarette vending machines: Evaluation of a city ordinance. *American Journal of Public Health, 82*(9), 1217–1219.

Forster, J. L., McGovern, P. G., Wagenaar, A. C., Wolfson, M., Perry, C. L., & Anstine, P. S. (1994). The ability of young people to purchase alcohol without age identification in northeastern Minnesota. *Addiction, 89,* 699–705.

Forster, J. L., Murray, D. M., Wolfson, M., & Wagenaar, A. C. (1995). Commercial availability of alcohol to young people: Results of alcohol purchase attempts. *Preventive Medicine, 24,* 342–347.

Forster, J. L., Wolfson, M., Murray, D. M., Blaine, T. M., Wagenaar, A. C., & Hennrikus, D. J. (1998). The effects of community policies to reduce youth access to tobacco. *American Journal of Public Health, 88*(8), 1193–1198.

Forster, J. L., Wolfson, M., Murray, D. M., Wagenaar, A. C., & Claxton, A. J. (1997). Perceived and measured availability of tobacco to youths in 14 Minnesota communities: The TPOP Study. *American Journal of Preventive Medicine, 13*(3), 167–174.

Foster, S. L., Biglan, A., & Katz, A. (2001, June). *Identifying what works: Issues and directions.* Washington, DC: Society for Prevention Research.

Foster, S. L., & Martinez, C. R. (1995). Ethnicity: Conceptual and methodological issues in child clinical research. *Journal of Clinical Child Psychology, 24*(2), 214–226.

Francis, D. D., Champagne, F. A., Liu, D., & Meaney, M. J. (1999). Maternal care, gene expression, and the development of individual differences in stress reactivity. In N. E. Adler, M. Marmot, B. S. McEwen, & J. Stewart (Eds.), *Socioeconomic status and health in industrial nations: Social, psychological, and biological pathways* (pp. 66–84). New York: New York Academy of Sciences.

Freeman, R. (1996). Why do so many young American men commit crimes and what might we do about it? *Journal of Economic Perspectives, 10*(1), 25–42.

Friedman, A. S., Granick, S., Bransfield, S., Kreisher, C., & Khalsa, J. (1995). Gender differences in early life risk factors for substance use/abuse: A study of an African American sample. *American Journal of Drug and Alcohol Abuse, 21*(4), 511–531.

Funk, J. B. (1993). Reevaluating the impact of video games. *Clinical Pediatrics, 32*(2), 86–90.

Futterman, D. D., Peralta, L., Rudy, B. J., Wolfson, S., Guttmacher, S., & Rogers, A.-S. (2001). The ACCESS (Adolescents Connected to Care, Evaluation, and Special Services) Project: Social marketing to promote HIV testing to adolescents, methods and first year results from a six city campaign. *Journal of Adolescent Health, 29*(Suppl. 3), 19–29.

Garnefski, N., & Diekstra, R. F. W. (1997). "Comorbidity" of behavioral, emotional, and cognitive problems in adolescence. *Journal of Youth and Adolescence, 26*(3), 321–338.

Gensheimer, L. K., Mayer, J. P., Gottschalk, R., & Davidson II, W. S. (1986). Diverting youth from the juvenile justice system: A meta-analysis of intervention efficacy. In S. J. Apter & A. P. Goldstein (Eds.), *Youth violence: Programs and prospects* (pp. 39–56). Elmsford Park, NY: Pergamon Press.

George, T. P., & Hartmann, D. P. (1996). Friendship networks of unpopular, average, and popular children. *Child Development, 67*(5), 2301–2316.

Gibson, C. L., Piquero, A. R., & Tibbetts, S. G. (2000). Assessing the relationship between maternal cigarette smoking during pregnancy and age at first police contact. *Justice Quarterly, 17,* 519–542.

Giesbrecht, N., & Grube, J. W. (2003). Information, education, and persuasion as strategies for reducing or preventing drinking-related problems. In T. Babor (Ed.), *Alcohol: No ordinary commodity. Research and public policy* (pp. 189–207). Oxford, UK: Oxford University Press.

Gilliam, W. S., & Zigler, E. F. (2000). A critical meta-analysis of all evaluations of state-funded preschool from 1977 to 1998: Implications for policy, service delivery, and program implementation. *Early Childhood Research Quarterly, 15*(4), 441–473.

Gillmore, M. R., Hawkins, J. D., Catalano, R. F., Day, L. E., Moore, M., & Abbott, R. (1991). Structure of problem behaviors in preadolescence. *Journal of Consulting and Clinical Psychology, 59*(4), 499–506.

Glantz, M. D., & Leshner, A. I. (2000). Drug abuse and developmental psychopathology. *Development and Psychopathology, 12*(4), 795–814.

Glantz, M. D., Weinberg, N. Z., Miner, L. L., & Colliver, J. D. (1999). The etiology of drug abuse: mapping the paths. In M. D. Glantz & C. R. Hartel (Eds.), *Drug abuse origins and interventions* (pp. 3–45). Washington, DC: American Psychological Association.

Glantz, S. A., & Parmley, W. W. (2001). Even a little secondhand smoke is dangerous. *Journal of the American Medical Association, 286*, 462–463.

Gliksman, L., McKenzie, D., Single, E., Douglas, R., Brunet, S., & Moffatt, K. (1993). The role of alcohol providers in prevention: An evaluation of a server intervention programme. *Addiction, 88*(9), 1195–1203.

Goeders, N. E. (1998). Stress, the hypothalamic–pituitary–adrenal axis, and vulnerability to drug abuse. *NIDA Research Monograph, 169*, 83–104.

Goeders, N. E. (2002). The HPA axis and cocaine reinforcement. *Psychoneuroendocrinology, 27*, 13–33.

Gold, M. R., Siegel, J. E., Russell, L. B., & Weinstein, M. C. (1996). *Cost-effectiveness in health and medicine*. New York: Oxford University Press.

Goldsmith, H. H., Lemery, K. S., Buss, K. A., & Campos, J. J. (1999). Genetic analyses of focal aspects of infant temperament. *Developmental Psychology, 35*(4), 972–985.

Gorman-Smith, D., & Tolan, P. (1998). The role of exposure to community violence and developmental problems among inner-city youth. *Development and Psychopathology, 10*(1), 101–116.

Gottlieb, G. (2000). Environmental and behavioral influences on gene activity. *Current Directions in Psychological Science, 9*, 93–102.

Grandy, G. S., Madsen, C. H., & De Mersseman, L. M. (1973). The effects of individual and interdependent contingencies on inappropriate classroom behavior. *Psychology in the Schools, 10*, 488–493.

Grant, B. F., & Dawson, D. A. (1997). Age at onset of alcohol use and its association with DSM-IV alcohol abuse and dependence: Results from National Longitudinal Alcohol Epidemiologic Survey. *Journal of Substance Abuse, 9*, 103–110.

Gray, D., Saggers, S., Atkinson, D., Sputore, B., & Bourbon, D. (2000). Beating the grog: an evaluation of the Tennant Creek liquor licensing restrictions. *Australian and New Zealand Journal of Public Health, 24*(1), 39–44.

Greenberg, M. T., Domitrovich, C. E., & Bumbarger, B. (1999). *Preventing mental disorders in school-age children: A review of the effectiveness of prevention programs*. White paper commissioned by the Center for Mental Health Services.

Greenberg, M. T., Domitrovich, C. E., & Bumbarger, B. (2001). The prevention of mental disorders in school-age children: Current state of the field. *Prevention and Treatment, 4*, Article 1. Available: *http://journals.apa.org/prevention/volume4/pre0040001a.html*.

Gregg, S. (1999). Creating effective alternatives for disruptive students. *The Clearing House, 73*(2), 107–113.

Griesler, P. C., Kandel, D. B., & Davies, M. (1998). Maternal smoking in pregnancy, child behavior problems, and adolescent smoking. *Journal of Research on Adolescence, 8*(2), 159–185.

Grimes, J. D., & Swisher, J. D. (1989). Educational factors influencing adolescent decision-making regarding use of alcohol and drugs. *Journal of Alcohol and Drug Education, 35,* 1–15.

Grossman, M., & Chaloupka, F. J. (1997). Cigarette taxes. The straw to break the camel's back. *Public Health Reports, 112,* 293–297.

Grossman, M., Chaloupka, F. J., Saffer, H., & Laixuthai, A. (1995). Effects of alcohol price policy on youth: A summary of economic research. In G. M. Boyd, J. Howard, & R. A. Zucker (Eds.), *Alcohol problems among adolescents: Current directions in prevention research* (pp. 225–242). Hillsdale, NJ: Erlbaum.

Grossman, M., Coate, D., & Arluck, G. M. (1987). Price sensitivity of alcoholic beverages in the US: Youth alcohol consumption. In H. Holder (Ed.), *Control issues in alcohol abuse prevention: Strategies for states and communities* (pp. 169–198). Greenwich, CT: JAI Press.

Grossman, M., & Markowitz, S. (in press). Alcohol regulation and violence on college campuses. In M. Grossman & C. R. Hsieh (Eds.), *The economics of substance use and abuse: The experiences of developed countries and lessons for developing countries.* Cheltenham, UK: Edward Elgar.

Grube, J. W. (1997). Preventing sales of alcohol to minors: Results from a community trial. *Addiction, 92,* S251–S260.

Grube, J. W., Madden, P. A., & Friese, B. (1996). *Television alcohol advertising increases adolescent drinking.* Poster presented at the annual meeting of the American Psychological Society, San Francisco.

Grube, J. W., & Wallack, L. (1994). Television beer advertising and drinking knowledge, beliefs, and intentions among schoolchildren. *American Journal of Public Health, 84*(2), 254–259.

Gruber, J. (2000). Risky behavior among youths: An economic analysis. *NBER Working Papers, 7781.* Cambridge, MA: National Bureau of Economic Research.

Gruenewald, P. J. (1991). Alcohol problems and the control of availability: Theoretical and empirical issues. Paper presented at the NIAAA Conference Economic & Socioeconomic Issues in the Prevention of Alcohol Related Problems, Bethesda, MD.

Gruenewald, P. J., Millar, A., Ponicki, W. R., & Brinkley, G. (2000). Physical and economic access to alcohol: The application of geostatistical methods to small area analysis in community settings. In R. Wilson & M. DuFour (Eds.), *The epidemiology of alcohol problems in small geographic areas* (NIAAA Monograph No. 36, pp. 163–212). Bethesda, MD: U.S. Department of Health and Human Services.

Gruenewald, P. J., Ponicki, W. R., & Holder, H. D. (1993). The relationship of outlet densities to alcohol consumption: A time series cross-sectional analysis. *Alcoholism: Clinical and Experimental Research, 17*(1), 38–47.

Grunbaum, J., Kann, L., Kinchen, S., Ross, J., Gowda, V., Collins, J., et al. (1999). Youth risk behavior surveillance—National Alternative High School Risk

Behavior Survey—United States, 1998. *Morbidity and Mortality Weekly Report, 48*(SS-07), 1–44.

Gunnar, M. R. (1998). Quality of early care and buffering of neuroendocrine stress reactions: Potential effects on the developing human brain. *Preventive Medicine, 27*(2), 208–211.

Gunnar, M. R., & Chisholm, K. (1999). *Effects of early institutional rearing and attachment quality on salivary cortisol levels in adopted Romanian children.* Poster presented at the meeting of the Society for Research in Child Development, Albuquerque, NM.

Halberstam, D. (1987). *The reckoning.* New York: Morrow Avon.

Haley, J. (1976). *Problem solving therapy.* San Francisco: Jossey-Bass.

Hanna, E. Z., Hsaio-ye, Y., & Dufour, M. (2000, June 24–29). *The relationship of drinking alone and other substance use alone and in combination to health and behavior problems among youth aged 12–16: Findings from the Third National Health and Nutrition Examination Survey (NHANES III).* Paper presented at the 23rd Annual Scientific Meeting of the Research Society on Alcoholism, Denver, CO.

Hansen, W. B., & Graham, J. W. (1991). Preventing alcohol, marijuana, and cigarette use among adolescents: peer pressure resistance training versus establishing conservative norms. *Preventive Medicine, 20*(3), 414–430.

Hanson, C. L., Henggeler, S. W., Haefele, W. F., & Rodnick, J. D. (1984). Demographic, individual, and family relationship correlates of serious and repeated crime among adolescents and their siblings. *Journal of Consulting and Clinical Psychology, 52,* 528–538.

Harris, J. R. (1998). *The nurture assumption: Why children turn out the way they do.* New York: Touchstone.

Harris, V. W., & Sherman, J. A. (1973). Use and analysis of the "good behavior game" to reduce disruptive classroom behavior. *Journal of Applied Behavior Analysis, 6*(3), 405–417.

Harwood, H. J., Fountain D., & Fountain, G. (1999). Economic cost of alcohol and drug abuse in the United States, 1992: A report. *Addiction, 94,* 631–635.

Harwood, H. J., Fountain, D., & Livermore, G. (1999). Cost estimates for alcohol and drug abuse. *Addiction, 94*(5), 631–647.

Hawkins, J. D. (1999). Preventing crime and violence through communities that care. *European Journal on Criminal Policy and Research, 7,* 443–458.

Hawkins, J. D., Abbott, R., Catalano, R. F., & Gillmore, M. R. (1991). Assessing effectiveness of drug abuse prevention: Implementation issues relevant to long-term effects and replication. In C. G. Leukefeld & W. J. Bukoski (Eds.), *Drug abuse prevention intervention research: Methodological issues* (DHHS Publication No. ADM 91-1761, pp. 195–212). Washington, DC: U.S. Government Printing Office.

Hawkins, J. D., & Catalano, R. F. (1992). *Communities that care: Action for drug abuse prevention.* San Francisco: Jossey-Bass.

Hawkins, J. D., Catalano, R. F., Kosterman, R., Abbott, R., & Hill, K. G. (1999). Preventing adolescent health-risk behaviors by strengthening protection during childhood. *Archives of Pediatrics and Adolescent Medicine, 153*(3), 226–234.

Hawkins, J., Catalano, R., Morrison, D., O'Donnell, J., Abbott, R., & Day, L. (1992). The Seattle Social Development Project: Effects of the first four years on protective factors and problem behaviors. In J. McCord & R. Tremblay (Eds.), *The prevention of antisocial behavior in children* (pp. 139–161). New York: Guilford Press.

Hawkins, J. D., von Cleve, E., & Catalano, R. F., Jr. (1991). Reducing early childhood aggression: results of a primary prevention program. *Journal of the American Academy of Child and Adolescent Psychiatry, 30*(2), 208–217.

He, J., Vupputuri, S., Allen, K., Prerost, M. R., Hughes, J., & Whelton, P. K. (1999). Passive smoking and risk of coronary heart disease: A meta-analysis of epidemiologic studies. *New England Journal of Medicine, 340*, 920–926.

Henggeler, S. W., Melton, G. B., Brondino, M. J., Scherer, D. G., & Hanley, J. H. (1997). Multisystemic therapy with violent and chronic juvenile offenders and their families: The role of treatment fidelity in successful dissemination. *Journal of Consulting and Clinical Psychology, 65*(5), 821–833.

Henggeler, S. W., Pickrel, S. G., & Brondino, M. J. (1999). Multisystemic treatment of substance abusing and dependent delinquents: Outcomes, treatment fidelity, and transportability. *Mental Health Services Research, 1*, 171–184.

Henggeler, S. W., Pickrel, S. G., Brondino, M. J., & Crouch, J. L. (1996). Eliminating (almost) treatment dropout of substance abusing or dependent delinquents through home-based multisystemic therapy. *American Journal of Psychiatry, 153*(3), 427–428.

Henggeler, S. W., Rowland, M. D., Pickrel, S. G., Miller, S. L., Cunningham, P. B., Santos, A. B., et al. (1997). Investigating family-based alternatives to institution-based mental health services for youth: Lessons learned from the pilot study of a randomized field trial. *Journal of Clinical Child Psychology, 26*, 226–233.

Henggeler, S. W., Schoenwald, S. K., Borduin, C. M., Rowland, M. D., & Cunningham, P. B. (1998). *Multisystemic treatment of antisocial behavior in children and adolescents.* New York: Guilford Press.

Henry, B., Caspi, A., Moffitt, T. E., & Silva, P. A. (1996). Temperamental and familial predictors of violent and nonviolent criminal convictions: Age 3 to age 18. *Developmental Psychology, 32*(4), 614–623.

Hinds, M. W. (1992). Impact of a local ordinance banning tobacco sales to minors. *Public Health Reports, 107*(3), 355–358.

Hingson, R. (1993). Prevention of alcohol-impaired driving. *Alcohol Health and Research World, 17*(1), 28–34.

Hingson, R. W., Heeren, T., Jamanka, A., & Howland, J. (2000). Age of drinking onset and unintentional injury involvement after drinking. *Journal of the American Medical Association, 284*, 1527–1533.

Hingson, R. W., Heeren, T., & Winter, M. (1994). Effects of lower legal blood alcohol limits for young and adult drivers. *Alcohol, Drugs and Driving, 10*, 243–252.

Hingson, R., Heeren, T., & Winter, M. (1996). Lowering state legal blood alcohol limits to 0.08%: The effect on fatal motor vehicle crashes. *American Journal of Public Health, 86*, 1297–1299.

Hingson, R. W., Howland, J., & Levenson, S. (1988). Effects of legislative reform to reduce drunken driving and alcohol-related traffic fatalities. *Public Health Reports, 103*(6), 659–667.

Hingson, R., McGovern, T., Howland, J., Heeren, T., Winter, M., & Zakocs, R. (1996). Reducing alcohol-impaired driving in Massachusetts: The Saving Lives Program. *American Journal of Public Health, 86,* 791–797.

Hogan, C. (1999). *Vermont communities count using results to strengthen services for families and children.* Waterbury, VT: Agency of Human Services.

Hogue, A. T., Liddle, H. A., Becker, D., & Johnson-Leckrone, J. (2002). Family-based prevention counseling for high-risk young adolescents: Immediate outcomes. *Journal of Community Psychology, 30*(1), 1–22.

Holder, H. D. (1998). *Alcohol and the community: A systems approach to prevention.* Cambridge, MA: Cambridge University Press.

Holder, H. D., & Blose, J. O. (1987). *Reduction of community alcohol problems: Computer simulation experiments in three counties.* Piscataway, NJ: Alcohol Research Documentation.

Holder, H. D., Gruenewald, P. J., Ponicki, W. R., Treno, A. J., Grube, J. W., Saltz, R. F., et al. (2000). Effect of community-based interventions on high-risk drinking and alcohol-related injuries. *Journal of the American Medical Association, 284*(18), 2341–2347.

Holder, W., Perry, C. L., & Pirie, P. L. (1988). *Evaluation report on the Unpuffables Pilot Project.* Unpublished report. Minneapolis, MN: University of Minnesota.

Holder, H. D., Saltz, R. F., Grube, J. W., Voas, R. B., Gruenewald, P. J., & Treno, A. J. (1997). A community prevention trial to reduce alcohol-involved accidental injury and death: overview. *Addiction, 92*(Suppl. 2), 155–171.

Holder, H. D., & Treno, A. J. (1997). Media advocacy in community prevention: News as a means to advance policy change. *Addiction, 92*(Suppl. 2), 189–199.

Holder, H. D., & Wagenaar, A. C. (1990). Effects of the elimination of a state monopoly on distilled spirits' retail sales: A time-series analysis of Iowa. *British Journal of Addiction, 85*(12), 1615–1625.

Holder, H. D., & Wagenaar, A. C. (1994). Mandated server training and reduced alcohol-involved traffic crashes: A time series analysis of the Oregon experience. *Accident Analysis and Prevention, 26*(1), 89–97.

Hollis, J. F., Lichtenstein, E., Vogt, T. M., Stevens, V. J., & Biglan, A. (1993). Nurse-assisted counseling for smokers in primary care. *Annals of Internal Medicine, 118,* 521–525.

Holtgrave, D. R., & Pinkerton, S. D. (1997). Updates of cost of illness and quality of life estimates for use in economic evaluations of HIV prevention programs. *Journal of Acquired Immune Deficiency Syndromes and Human Retrovirology, 16,* 54–62.

Homel, R. (1986). *Policing the drinking driver: Random breath testing and the process of deterrence.* Canberra, Australia: Federal Office of Road Safety.

Homel, R. (1990). Random breath testing and random stopping programs in Australia. In R. J. Wilson & R. E. Mann (Eds.), *Drinking and driving: Advances in research and prevention* (pp. 159–202). New York: Guilford Press.

Horner, R. H., Sugai, G., Lewis-Palmer, T., & Todd, A. W. (2001). Teaching school-wide behavioral expectations. *Report on Emotional and Behavioral Disorders in Youth, 1*(4), 77–79 & 93–96.

Houck, G. M. (1999). The measurement of child characteristics from infancy to toddlerhood: temperament, developmental competence, self-concept, and social competence. *Issues in Comprehensive Pediatric Nursing, 22*(2–3), 101–127.

Howard, M. O., Walker, R. D., Walker, P. S., Cottler, L. B., & Compton, W. M. (1999). Inhalant use among urban American Indian youth. *Addiction, 94*(1), 83–95.

Howes, C. (1988). Relations between early childcare and schooling. *Developmental Psychology, 24*(1), 53–57.

Huber, H. (1979). The value of a behavior modification programme, administered in a fourth grade class of a remedial school. *Praxis der Kinderpsychologie und Kinderpsychiatrie, 28*(2), 73–79.

Huesmann, L. R., Moise, J. F., & Podolski, C. L. (1997). The effects of media violence on the development of antisocial behavior. In D. M. Stoff, J. Breiling, & J. D. Maser (Eds.), *Handbook of antisocial behavior* (pp. 181–193). New York: Wiley.

Huitfeldt, B., & Jorner, U. (1972) Demand for alcoholic beverages in Sweden: An econometric study of the development of consumption following the abolishment of the personal ration book. *SOU, 91 [Rapport från Alkoholpolitiska utredningen* (APU)].

Huizinga, D., Loeber R., & Thornberry, T. P. (1993). Longitudinal study of delinquency, drug use, sexual activity, and pregnancy among children and youth in three cities. *Public Health Reports, 108*(Suppl. 1), 90–96.

Huttunen, M. O., & Niskanen, P. (1978). Prenatal loss of father and psychiatric disorders. *Archives of General Psychiatry, 35*(4), 429–431.

Institute of Medicine. (1996). *Pathways of addiction: Opportunities in drug abuse research*. Washington, DC: National Academy Press.

International drug supply, control, and interdiction: Hearing before the Subcommittee on Crime and Criminal Justice, of the House Committee on the Judiciary, 103rd Cong. (1993).

Irvine, A. B., Biglan, A., Smolkowski, K., Metzler, C. W., & Ary, D. V. (1999). The effectiveness of a parenting skills program for parents of middle school students in small communities. *Journal of Consulting and Clinical Psychology, 67*(6), 811–825.

Isohanni, M., Moilanen, I., & Rantakallio, P. (1991). Determinants of teenage smoking, with special reference to non-standard family background. *British Journal of Addiction, 86*, 391–398.

Jacob, T., & Leonard, K. (1986). Psychosocial functioning in children of alcoholic fathers, depressed fathers, and control fathers. *Journal of Studies on Alcohol, 47*(5), 373–380.

James, L., & Biglan, A. (2000). *Assessment of the effectiveness of a positive reinforcement approach to reducing illegal sales of tobacco to young people*. Unpublished manuscript.

Jason, L. A., Berk, M., Schnopp-Wyatt, D. L., & Talbot, B. (1999). Effects of enforcement of youth access laws on smoking prevalence. *American Journal of Community Psychology, 27*(2), 143–160.

Jason, L. A., Ji, P. Y., Anes, M. D., & Birkhead, S. H. (1991). Active enforcement of cigarette control laws in the prevention of cigarette sales to minors. *Journal of the American Medical Association, 266*(22), 3159–3161.

Jemmott, J. B., Jemmott, L. S., & Fong, G. T. (1998). Abstinence and safer sex HIV risk-reduction interventions for African American adolescents: A randomized controlled trial. *Journal of the American Medical Association, 279*(19), 1529–1536.

Jessor, R., & Jessor, S. L. (1977). *Problem behavior and psychosocial development: A longitudinal study of youth.* New York: Academic Press.

Johnson, C. A., Pentz, M. A., Weber, M. D., Dwyer, J. H., Baer, N., MacKinnon, D. P., et al. (1990). Relative effectiveness of comprehensive community programming for drug abuse prevention with high-risk and low-risk adolescents. *Journal of Consulting and Clinical Psychology, 58,* 447–456.

Johnston, L. D., O'Malley, P. M., & Bachman, J. G. (1999). *National survey results on drug use from the Monitoring the Future study, 1975–1998: Vol. I. Secondary school students* (NIH Publication No. 99-4660). Bethesda, MD: National Institute on Drug Abuse.

Johnston, L. D., O'Malley, P. M., & Bachman, J. G. (2000a). *Monitoring the Future national survey results on drug use, 1975–1999: Vol. I: Secondary school students* (NIH Publication No. 00-4802). Bethesda, MD: National Institute on Drug Abuse.

Johnston, L. D., O'Malley, P. M., & Bachman, J. G. (2000b). *Monitoring the Future national survey results on drug use, 1975–1999: Vol. II: College students and young adults.* (NIH Publication No. 00-4803). Bethesda, MD: National Institute on Drug Abuse.

Johnston, L. D., O'Malley, P. M., & Bachman, J. G. (2000c). *The Monitoring the Future national survey results on adolescent drug use: Overview of key findings, 1999* (NIH Publication No. 00-4690). Bethesda, MD: National Institute on Drug Abuse.

Johnston, L. D., O'Malley, P. M., & Bachman, J. G. (2001). *The Monitoring the Future National survey results on adolescent drug use: Overview of key findings, 2000* (NIH Publication No. 01-4923). Bethesda, MD: National Institute on Drug Abuse.

Johnston, L. D., O'Malley, P. M., & Bachman, J. G. (2003). *The Monitoring the Future national survey results on adolescent drug use: Overview of key findings, 2002* (NIH Publication No. 03-5374). Bethesda, MD: National Institute on Drug Abuse.

Kandel, D. B. (2002). *Stages and pathways of drug involvement: Examining the gateway hypothesis.* Cambridge, UK: Cambridge University Press.

Kann, L., Kinchen, S. A., Williams, B. I., Ross, J. G., Lowry, R., Grunbaum, J. A., et al. (2000). Youth Risk Behavior Surveillance—United States, 1999. *Morbidity and Mortality Weekly Report, 49*(SS-5), 1–94.

Kaplan, S. L., Busner, J., Kupietz, S., Wassermann, E., & Segal, B. (1990). Effects of methylphenidate on adolescents with aggressive conduct disorder and ADDH:

A preliminary report. *Journal of the American Academy of Child and Adolescent Psychiatry, 29*(5), 719–723.

Kazdin, A. E., Siegel, T. C., & Bass, D. (1992). Cognitive problem-solving skills training and parent management training in the treatment of antisocial behavior in children. *Journal of Consulting and Clinical Psychology, 60*(5), 733–747.

Kelder, S. H., Maibach, E., Worden, J. K., Biglan, A., & Levitt, A. (2000). Planning and initiation of the ONDCP National Youth Anti-Drug Media Campaign. *Journal of Public Health Management and Practice, 6*(3), 14–26.

Kellam, S. G. (1990). Developmental epidemiological framework for family research on depression and aggression. In G. R. Patterson (Ed.), *Depression and aggression in family interaction* (pp. 11–48). Hillsdale, NJ: Erlbaum.

Kellam, S. G., & Anthony, J. C. (1998). Targeting early antecedents to prevent tobacco smoking: Findings from an epidemiologically based randomized field trial. *American Journal of Public Health, 88*(10), 1490–1495.

Kellam, S. G., Brown, C., Rubin, B., & Ensminger, M. (1983). Paths leading to teenage psychiatric symptoms and substance use: Developmental epidemiologic studies in Woodlawn. In S. B. Guze, F. J. Earls, & J. E. Barrett (Eds.), *Childhood Psychopathology and Development* (pp. 17–51). New York: Raven Press.

Kellam, S. G., Ling, X., Merisca, R., Brown, C. H., & Ialongo, N. (1998). The effect of the level of aggression in the first grade classroom on the course and malleability of aggressive behavior into middle school. *Development and Psychopathology, 10*(2), 165–185.

Kellam, S. G., Mayer, L. S., Rebok, G. W., & Hawkins, W. E. (1998). Effects of improving achievement on aggressive behavior and of improving aggressive behavior on achievement through two preventive interventions: An investigation of causal paths. In B. Dohrenwend (Ed.), *Adversity, stress, and psychopathology* (pp. 486–505). New York: Oxford University Press.

Kellam, S. G., & Rebok, G. W. (1992). Building developmental and etiological theory through epidemiologically based preventive intervention trials. In J. McCord & R. E. Tremblay (Eds.), *Preventing antisocial behavior: Interventions from birth through adolescence* (pp. 162–195). New York: Guilford Press.

Kellam, S. G., & Van Horn, Y. V. (1997). Life course development, community epidemiology, and preventive trials: A scientific structure for prevention research. *American Journal of Community Psychology, 25,* 177–188.

Kelling, G. L., & Coles, C. M. (1996). *Fixing broken windows: Restoring order and reducing crime in our communities.* New York: Martin Kessler.

Kelly, J. A., St. Lawrence, J. S., Hood, H. V., & Brasfield, T. L. (1989). Behavioral intervention to reduce AIDS risk activities. *Journal of Consulting and Clinical Psychology, 57*(1), 60–67.

Kelly, J. G. (1988). *A guide to conducting prevention research in the community: First steps.* New York: Haworth.

Kendler, K. S., Karkowski, L. M., Neale, M. C., & Prescott, C. A. (2000). Illicit psychoactive substance use, heavy use, abuse, and dependence in a US population-based sample of male twins. *Archives of General Psychiatry, 57,* 261–269.

Kenkel, D. S. (1993). Drinking, driving, and deterrence: The effectiveness and social costs of alternative policies. *Journal of Law and Economics, 36*(2), 877–913.

Kilpatrick, D. G., Acierno, R., Saunders, B., Resnick, H. S., Best, C. L., & Schnurr, P. P. (2000). Risk factors for adolescent substance abuse and dependence: Data from a national sample. *Journal of Consulting and Clinical Psychology, 68*(1), 19–30.

King, C. I., Siegel, M., Celebucki, C., & Connolly, G. N. (1998). Adolescent exposure to cigarette advertising in magazines. An evaluation of brand-specific advertising in relation to youth readership. *Journal of the American Medical Association, 279*(7), 516–520.

King, J. A. (1996). Perinatal stress and impairment of the stress response: Possible link to non-optimal behavior. In C. F. Ferris & T. Grisso (Eds.), *Understanding aggressive behavior in children. Annals of the New York Academy of Sciences, Vol. 794.* (Academy volume 426, pp. 104–112). New York: New York Academy of Sciences.

Kirby, D. (2000). School-based interventions to prevent unprotected sex and HIV among adolescents. In J. L. Peterson & R. J. DiClemente (Eds.), *Handbook of HIV prevention* (pp. 83–101). New York: Kluwer Academic/Plenum.

Kirby, D. (2001). *Emerging answers: Research findings on programs to reduce teen pregnancy.* Washington, DC: National Campaign to Prevent Teen Pregnancy.

Kirby, D., Korpi, M., Barth, R., & Cagampang, H. (1995). *Evaluation of Education Now and Babies Later (ENABL): Final report.* Berkeley: University of California, School of Social Welfare.

Kitzman, H., Olds, D. L., Sidora, K., Henderson, C. R., Hanks, C., Cole, R., et al. (2000). Enduring effects of nurse home visitation on maternal life course: A 3-year follow-up of a randomized trial. *Journal of the American Medical Association, 283*(15), 1983–1989.

Klein, N. C., Alexander, J. F., & Parsons, B. V. (1977). Impact of family systems intervention on recidivism and sibling delinquency: A model of primary prevention and program evaluation. *Journal of Consulting and Clinical Psychology, 45*(3), 469–474.

Klorman, R., Brumaghim, J. T., Salzman, L. F., Strauss, J., Borgstedt, A. D., McBride, M. C., et al. (1988). Effects of methylphenidate on attention-deficit hyperactivity disorder with and without aggressive/noncompliant features. *Journal of Abnormal Psychology, 97*(4), 413–422.

Kowaleski-Jones, L., & Mott, F. L. (1998). Sex, contraception, and childbearing among high-risk youth: Do different factors influence males and females? *Family Planning Perspectives 30,* 163–169.

Ku, L., Sonenstein, F. L., & Pleck, J. H. (1993). Neighborhood, family and work: Influences on the premarital behavior of adolescent males. *Social Forces, 72,* 479–503.

Lacey, J. H., Jones, R. K., & Smith, R. G. (1999). *Evaluation of checkpoint Tennessee: Tennessee's statewide sobriety checkpoint program.* Washington, DC: National Highway Traffic Safety Administration.

Ladd, G. W. (1983). Social networks of popular, average, and rejected children in school settings. *Merrill-Palmer Quarterly, 29*(3), 283–307.

Laixuthai, A., & Chaloupka, F. J. (1993). Youth alcohol use and public policy. *Contemporary Policy Issues, 11,* 70–81.

Landrine, H., Klonoff, E. A., & Reina-Patton, A. (2000). Minors' access to tobacco before and after the California STAKE Act. *Tobacco Control, 9*(S11), ii15–ii17.

Landsburg, S. E. (1993). *The armchair economist. Economics and everyday life.* New York: Free Press.

Lang, E., Stockwell, T., Rydon, P., & Beel, A. (1996). Use of pseudo-patrons to assess compliance with laws regarding under- age drinking. *Australian and New Zealand Journal of Public Health, 20*(3), 296–300.

Lang, E., Stockwell, T., Rydon, P., & Beel, A. (1998). Can training bar staff in responsible serving practices reduce alcohol-related harm? *Drug and Alcohol Review, 17*(1), 39–50.

Lantz, P. M., Jacobson, P. D., Warner, K. E., Wasserman, J., Pollack, H., Berson, J., et al. (2000). Investing in youth tobacco control: A review of smoking prevention and control strategies. *Tobacco Control, 9,* 47–63.

Larson, R., & Richards, M. H. (1994). *Divergent realities: the emotional lives of mothers, fathers, and adolescents.* New York: Basic Books.

Lawrence, B. M., Miller, T. R., Jensen, A. F., Fisher, D. A., & Zamula, W. F. (2000). Estimating the costs of nonfatal consumer product injuries in the United States. *Journal for Injury and Safety Promotion, 7,* 97–113.

Leadership to Keep Children Alcohol Free. (2001). Retrieved July 15, 2002, from *http://www.alcoholfreechildren.org/gs/stats/health.cfm.*

Legrand, L. N., McGue, M., & Iacono, W. G. (1999). Searching for interactive effects in the etiology of early-onset substance use. *Behavior Genetics, 29,* 433–443.

Levanthal, T., & Brooks-Gunn, J. (2000). The neighborhoods they live in: The effects of neighborhood residence on child and adolescent outcomes. *Psychological Bulletin, 126,* 309–337.

Levitsky, D. A., & Strupp, B. J. (1995). Malnutrition and the brain: Changing concepts, changing concerns. *Journal of Nutrition, 125*(8, Suppl.), 2212S–2220S.

Levy, D. T., Friend, K., Holder, H., & Carmona, M. (2001). The effect of policies directed at youth access to smoking: Results from the *SimSmoke* computer simulation model. *Tobacco Control, 10,* 108–116.

Levy, D. T., Miller, T. R., & Cox, K. C. (1999). *Costs of underage drinking.* Washington, DC: Office of Juvenile Justice and Delinquency Prevention.

Levy, D. T., Miller, T. R., Cox, K. C., & Spicer, R. S. (2001). *Costs of underage drinking.* Working paper. Calverton, MD: Pacific Institute for Research and Evaluation.

Levy, D., & Sheflin, N. (1983). New evidence on controlling alcohol use through price. *Journal of Studies on Alcohol, 44,* 920–937.

Lewinsohn, P. M., Rohde, P., Brown, R. A. (1999). Level of current and past adolescent cigarette smoking as predictors of future substance use disorders in young adulthood. *Addiction, 94*(6), 913–921.

Lewit, E. M., & Coate, D. (1982). The potential for using excise taxes to reduce smoking. *Journal of Health Economics, 1,* 121–145.

Lewit, E. M., Coate, D., & Grossman, M. (1981). The effects of government regulation on teenage smoking. *Journal of Law and Economics, 24,* 545–569.

Lewit, E. M., Hyland, A., Kerrebrock, N., & Cummings, K. M. (1997). Price, public policy, and smoking in young people. *Tobacco Control, 7*(Suppl. 2), S17–S24.

Liddle, H. A., Dakof, G. A., & Henderson, C. E. (2002, June). *A family-based, intensive outpatient alternative to residential drug treatment for co-morbid adolescent substance abusers.* Poster presented at the 64th annual meeting of the CPDD, Quebec City, Quebec, Canada.

Liddle, H. A., Henderson, C. E., Rowe, C., & Dakof, G. A. (2001, June). *Multidimensional family therapy for adolescent drug abuse: Major findings from a clinical research program.* Poster presented at the annual conference of the American Family Therapy Academy, Miami Beach, FL.

Lindberg, L. D., Boggess, S., & Williams, S. (1999). Multiple threats: The co-occurrence of teen health risk behaviors. In *Trends in the well-being of America's children and youth* (HHS-100-95-0021). Washington, DC: USDHHS, Office of the Assistant Secretary for Planning and Evaluation.

Lindenmayer, J. P., & Kotsaftis, A. (2000). Use of sodium valproate in violent and aggressive behaviors: A critical review. *Journal of Clinical Psychiatry, 61*(2), 123–128.

Lipsey, M. W., & Derzon, J. H. (1998). Predictors of violent or serious delinquency in adolescence and early adulthood: A synthesis of longitudinal research. In R. Loeber & D. P. Farrington (Eds.), *Serious and violent juvenile offenders: Risk factors and successful interventions.* (pp. 86–105). Thousand Oaks, CA: Sage.

Lipsey, M. W., & Wilson, D. B. (1998). Effective intervention for serious juvenile offenders. In R. Loeber & D. P. Farrington (Eds.), *Serious and violent juvenile offenders* (pp. 313–45). Thousand Oaks, CA: Sage.

Loeber, R., Farrington, D. P., Stouthamer-Loeber, M., & Van Kammen, W. B. (1998a). Multiple risk factors for multiproblem boys: Co-occurrence of delinquency, substance use, attention deficit, conduct problems, physical aggression, covert behavior, depressed mood, and shy/withdrawn behavior. In R. Jessor (Ed.), *New perspectives on adolescent risk behavior* (pp. 90–149). Cambridge, MA: Cambridge University Press.

Loeber, R., Farrington, D. P., Stouthamer-Loeber, M., & Van Kammen, W. B. (1998b). *Antisocial behavior and mental health problems: Explanatory factors in childhood and adolescence.* Mahwah, NJ: Erlbaum.

Loeber, R., Stouthamer-Loeber, M., & White, H. R. (1999). Developmental aspects of delinquency and internalizing problems and their association with persistent juvenile substance use between ages 7 and 18. *Journal of Clinical Child Psychology, 28,* 322–332.

Lonczak, H. S., Abbott, R. D., Hawkins, J. D., Kosterman, R., & Catalano, R. F. (2002). Effects of the Seattle Social Development Project on sexual behavior, pregnancy, birth, and sexually transmitted disease outcomes by age 21 years. *Archives of Pediatrics and Adolescent Medicine, 156*(5), 438–447.

Lynam, D., Moffitt, T. E., & Stouthamer-Loeber, M. (1993). Explaining the relation between IQ and delinquency: Class, race, test motivation, school failure, or self-control? *Journal of Abnormal Psychology, 102*(2), 187–196.

Lynskey, M. T., & Fergusson, D. M. (1997). Factors protecting against the development of adjustment difficulties in young adults exposed to childhood sexual abuse. *Child Abuse and Neglect, 21*(12), 1177–1190.

Lyons-Ruth, K., Easterbrook, M. A., & Cibelli, C. D. (1997). Infant attachment strategies, infant mental lag, and maternal depressive symptoms: Predictors of internalizing and externalizing problems at age 7. *Developmental Psychology, 33*, 681–692.

MacKinnon, D. P., Pentz, M. A., & Stacy, A. W. (1993). The alcohol warning label and adolescents: The first year. *American Journal of Public Health, 83*(4), 585–587.

Malmquist, S. (1948). *A statistical analysis of demand for liquor in Sweden: A study of the demand for a rationed commodity.* Uppsala, S.N.: Institute of Statistics.

Malone, R. P., Delaney, M. A., Luebbert, J. F., Cater, J., & Campbell, M. (2000). A double-blind placebo-controlled study of lithium in hospitalized aggressive children and adolescents with conduct disorder. *Archives of General Psychiatry, 57*(7), 649–654.

Malow, R., Gustan, S., Ziskind, D., McMahon, R., & St. Lawrence, J. (1998). Evaluating HIV prevention interventions among drug abusers: Validity issues. *Journal of HIV/AIDS Prevention and Education for Adolescents and Children, 2*, 21–40.

Manning, W. G., Keeler, E. B., Newhouse, J. P., Sloss, E. M. S., & Wasserman, J. (1991). *The costs of poor health habits. A RAND study.* Cambridge, MA: Harvard University Press.

Markowitz, S. (2000a). The price of alcohol, wife abuse, and husband abuse. *Southern Economic Journal, 67*, 279–303.

Markowitz, S. (2000b). *The role of alcohol and drug consumption in determining physical fights and weapon carrying by teenagers.* NBER working paper #7500.

Markowitz, S. (2000c). Criminal violence and alcohol beverage control: Evidence from an international study. In: M. Grossman & C. R. Hsieh (Eds.), *The economic analysis of substance use and abuse: The experience of developed countries and lessons for developing countries.* Cheltenham, UK: Edward Elgar.

Markowitz, S., & Grossman, M. (1998). Alcohol regulation and violence towards children. *Contemporary Economic Policy, 16*(3), 309–320.

Martin, S. E., Grube, J., Voas, R. B., Baker, J., & Hingson R. (1996). Zero tolerance laws: Effective public policy? *Alcoholism: Clinical and Experimental Research, 20*(S8), 147A–150A.

Mayer, G. R. (1972). Behavioral consulting: Using behavior modification procedures in the consulting relationship. *Elementary School Guidance and Counseling, (2)*, 114–119.

Mayer, G. R. (1999). Constructive discipline for school personnel. *Education and Treatment of Children, 22*(1), 36–54.

Mayer, G. R., Butterworth, T., Nafpaktitis, M., & Sulzer-Azaroff, B. (1983). Preventing school vandalism and improving discipline: A three-year study. *Journal of Applied Behavior Analysis, 16,* 355–369.

Mayer, G. R., Mitchell, L. K., Clementi, T., Clement-Robertson, E., Myatt, R., & Bullara, D. T. (1993). A dropout prevention program for at-risk high school students: Emphasizing consulting to promote positive classroom climates. *Education and Treatment of Children, 16,* 135–146.

Mayer, J. P., Gensheimer, L. K., Davidson, W. S. II, & Gottschalk, R. (1986). Social learning treatment within juvenile justice: A meta-analysis of impact in the natural environment. In S. J. Apter & A. P. Goldstein (Eds.), *Youth violence: Programs and prospects: Pergamon general psychology series* (Vol. 135, pp. 24–38). Elmsford, NY: Pergamon Press.

Maynard, A. (1996). Evidence based medicine. Cost effectiveness and equity are ignored. *British Medical Journal, 313,* 170–171.

McCord, J. (1992). The Cambridge–Somerville Study: A pioneering longitudinal–experimental study of delinquency prevention. In J. McCord & R. E. Tremblay (Eds.), *Preventing antisocial behavior: Interventions from birth through adolescence* (pp. 196–206). New York: Guilford Press.

McGee, L., & Newcomb, M. D. (1992). General deviance syndrome: Expanded hierarchical evaluations at four ages from early adolescence to adulthood. *Journal of Consulting and Clinical Psychology, 60*(5), 766–776.

McLoyd, V. C. (1990). The impact of economic hardship on Black families and development. *Child Development, 61,* 311–346.

McLoyd, V. C. (1995). Poverty, parenting, and policy: Meeting the support needs of poor parents. In H. E. Fitzgerald & B. M. Lester (Eds.), *Children of poverty: Research, health, and policy issues* (pp. 269–303). New York: Garland.

McMahon, R. J., & Forehand, R. (2003). *Helping the noncompliant child* (2nd ed.): *Family-based treatment for oppositional behavior.* New York: Guilford Press.

Mercer, G. W. (1985). The relationships among driving while impaired charges, police drinking-driving roadcheck activity, media coverage and alcohol-related casualty traffic accidents. *Accident Analysis and Prevention, 17*(6), 467–474.

Meschke, L. L., Bartholomae, S., & Zentall, S. R. (2000). Adolescent sexuality and parent–adolescent processes: Promoting healthy teen choices. *Family Relations, 49,* 143–154.

Metzler, C. W., Biglan, A., Ary, D. V., & Li, F. (1998). The stability and validity of early adolescents' reports of parenting constructs. *Journal of Family Psychology, 12*(4), 600–619.

Metzler, C. W., Biglan, A., Noell, J., Ary, D. V., & Ochs, L. (2000). A randomized controlled trial of a behavioral intervention to reduce high-risk sexual behavior among adolescents in STD clinics. *Behavior Therapy, 31,* 27–54.

Metzler, C. W., Biglan, A., Rusby, J. C., & Sprague, J. R. (2001). Evaluation of a comprehensive behavior management program to improve school-wide positive behavior support. *Education and Treatment of Children, 24*(4), 448–479.

Metzler, C. W., Noell, J. W., Biglan, A., Ary, D. V., & Smolkowski, K. (1994). The social context for risky sexual behavior among adolescents. *Journal of Behavioral Medicine, 17*(4), 419–438.

Miller, L. S., Wasserman, G. A., Neugebauer, R., Gorman-Smith, D., & Kamboukos, D. (1999). Witnessed community violence and antisocial behavior in high-risk, urban boys. *Journal of Clinical Child Psychology, 28,* 2–11.

Miller, P. M., Smith, G. T., & Goldman, M. S. (1990). Emergence of alcohol expectancies in childhood: A possible critical period. *Journal of Studies on Alcohol, 51*(4), 343–349.

Miller, T. R. (1990). The plausible range for the value of life: Red herrings among the mackerel. *Journal of Forensic Economics, 3*(3), 75–89.

Miller, T. R. (1993). Costs and functional consequences of U.S. roadway crashes. *Accident Analysis and Prevention, 25*(5), 593–607.

Miller, T. R. (2000). Variations between countries in values of statistical life. *Journal of Transport Economics and Policy, 34*(2), 169–188.

Miller, T. R., Calhoun, C., & Arthur, W. B. (1989). Utility-adjusted impairment years: A low cost approach to morbidity valuation. In *Estimating and valuing morbidity in a policy context: Proceedings of Association of Environmental and Resource Economists Workshop* (Rep. No. EPA-23-08-89-05). Washington, DC: U.S. Environmental Protection Agency.

Miller, T. R., Cohen, M. A., & Wiersema, B. (1996). *Victim costs and consequences: a new look.* (Research report). Washington, DC: National Institute of Justice.

Miller, T. R., Fisher, D. A., & Cohen, M. A. (2001). Costs of juvenile violence: Policy implications. *Pediatrics, 107*(1), electronic edition, e3, 1–7.

Miller, T. R., Lestina, D. C., & Spicer, R. S. (1998). Highway crash costs in the United States by driver age, blood alcohol level, victim age, and restraint use. *Accident Analysis and Prevention, 30*(2), 137–150.

Miller, T. R., Levy, D. T., Cohen, M. A., & Cox, K. C. (2001). *The costs of alcohol- and drug-involved crime.* Working paper, Pacific Institute for Research and Evaluation, Calverton, MD.

Miller, T. R., Pindus, N. M., Douglass, J. B., & Rossman, S. B. (1995). *Data book on nonfatal injury—Incidence, costs, and consequences.* Washington, DC: Urban Institute Press.

Miller, T. R., Romano, E. O., & Spicer, R. S. (2000). The cost of unintentional childhood injuries and the value of prevention. *The Future of Children, 10*(1), 137–163.

Miller Brewing Company. (2000). *Beer is volume with profit 2000.* Milwaukee WI: Author.

Minuchin, S. (1974). *Families and family therapy.* Cambridge, MA: Harvard University Press

Moberg, D. P., & Piper, D. L. (1998). The Healthy for Life project: Sexual risk behavior outcomes. *AIDS Education and Prevention, 10*(2), 128–148.

Modzeleski, W., Small, M. L., & Kann, L. (1999). Alcohol and other drug prevention policies and education in the United States. *Journal of Health Education, 30*(Suppl. 5), S42–S49.

Moffitt, T. E. (1990). Juvenile delinquency and attention deficit disorder: Boys' developmental trajectories from age 3 to age 15. *Child Development, 61,* 893–910.

Moffitt, T. E. (1993). Adolescence-limited and life-course-persistent antisocial behavior: A developmental taxonomy. *Psychology Review, 100*(4), 674–701.

Moffitt, T. E., Lynam, D. R., & Silva, P. A. (1994). Neuropsychological tests predicting persistent male delinquency. *Criminology, 32,* 277–300.

Monitoring the future. (2003). Retrieved March 28, 2003, from *http://www.monitoringthefuture.html.*

Moore, V., Barker, J., Ryan, A., & McLean, J. (1993). Effect of random breath testing on perception of likelihood of apprehension and on illegal drunk driving. *Drug and Alcohol Review, 12*(3), 251–258.

Moynihan, D. P. (1996). *Miles to go: A personal history of social policy.* Boston: Harvard University Press.

Mrazek, P. J., & Brown, C. H. (1999). *An evidence-based literature review regarding outcomes in psychosocial prevention and early intervention in young children.* Toronto: Invest in Kids Foundation.

Mrazek, P. J., & Haggerty, R. J. (1994). *Reducing risks for mental disorders: Frontiers for preventive intervention research.* Washington, DC: National Academy Press.

Murray, D. M., Moskowitz, J. M., & Dent, C. W. (1996). Design and analysis issues in community-based drug abuse prevention. *American Behavioral Scientist, 39*(7), 853–867.

Nansel, T. R., Overpeck, M., Pilla, R. S., Ruan, W. J., Simons-Morton, B., & Scheidt, P. (2001). Bullying behaviors among US youth: Prevalence and association with psychosocial adjustment. *Journal of the American Medical Association, 285*(16), 2094–2100.

National Center for Health Statistics. (1997). *Multiple cause of death public use data file.* Hyattsville, MD: U.S. Department of Health and Human Services, Centers for Disease Control, Division of Data Services.

National Highway Traffic Safety Administration. (1998). *Traffic safety facts 1997: Alcohol.* Washington, DC: U.S. Department of Transportation, National Center for Statistics and Analysis.

National Highway Traffic Safety Administration. (2001). *Traffic safety facts 2000—Children.* Washington, DC: U.S. Department of Transportation.

National Institute of Child Health and Human Development Early ChildCare Research Network. (2001). Childcare and children's peer interaction at 24 and 36 months: NICHD Study of Early ChildCare. *Child Development, 72*(5), 1478–1500.

National Institute on Alcohol Abuse and Alcoholism. (1996). *State trends in alcohol mortality, 1979–1992* (U.S. alcohol epidemiologic data reference manual, 5). Rockville, MD: Author.

National Institutes on Drug Abuse. (2003). Clinical trials network. Retrieved March 3, 2003, from *http://www.nida.nih.gov/CTN/index.htm.*

Nelson, J. P., & Moran, J. R. (1995). Advertising and US alcoholic beverage demand: system-wide estimates. *Applied Economics, 27,* 1225–1236.

Newcomb, A. F., Bukowski, W. M., & Pattee, L. (1993). Children's peer relations:

A meta-analytic review of popular, rejected, controversial, and average sociometric status. *Psychological Bulletin, 113*, 91–128.

O'Brien, C. P. (1997). A range of research-based pharmacotherapies for addiction. *Science, 278*, 66–70.

Oden, S., Schweinhart, L. J., Weikart, D. P., Marcus, S. M., & Xie, Y. (2000). *Into adulthood: A study of the effects of Head Start.* Ypsilanti, MI: High/Scope Press.

O'Donnell, C. R. (1996). The interplay of theory and practice in delinquency prevention: From behavior modification to activity settings. In J. McCord & R. E. Tremblay (Eds.), *Preventing antisocial behavior: Interventions from birth through adolescence* (pp. 209–232). New York: Guilford Press.

O'Donnell, J., Hawkins, J. D., Catalano, R. F., Abbott, R. D., & Day, L. E. (1995). Preventing school failure, drug use, and delinquency among low-income children: Long-term intervention in elementary schools. *American Journal of Orthopsychiatry, 65*(1), 87–100.

Office of Applied Studies. (1995). *Preliminary estimates from the 1994 National Household Survey on Drug Abuse.* Rockville, MD: U.S. Department of Health and Human Services, Substance Abuse and Mental Health Services Administration.

Office of Juvenile Justice and Delinquency Prevention. (2000). *OJJDP Statistical Briefing Book.* Retrieved January 20, 2002, from *http://ojjdp.ncjrs.org/ ojstatbb/html/qa253.html.*

O'Grady, B., Asbridge, M., & Abernathy, T. (1999). Analysis of factors related to illegal tobacco sales to young people in Ontario. *Tobacco Control, 8*(3), 301–305.

Olds, D. L. (1988). The Prenatal/Early Infancy Project. In R. H. Price, E. L. Cowen, R. P. Lorion & J. R. Ramos-McKay: *Fourteen ounces of prevention: A casebook for practitioners* (pp. 9–23). Washington, DC: American Psychological Association.

Olds, D. L., Henderson, C. R., Jr., Cole, R. E., Eckenrode, J., Kitzman, H. J., Luckey, D., et al. (1998). Long-term effects of nurse home visitation on children's criminal and antisocial behavior: 15-year follow-up of a randomized trial. *Journal of the American Medical Association, 280*, 1238–1244.

Olds, D. L., Henderson, C. R., Jr., Kitzman, H. J., Eckenrode, J., Cole, R. E., & Tatelbaum, R. (1998). The promise of home visitation: Results of two randomized trials. *Journal of Community Psychology, 26*(1), 5–21.

Olds, D. L., Henderson, C. R., Jr., Phelps, C., Kitzman, H., & Hanks, C. (1993). Effect of prenatal and infancy nurse home visitation on government spending. *Medical Care, 31*(2), 155–174.

Olds, D. L., & Kitzman, H. (1993). Review of research on home visiting for pregnant women and parents of young children. *The Future of Children, 3*(3), 53–92.

Ornstein, S. I., & Levy, D. (1983). Price and income elasticities and the demand for alcoholic beverages. In M Galanter (Ed.), *Recent developments in alcoholism* (pp. 303–345). New York: Plenum Press.

Osgood, D. W., Johnston, L. D., O'Malley, P. M., & Bachman, J. G. (1988). The generality of deviance in late adolescence and early adulthood. *American Sociological Review, 53*(1), 81–93.

Ozechowski, T., & Liddle, H. A. (2000). Family-based therapy for adolescent drug abuse: Knowns and unknowns. *Clinical Child and Family Psychology Review, 3*(4), 269–298.

Pacula, R. L. (1998). Does increasing the beer tax decrease marijuana consumption? *Journal of Health Economics, 17,* 557–585.

Pacula, R. L., Grossman, M., Chaloupka, F. J., O'Malley, P. M., & Johnston, L. D. (2001). *Marijuana and youth.* Washington, DC: Society for Prevention Research.

Paikoff, R. L., & Brooks-Gunn, J. (1991). Do parent–child relationships change during puberty? *Psychological Bulletin, 110*(1), 47–66.

Palmgreen, P., Donohew, L., Lorch, E. P., Hoyle, R. H., & Stephenson, M. T. (2002). Television campaigns and sensation seeking targeting of adolescent marijuana use: A controlled time-series approach. In R. Hornik (Ed.), *Public health communication: Evidence for behavior change* (35–56). Mahway, NJ: Erlbaum.

Patterson, G. R., DeBaryshe, B. D., & Ramsey, E. (1989). A developmental perspective on antisocial behavior. Special Issue: Children and their development: Knowledge base, research agenda, and social policy application. *American Psychologist, 44*(2), 329–335.

Patterson, G. R., & Dishion, T. J. (1985). Contributions of families and peers to delinquency. *Criminology, 23,* 63–79.

Patterson, G. R., & Dishion, T. J. (1988). Multilevel family process models: Traits, interactions and relationships. In R. A. Hinde & J. Stevenson-Hinde (Eds.), *Relationships within families: Mutual influences* (pp. 283–310). Oxford, UK: Clarendon Press.

Patterson, G. R., Dishion, T. J., & Yoerger, K. (2000). Adolescent growth in new forms of problem behavior: Macro- and micro-peer dynamics. *Prevention Science, 1,* 3–13.

Patterson, G. R., Forgatch, M. S., Yoerger, K. L., & Stoolmiller, M. (1998). Variables that initiate and maintain an early-onset trajectory for juvenile offending. *Development and Psychopathology, 10*(3), 531–547.

Patterson, G. R., Reid, J. B., & Dishion, T. J. (1992). *Antisocial boys: A social interactional approach* (Vol. 4). Eugene, OR: Castalia.

Patterson, G. R., Reid, J. B., & Dishion, T. J. (1998). Antisocial boys. In J. M. Jenkins, K. Oatley, & N. L. Stein (Eds.), *Human emotions: A reader* (pp. 330–336). Malden, MA: Blackwell.

Peisner-Feinberg, E. S., Burchinal, M. R., Clifford, R. M., Culkin, M. L., Howes, C., Kagan, S. L., et al. (1999). *The children of the cost, quality, and outcomes study go to school: Executive summary.* Chapel Hill: University of North Carolina, Frank Porter Graham Child Development Center.

Peisner-Feinberg, E. S., Burchinal, M. R., Clifford, R. M., Culkin, M. L., Howes, C., Kagan, S. L., et al. (2001). The relation of preschool child-care quality to children's cognitive and social developmental trajectories through second grade. *Child Development, 72*(5), 1534–1553.

Pentz, M. A., Brannon, B. R., Charlin, V. L., Barrett, E. J., MacKinnon, D. P., & Flay, B. R. (1989). The power of policy: The relationship of smoking policy to adolescent smoking. *American Journal of Public Health, 79*(7), 857–862.

Pentz, M. A., Dwyer, J. H., Johnson, C. A., Flay, B. R., Hansen, W. B., MacKinnon, D. P., et al. (1994). *Long-term follow-up of a multicommunity trial for prevention of tobacco, alcohol, and drug use.* Unpublished manuscript.

Pentz, M. A., Dwyer, J. H., MacKinnon, D. P., Flay, B. R., Hansen, W. B., Wang, E., et al. (1989). A multicommunity trial for primary prevention of adolescent drug abuse: Effects on drug use prevalence. *Journal of American Medical Association, 261,* 3259–3266.

Pentz, M. A., MacKinnon, D. P., Flay, B. R., Hansen, W. B., Johnson, C. A., & Dwyer, J. H (1989). Primary prevention of chronic diseases in adolescence: Effects of the Midwestern Prevention Project (MPP) on tobacco use. *American Journal of Epidemiology, 130,* 713–724.

Pentz, M. A., Trebow, E. A., Hansen, W. B., & MacKinnon, D. P. (1990). Effects of program implementation on adolescent drug use behavior: The Midwestern Prevention Project. *Evaluation Review, 14,* 264–289.

Perry, C. L., Luepker, R. V., Murray, D. M., Kurth, C., Mullis, R., Crockett, S. J., et al. (1988). Parent involvement with children's health promotion: The Minnesota home team. *American Journal of Public Health, 78*(9), 1156–1160.

Perry, C. L., Williams, C. L., Forster, J. L., Wolfson, M., Wagenaar, A. C., Finnegan, J. R., et al. (1993). Background, conceptualization, and design of a community-wide research program on adolescent alcohol use: Project Northland. *Health Education Research, 8,* 125–136.

Perry, C. L., Williams, C. L., Komro, K. A., Veblen-Mortenson, S., Forster, J. L., Bernstein-Lachter, R., et al. (1998, February). *Project Northland-II: Community action to reduce adolescent alcohol use.* Paper presented at the Fourth Symposium on Community Action Research and the Prevention of Alcohol and other Drug Problems, Russell, NZ.

Perry, C. L., Williams, C. L., Komro, K. A., Veblen-Mortenson, S., Forster, J. L., Bernstein-Lachter, R., et al. (2000). Project Northland high school interventions: Community action to reduce adolescent alcohol use. *Health Education and Behavior, 27,* 29–49.

Perry, C. L., Williams, C. L., Komro, K. A., Veblen-Mortenson, S., Stigler, M. H., Munson, K. A., et al. (2002). Project Northland: Long-term outcomes of community action to reduce adolescent alcohol use. *Health Education Research, 17*(1), 117–132.

Perry, C. L., Williams, C. L., Veblen-Mortenson, S., Toomey, T.L., Komro, K. A., Anstine, P. S., et al. (1996). Project Northland: Outcomes of a community-wide alcohol use prevention program during early adolescence. *American Journal of Public Health, 86*(7), 956–965.

Personal Improvement Computer Systems. (2001). *The Health Authority: Changing behaviors to improve health. Tobacco dependence.* Retrieved March 7, 2003, from *http://www.healthauthority.com/tobaccodependence.htm.*

Phillips, D., McCartney, K., & Scarr, S. (1987). Child-care quality and children's social development. *Developmental Psychology, 23,* 537–543.

Phillips, K., & Matheny, A. P., Jr. (1997). Evidence for genetic influence on both cross-situation and situation-specific components of behavior. *Journal of Personality and Social Psychology, 73*(1), 129–138.

Pierce, J. P., Choi, W. S., Gilpin, E. A., Farkas, A. J., & Berry, C. C. (1998). Tobacco industry promotion of cigarettes and adolescent smoking. *Journal of the American Medical Association, 279*(7), 511–515.

Pierce, J. P., & Gilpin, E. A. (1995). A historical analysis of tobacco marketing and the uptake of smoking by youth in the United States: 1890–1977. *Health Psychology, 14*(6), 500–508.

Pierce, J. P., Giovino, G., Hatziandreu, E., & Shopland, D. (1989). National age and sex differences in quitting smoking. *Journal of Psychoactive Drugs, 21,* 293–298.

Pierce, J. P., Gilpin, E. A., & Choi, W. S. (1999). Sharing the blame: smoking experimentation and future smoking-attributable mortality due to Joe Camel and Marlboro advertising and promotions. *Tobacco Control, 8*(1), 37–44.

Pierre, N., Shrier, L. A., Emans, S. J., & DuRant, R. H. (1998). Adolescent males involved in pregnancy: associations of forced sexual contact and risk behaviors. *Journal of Adolescent Health, 23*(6), 364–369.

Pihl, R. O., & Peterson, J. B. (1991). Attention deficit hyperactivity disorder, childhood conduct disorders and alcoholism: Is there an association? *Alcohol Health and Research World, 15,* 25–31.

Pinkerton, S. D., Holtgrave, D. R., DiFranceisco, W. J., Stevenson, L. Y., & Kelly, J. A. (1998). Cost-effectiveness of a community-level HIV risk reduction intervention. *American Journal of Public Health, 88,* 1239–1242.

Poon, E., Ellis, D. A., Fitzgerald, H. E., & Zucker, R. A. (2000). Intellectual, cognitive, and academic performance among sons of alcoholics during the early school years: Differences related to subtypes of familial alcoholism. *Alcoholism: Clinical and Experimental Research, 24,* 1020–1027.

Preusser, D. F., & Williams, A. F. (1992). Sales of alcohol to underage purchasers in three New York counties and Washington DC. *Journal of Public Health Policy, 13,* 306–317.

Raine, A., Brennan, P., & Mednick, S. A. (1994). Birth complications combined with early maternal rejection predispose to adult violent crime. *Archives of General Psychiatry, 51,* 984–988.

Raine, A., Venables, P. H., Dalais, C., Mellingen, K., Reynolds, C., & Mednick, S. A. (2001). Early educational and health enrichment at age 3–5 years is associated with increased autonomic and central nervous system arousal and orienting at age 11 years: Evidence from the Mauritius Child Health Project. *Psychophysiology, 38*(2), 254–266.

Rappaport, J. (1987). Terms of empowerment/exemplars of prevention: Toward a theory for community psychology. *American Journal of Community Psychology, 15,* 121–148.

Reid, J. B., Eddy, J. M., Fetrow, R. A., & Stoolmiller, M. (1999). Description and immediate impacts of a preventive intervention for conduct problems. Special Issue: Prevention science, part 1. *American Journal of Community Psychology, 27*(4), 483–517.

Reid, J. B., & Patterson, G. R. (1991). Early prevention and intervention with conduct problems: A social interactional model for the integration of research and practice. In G. Stoner, M. Shinn, & H. Walker (Eds.), *Interventions for achievement and behavior problems* (pp. 715–739). Silver Spring, MD: National Association of School Psychologists.

Reiss, D., & Neiderhiser, J. M. (2000). The interplay of genetic influences and social processes in developmental theory: specific mechanisms are coming into view. *Development and Psychopathology, 12*(3), 357–374.

Reiss, D., Neiderhiser, J. M., Hetherington, E. M., & Plomin, R. (2000). *The relationship code: Deciphering genetic and social influences on adolescent development.* Cambridge, MA: Cambridge University Press.

Richardson, J. L., Dwyer, K. M., McGuigan, K., Hansen, W. B., Dent, C. W., Johnson, C. A., et al. (1989). Substance use among eighth-grade students who take care of themselves after school. *Pediatrics, 84*(3), 556–566.

Richardson, J. L., Radziszewska, B., Dent, C. W., & Flay, B. R. (1993). Relationship between after-school care of adolescents and substance use, risk taking, depressed mood, and academic achievement. *Pediatrics, 92*(1), 32–38.

Rigotti, N. A., DiFranza, J. R., Chang, Y., Tisdale, T., Kemp, B., & Singer, D. E. (1997). The effect of enforcing tobacco-sales laws on adolescents' access to tobacco and smoking behavior. *New England Journal of Medicine, 337*(15), 1044–1051.

Riley, D., Meinhardt, G., Nelson, C., Salisbury, M., & Winnett, T. (1991). How effective are age-paced newsletters for new parents? A replication and extension of earlier studies. *Family Relations, 40,* 247–253.

Rind, B., & Tromovitch, P. (1997). A meta-analytic review of findings from national samples on psychological correlates of child sexual abuse. *Journal of Sex Research, 34*(3), 237–255.

Roberts, S. J., Sorensen, L., Patsdaughter, C. A., & Grindel, C. (2000). Sexual behaviors and sexually transmitted diseases in lesbians: Results of the Boston Lesbian Health Project. *Journal of Lesbian Studies, 4*(3), 47–70.

Robins, L. N., & McEvoy, L. (1990). Conduct problems as predictors of substance abuse. In L. N. Robins & M. Rutter (Eds.), *Straight and devious pathways from childhood to adulthood.* (pp. 182–204). Cambridge, MA: Cambridge University Press.

Rodgers, G. B. (1993). Estimating jury compensation for pain and suffering in product liability cases involving nonfatal personal injury. *Journal of Forensic Economics, 6,* 251–262.

Rosenstein, D. S., & Horowitz, H. A. (1996). Adolescent attachment and psychopathology. *Journal of Consulting and Clinical Psychology, 64,* 244–253.

Ross, H. L. (1982). *Deterring the drinking driver: Legal policy and social control.* Lexington, MA: D.C. Heath.

Ross, H. L. (1988a). British drunk-driving policy. *British Journal of Addiction, 83*(8), 863–865.

Ross, H. L. (1988b). Deterrence-based policies in Britain, Canada and Australia. In M. D. Laurence, J. R. Snortum, & F. E. Zimring (Eds.), *The social control of drinking and driving* (pp. 64–78). Chicago: University of Chicago Press.

Ross, H. L. (1991). *Administrative license revocation for drunk drivers: Options and choices in three states.* Washington, DC: AAA Foundation for Traffic Safety.

Rotheram-Borus, M. J. (2000). Expanding the range of interventions to reduce HIV among adolescents. *AIDS, 14,* S33–S40.

Rotheram-Borus, M. J., O'Keefe, Z., Kracker, R., & Foo, H-H. (2000). Prevention of HIV among adolescents. *Prevention Science, 1,* 15–30.

Roussos, S. T., & Fawcett, S. B. (2000). A review of collaborative partnerships as a strategy for improving community health. *Annual Review of Public Health, 21,* 369–402.

Rueter, M. A., & Conger, R. D. (1995). Interaction style, problem-solving behavior, and family problem-solving effectiveness. *Child Development, 66*(1), 98–115.

Ruhm, C. J. (1996). Alcohol policies and highway vehicle fatalities. *Journal of Health Economics, 15,* 435–454.

Rusby, J. C., Forrester, K. K., & Biglan, A. (2002). *Relationships between victimization and problem behavior in adolescence.* Manuscript submitted for publication.

Rushton, J. L., Clark, S. J., & Freed, G. L. (2000). Pediatrician and family physician prescription of selective serotonin reuptake inhibitors. *Pediatrics, 105*(6), E82.

Rutter, M. (1979). Protective factors in children's responses to stress and disadvantage. In M. W. Kent & J. E. Rolf (Eds.), *Primary prevention of psychopathology, 3: Social competence in children* (pp. 49–74). Hanover, NH: University Press of New England.

Rydell, C. P., & Everingham, S. S. (1994). *Controlling cocaine: Supply versus demand programs.* Santa Barbara, CA: Rand.

Saffer, H. (1997). Alcohol advertising and motor vehicle fatalities. *Review of Economics and Statistics, 79,* 431–442.

Saffer, H., & Chaloupka F. (2000). The effect of tobacco advertising bans on tobacco consumption, *Journal of Health Economics, 19*(6), 1117–1137.

Saffer, H., & Grossman, M. (1987a). Beer taxes, the legal drinking age, and youth motor vehicle fatalities. *Journal of Legal Studies, 16,* 351–374.

Saffer, H., & Grossman, M. (1987b). Drinking age laws and highway mortality rates: Cause and effect. *Economic Inquiry, 25,* 403–417.

Saigh, P. A., & Umar, A. M. (1983). The effects of a Good Behavior Game on the disruptive behavior of Sudanese elementary school students. *Journal of Applied Behavior Analysis, 16,* 339–344.

Salend, S. J., Reynolds, C. J., & Coyle, E. M. (1989). Individualizing the Good Behavior Game across type and frequency of behavior with emotionally disturbed adolescents. *Behavior Modification, 13*(1), 108–126.

Saltz, R. F. (1987). The roles of bars and restaurants in preventing alcohol-impaired driving: An evaluation of server intervention. *Evaluation and Health Professions, 10*(1), 5–27.

Saltz, R. F. (1989). Server intervention and responsible beverage service programs. In *Surgeon General's workshop on drunk driving* (pp. 169–179). Rockville, MD: U.S. Department of Health and Human Services.

Saltz, R. F., & Hennessy, M. (1990a). *The efficacy of Responsible Beverage Service programs in reducing intoxication.* Berkeley, CA: Prevention Research Center.

Saltz, R. F., & Hennessy, M. (1990b). *Reducing intoxication in commercial establishments: An evaluation of Responsible Beverage Service practices.* Berkeley, CA: Prevention Research Center.

Sameroff, A. J. (1998). Environmental risk factors in infancy. *Pediatrics, 102,* 1287–1292.

Sameroff, A. J. (2001). *Individual and contextual influences on adolescent competence.* Paper presented at the biennial meeting of the Society for Research on Child Development, Minneapolis, MN.

Sampson, R. J. (1997). Collective regulation of adolescent misbehavior: Validation results from eighty Chicago neighborhoods. *Journal of Adolescent Research, 12*(2), 227–244.

Sampson, R. J., & Groves, W. B. (1989). Community structure and crime: Testing social-disorganization theory. *American Journal of Sociology, 94,* 774–780.

Sampson, R. J., & Laub, J. H. (1994). Urban poverty and the family context of delinquency: A new look at structure and process in a classic study. *Child Development, 65,* 523–540.

Sampson, R. J., & Laub, J. H. (1997). A life course theory of cumulative disadvantage and the stability of delinquency. In T. P. Thornberry (Ed.), *Developmental theories of crime and delinquency* (pp. 133–61). New Brunswick, NJ: Transaction.

Sampson, R. J., & Raudenbush, S. (1999). Systematic social observation of public spaces: A new look at disorder in urban neighborhoods. *American Journal of Sociology, 105,* 603–651.

Sampson, R. J., Raudenbush, S. W., & Earls, F. (1997). Neighborhoods and violent crime: A multilevel study of collective efficacy. *Science, 277*(5328), 918–924.

Sanders, M. R. (1996). New directions in behavioral family intervention with children. In T. H. Ollendick & R. J. Prinz (Eds.), *Advances in clinical child psychology* (pp. 283–330). New York: Plenum Press.

Sanders, M. R. (1999). Triple P-Positive Parenting Program: Towards an empirically validated multilevel parenting and family support strategy for the prevention of behavior and emotional problems in children. *Clinical Child and Family Psychology Review, 2*(2), 71–90.

Sanders, M. R., Dadds, M. R., Johnson, B. M., & Cash, R. (1992). Childhood depression and Conduct Disorder: I. Behavioral, affective, and cognitive aspects of family problem-solving interactions. *Journal of Abnormal Psychology, 101,* 495–504.

Sanders, M. R., Markie-Dadds, C., Tully, L. A., & Bor, W. (2000). The Triple P-Positive Parenting Program: A comparison of enhanced, standard, and self-directed behavioral family intervention. *Journal of Consulting and Clinical Psychology, 68,* 624–640.

Sanders, M. R., Montgomery, D. T., & Brechman-Toussaint, M. L (2000). The mass media and the prevention of child behavior problems: The evaluation of a television series to promote positive outcomes for parents and their children. *Journal of Child Psychology and Psychiatry, 41,* 939–948.

Sargent, J. D., Dalton, M., Beach, M., Bernhardt, A., Heatherton, T., & Stevens, M. (2000). Effect of cigarette promotions on smoking uptake among adolescents. *Preventive Medicine, 30*(4), 320–327.

Scales, P. C., & Leffert, N. (1999). *Developmental assets: A synthesis of the scientific research on adolescent development.* Minneapolis, MN: Search Institute.

Schillo, B. A., Monaghan, T. M., & Davidson, W. S. (1996). *The adolescent diver-*

sion project: An alternative to traditional court services for youthful offenders. Ann Arbor: Michigan State University.

Schmitz, S., Saudino, K. J., Plomin, R., Fulker, D. W., & DeFries, J. C. (1996). Genetic and environmental influences on temperament in middle childhood: Analyses of teacher and tester ratings. *Child Development, 67*(2), 409–422.

Schonfeld, I. S., Shaffer, D., O'Connor, P., & Portnoy, S. (1988). Conduct disorder and cognitive functioning: Testing three causal hypotheses. *Child Development, 59*(4), 993–1007.

Schuhmann, E. M., Foote, R. C., Eyberg, S. M., Boggs, S. R., & Algina, J. (1998). Efficacy of parent–child interaction therapy: Interim report of a randomized trial with short-term maintenance. *Journal of Clinical Child Psychology, 27*(1), 34–45.

Schweinhart, L. J., Barnes, H. V., & Weikart, D. P. (1993). Significant benefits: The High/Scope Perry Preschool Study through age 27. *Monographs of the High/Scope Educational Research Foundation, 10*. Ypsilanti, MI: High/Scope Press.

Schweinhart, L. J., Berrueta-Clement, J. R., Barnett, W. S., Epstein, A. S., & Weikart, D. P. (1985). Effects of the Perry Preschool Program on youth through age 19: A summary. *Topics in Early Childhood Education, 5*(2), 26–35.

Seifer, R. (2000). Temperament and goodness of fit. In A. J. Sameroff, M. Lewis & S. M. Miller (Eds.), *Handbook of developmental psychology* (pp. 257–276). New York: Kluwer Press.

Sherman, L. W., Gottfredson, D. C., MacKenzie, D. L., Eck, J., Reuter, P., & Bushway, S. D. (1998 July). *Preventing crime: What works, what doesn't, what's promising* [National Institute of Justice, Research in Brief]. Washington, DC: U.S. Department of Justice, National Institute of Justice.

Shonkoff, J. P., & Phillips, D. A. (2000). *From neurons to neighborhoods: The science of early childhood development*. Washington, DC: National Academy Press.

Siegel, A. W., & Scovill, L. C. (2000). Problem behavior: The double symptom of adolescence. *Development and Psychopathology, 12*(4), 763–793.

Silbereisen, R. K., & Noack, P. (1988). On the constructive role of problem behavior in adolescence. In N. Bolger, A, Caspi, G, Downey, & M. Moorehouse (Eds.), *Persons in context: Developmental processes* (pp. 152–180). Cambridge, MA: Cambridge University Press.

Silbereisen, R. K., Petersen, A. C., Albrecht, H. T., & Kracke, B. (1989). Maturational timing and the development of problem behavior: Longitudinal studies in adolescence. *Journal of Early Adolescence, 9*, 247–268.

Sing, C. F., Haviland, M. B., & Reilly, S. L. (1996). Genetic architecture of common multifactorial diseases. *Ciba Foundation Symposium, 197*, 211–229.

Sing, C. F., Haviland, M. B., Templeton, A. R., Zerba, K. E., & Reilly, S. L. (1992). Biological complexity and strategies for finding DNA variations responsible for inter-individual variation in risk of a common chronic disease, coronary artery disease. *Annals of Medicine, 24*(6), 539–547.

Singh, S. (1986). Adolescent pregnancy in the United States: An interstate analysis. *Family Planning Perspectives, 18*(5), 210–220.

Sloan, F. A., Reilly, B. A., & Schenzler, C. (1994). Effects of prices, civil and criminal sanctions, and law enforcement on alcohol-related mortality. *Journal of
Studies on Alcohol, 55*, 454–465.

Slovic, P. (2000). *Perception of risk.* London: Earthscan.

Smith, D. I. (1990). Effect on casualty traffic accidents of changing Sunday alcohol
sales legislation in Victoria, Australia. *Journal of Drug Issues, 20*(3), 417–
426.

Smith, S. V. (1998). Why juries can be trusted. *Voir Dire, 5,* 19–21.

Smoking-related deaths and financial costs: Office of technology assessment estimates for 1990: Hearing before the Senate Special Committee on Aging,
103rd Cong. (1993) (testimony of Roger Herdman, Maria Hewitt, and Mary
Laschober).

Snyder, H. N., & Sickmund, M. (1999). *Juvenile offenders and victims: 1999 National Report* (NCJ 178257). Washington, DC: Office of Juvenile Justice &
Delinquency Prevention.

Snyder, L. B., & Blood, D. J. (1992). Caution: Alcohol advertising and the Surgeon
General's alcohol warnings may have adverse effects on young adults. *Journal
of Applied Communication Research, 20*(1), 37–53.

Spoth, R., Guyll, M., & Day, S. X. (2002). Universal family-focused interventions
in alcohol-use disorder prevention: Cost-effectiveness and cost-benefit analyses of two interventions. *Journal of Studies on Alcohol, 63,* 219–228.

Spoth, R., Redmond, C., & Lepper, H. (1999, March). Alcohol initiation outcomes of universal family-focused preventive interventions: one- and two-
year follow-ups of a controlled study. *Journal of Studies on Alcohol* (Suppl.
13), 103–111.

Spoth, R., Redmond, C., & Shin, C. (1998). Direct and indirect latent variable par-
enting outcomes of two universal family-focused preventive interventions:
Extending a public health-oriented research base. *Journal of Consulting and
Clinical Psychology, 66,*(2), 385–399.

Spoth, R. L., Redmond, C., & Shin, C. (2000). Reducing adolescents' aggressive
and hostile behaviors: Randomized trial effects of a brief family intervention
four years past baseline. *Archives of Pediatric and Adolescent Medicine,
154*(12), 1248–1257.

Spoth, R. L., Redmond, C., & Shin, C. (2001). Randomized trial of brief family interventions for general populations: Adolescent substance use outcomes four
years following baseline. *Journal of Consulting and Clinical Psychology,
69*(4), 627–642.

St. Lawrence, J. S., Brasfield, T. L., Jefferson, K. W., Alleyne, E., O'Bannon, R. E.,
& Shirley, A. (1995). Cognitive-behavioral intervention to reduce African-
American adolescents' risk for HIV infection. *Journal of Consulting and
Clinical Psychology, 63*(2), 221–237.

St. Lawrence, J. S., Jefferson, K. W., Alleyne, E., & Brasfield, T. L. (1995). Comparison of education versus behavioral skills training interventions in lowering
sexual HIV-risk behavior of substance- dependent adolescents. *Journal of
Consulting and Clinical Psychology, 63*(1), 154–157.

Stark, M. J. (1992). Dropping out of substance abuse treatment: A clinically oriented review. *Clinical Psychology Review, 12*(1), 93–116.

Stewart, L., & Casswell, S. (1993). Media advocacy for alcohol policy support: Results from the New Zealand Community Action Project. *Health Promotion International, 8*(3), 167–175.

Stice, E., Myers, M. G., & Brown, S. A. (1998). Relations of delinquency to adolescent substance use and problem use: A prospective study. *Psychology of Addictive Behaviors, 12*(2), 136–146.

Stoddard, J. J., & Gray, B. (1997). Maternal smoking and medical expenditures for childhood respiratory illness. *American Journal of Public Health, 87,* 205–209.

Stuster, J. W., & Blowers, P. A. (1995). *Experimental evaluation of sobriety checkpoint programs.* Washington, DC: National Highway Traffic Safety Administration.

Substance Abuse and Mental Health Services Administration. (1998). *National Household Survey on Drug Abuse: Population estimates 1997.* Washington, DC: U.S. Department of Health and Human Services.

Substance Abuse and Mental Health Services Administration. (1999). *The relationship between mental health and substance abuse among adolescents.* Rockville, MD: Author.

Substance Abuse Prevention and Treatment Block Grants: Sale or Distribution of Tobacco Products to Individuals Under 18 Years of Age, 58 Fed. Reg. 45156–45174 (1993).

Sue, S. (1977). Community mental health services to minority groups: Some optimism, some pessimism. *American Psychologist, 32*(8), 616–624.

Sue, S., & Morishima, J. K. (1982). *The mental health of Asian Americans.* San Francisco: Jossey-Bass.

Susman, E. J., Nottelmann, E. D., Dorn, L. D., Inoff-Germain, G., & Chrousos, G. P. (1988). Physiological and behavioral aspects of stress in adolescence. In G. P. Chrousos, D. L. Loriaux, & P. W. Gold (Eds.), *Mechanisms of physical and emotional stress* (pp. 341–352). New York: Plenum Press.

Sussman, S., Lichtman, K., Ritta, A., & Pallonen, U. E. (1999). Effects of thirty-four adolescent tobacco use cessation and prevention trials on regular users of tobacco products. *Substance Use and Misuse, 34*(11), 1469–1503.

Sussman, S. Y., Dent, C. W., Burton, D., Stacy, A. W., & Flay, B. R. (1995). *Developing school-based tobacco use prevention and cessation programs.* Thousand Oaks, CA: Sage.

Swiezy, N. B., Matson, J. L., & Box, P. (1992). The Good Behavior Game: A token reinforcement system for preschoolers. *Child and Family Behavior Therapy, 14*(3), 21–32.

Tarnowski, K. J. (1991). Disadvantaged children and families in pediatric primary care settings: I. Broadening the scope of integrated mental health service. *Journal of Clinical Child Psychology, 20*(4), 351–359.

Tarter, R., Vanyukov, M., Giancola, P., Dawes, M., Blackson, T., Mezzich, A., et al. (1999). Etiology of early age onset substance use disorder: A maturational perspective. *Development and Psychopathology, 11*(4), 657–683.

Taylor-Greene, S., Brown, D., Nelson, L., Longton, J., Gassman, T., Cohen, J., et al. (1997). School-wide behavioral support: Starting the year off right. *Journal of Behavioral Education, 7,* 99–112.

Thornton, T. N., Craft, C. A., Dahlberg, L. L., Lynch, B. S., & Baer, K. (2000). *Best practices of youth violence prevention: A sourcebook for community action.* Atlanta: Centers for Disease Control and Prevention, National Center for Injury Prevention and Control.

Tildesley, E. A., Hops, H., Ary, D., & Andrews, J.A. (1995). Multitrait-multimethod model of adolescent deviance, drug use, academic, and sexual behaviors. *Journal of Psychopathology and Behavioral Assessment, 17*(2), 185–215.

Tobler, N. S., Roona, M. R., Ochshorn, P., Marshall, D. G., Streke, A. V., & Stackpole, K. M. (2000). School-based adolescent drug prevention programs: 1998 meta-analysis. *Journal of Primary Prevention 20*(4), 275–336.

Tolley, G., Kenkel, D., & Fabian, R. (1994). *Valuing health for policy: An economic approach.* Chicago: University of Chicago Press.

Tonry, M., & Lynch, M. (1996). Intermediate sanctions. *Crime and justice: A review of the research, 20,* 99–144.

Tortu, S., & Botvin, G. (1989). School-based smoking prevention: The teacher training process. *Preventive Medicine, 18,* 280–289.

Tremblay, R. E., Pagani-Kurtz, L., Masse, L. C., Vitaro, F., & Pihl, R. O. (1995). A bi-modal preventive intervention for disruptive kindergarten boys: Its impact through mid-adolescence. *Journal of Consulting and Clinical Psychology, 63*(4), 560–568.

Tremblay, R. E., & Schaal, B. (1996). Physically aggressive boys from age 6 to 12 years: Their biopsychosocial status at puberty. *Annals of the New York Academy of Sciences, 794,* 192–207.

Trumbull, W. N. (1990). Who has standing in cost-benefit analysis? *Journal of Policy Analysis and Management, 9,* 201–218.

Trussell, J., Koenig, J., Stewart, F, & Darroch, J. E. (1997). Medical care cost savings from adolescent contraceptive use. *Family Planning Perspectives, 29,* 248–255.

U.S. Census Bureau. (1995). *Statistical abstract of the United States* (115th ed.). Washington, DC: Author.

U.S. Census Bureau. (1998, October). *Statistical abstract of the United States.* Washington, DC: Author.

U.S. Department of Education. (1999). *Statement of Pascall D. Forgione, Jr., Commissioner of Education Statistics, National Center for Education Statistics.*U.S. Department of Education [On-line]. Available *http://nces.ed.gov/ Pressrelease/tq.html.*

U.S. Department of Health and Human Services. (1994). *Preventing tobacco use among young people: A report of the Surgeon General.* Atlanta: Author, Public Health Service, Centers for Disease Control & Prevention, National Center for Chronic Disease Prevention & Health Promotion, Office of Smoking & Health.

U.S. Department of Health and Human Services (2000a). The 1999 National Household Survey on Drug Abuse Summary Findings. Retrieved January 2003, from *http://www.drugabusestatistics.samhsa.gov/.*

U.S. Department of Health and Human Services (2000b). *Summary of Findings from the 1999 National Household Survey on Drug Abuse.* Rockville: MD: Office of Applied Studies. Substance Abuse and Mental Health Services Administration. Available online at: *http//:www.health.org/govstudy/bkd376/ TableofContents.htm.*

U.S. Department of Health and Human Services. (2001). *Women and smoking: A report of the Surgeon General.* Rockville, MD: Author, Public Health Service, Office of the Surgeon General.

U.S. Department of Justice, Bureau of Justice Statistics. (1999). *Census of State and Federal Correctional Facilities, 1997.* Washington, DC: U.S. Government Printing Office.

U.S. Department of Justice, Office of Juvenile Justice and Delinquency Prevention. (1994). *Census of public and private juvenile detention, correctional, and shelter facilities, 1986–1987: United States* [Computer file]. Conducted by the U.S. Department of Commerce, Bureau of the Census. ICPSR ed. Ann Arbor, MI: Inter-university Consortium for Political and Social Research.

U.S. General Accounting Office. (1987). *Drinking age laws: an evaluation synthesis of their impact on highway safety.* Report to the Chair, Subcommittee on Investigations and Oversight, Committee on Public Works and Transportation, House of Representatives. Washington, DC: Author.

U.S. General Accounting Office. (1993). *Confronting the drug problem: Debate persists on enforcement and alternative approaches.* Washington, DC: Author.

U.S. Government Printing Office. (2000). *National Crime Victimization Survey Web tables: Sourcebook of Criminal Justice Statistics 1999.* Washington DC: U.S. Government Printing Office.

U.S. Office of Management and Budget. (2000). *Economic report of the President.* Washington, DC: U.S. Government Printing Office.

University of Kansas. (2003). *Community Toolbox.* Retrieved March 4, 2000, from *http://ctb.ku.edu/.*

Valli, R. (1998). Changes in young people's alcohol consumption with improved availability of medium strength beer: The case of Pietarsaari. *Nordic Alcohol and Drug Studies, 15*(3), 168–175.

Veblen-Mortenson, S., Rissel, C., Perry, C. L., Forster, J., Wolfson, M., & Finnegan, J. R. (1999). Lessons learned from Project Northland: Community organization in rural communities. In N. Bracht (Ed.), *Health promotion at the community level 2: New advances* (pp. 105–117). Thousand Oaks, CA: Sage.

Vernon, S. W., & Roberts, R. E. (1982). Prevalence of treated and untreated psychiatric disorders in three ethnic groups. *Social Science and Medicine, 16*(17), 1575–1582.

Vingilis, E., & Coultes, B. (1990). Mass communications and drinking-driving: Theories, practices, and results. *Alcohol, Drugs, and Driving, 6*(2), 61–81.

Viscusi, W. K. (1988). Pain and suffering in product liability cases: Systematic compensation or capricious awards? *International Review of Law and Economics, 8,* 203–220.

Viscusi, W. K. (1993). The value of risks to life and health. *Journal of Economic Literature, 31,* 1912–1946.

Voas, R. B., Holder, H. D., & Gruenewald, P. J. (1997). The effect of drinking and driving interventions on alcohol-involved traffic crashes within a comprehensive community trial. *Addiction, 92*(Suppl. 2), 221–236.

Voas, R. B., Tippetts, A. S., & Fell, J. (1999). Minimum legal drinking age and zero tolerance laws: do they reduce alcohol-related crashes? *Forty-third Annual Proceedings, Association for Advancement of Automotive Medicine, 265–278.*

Vogt, T. M., Lichtenstein, E., Ary, D. V., & Biglan, A. (1989). Integrating tobacco intervention into a health maintenance organization: The TRACC program. *Health Education Research, 4*(1), 125–135.

Wachs, T. D. (2000). *Necessary but not sufficient: The respective roles of single and multiple influences on individual development.* Washington, DC: American Psychological Association.

Wagenaar, A. C., Gehan, J. P., Jones-Webb, R., Wolfson, M., Toomey, T. L., Forster, J. L., et al. (1999). Communities mobilizing for change on alcohol: Lessons and results from a 15-community randomized trial. *Journal of Community Psychology, 27,* 315–326.

Wagenaar, A. C., & Holder, H. D. (1995). Changes in alcohol consumption resulting from the elimination of retail wine monopolies: Results from five US states. *Journal of Studies on Alcohol, 10*(1), 566–572.

Wagenaar, A. C., Murray, D. M., Gehan, J. P., Wolfson, M., Forster, J. L., Toomey, T. L., et al.(2000). Communities mobilizing for change on alcohol: Outcomes from a randomized community trials. *Journal of Studies on Alcohol, 61,* 85–94.

Wagenaar, A. C., Murray, D. M., & Toomey, T. L. (2000). Communities mobilizing for change on alcohol (CMCA): Effects of a randomized trial on arrests and traffic crashes. *Addiction, 95*(2), 209–217.

Wagenaar, A. C., Murray, D. M., Wolfson, M., & Forster, J. L. (1994). Communities mobilizing for change on alcohol: Design of a randomized community trial. *Journal of Community Psychology, 19,* 94–101.

Wagenaar, A., O'Malley, P., & LaFond, C. (2001). Effects of lowered legal blood alcohol limits for young drivers: Effects on drinking, driving, and driving after drinking behaviors in 30 states. *American Journal of Public Health 91*(5), 801–880.

Wagenaar, A. C., & Toomey, T. L. (2000). *Effects of minimum drinking age laws: Review and analyses of the literature.* Paper prepared for Advisory Council Subcommittee, Rockville, MD.

Wagenaar, A. C., & Wolfson, M. (1994). Enforcement of the legal minimum drinking age in the United States. *Journal of Public Health Policy, 15,* 37–53.

Wagenaar, A. C., & Wolfson, M. (1995). Deterring sales and provision of alcohol to minors: A study of enforcement in 295 counties in four states. *Public Health Reports, 110,* 419–427.

Wakefield, M., & Chaloupka, F. J. (2000). Effectiveness of comprehensive tobacco control programmes in reducing teenage smoking in the USA. *Tobacco Control, 9,* 177–186.

Wakefield, M., Flay, B., Nichter, M., & Giovino, G. (2001). *Role of media in influencing trajectories of youth smoking.* Chicago: Health Research and Policy Centers, University of Illinois.

Wakefield, M., Flay, B., Nichter, M., & Giovino, G. (2003). Role of media in influencing trajectories of youth smoking, *Addiction, 98*(51), 79.

Wakschlag, L. S., Lahey, B. B., Loeber, R., Green, S. M., Gordon, R. A., & Leventhal, B. L. (1997). Maternal smoking during pregnancy and the risk of conduct disorder in boys. *Archives of General Psychiatry, 54*(7), 670–676.

Waldron, H. B., Slesnick, N., Brody, J. L., Turner, C. W., & Peterson, T. R. (2001). Treatment outcomes for adolescent substance abuse at 4- and 7-month assessments. *Journal of Consulting and Clinical Psychology, 69*(5), 802–813.

Walker, H. M., Colvin, G., & Ramsey, E. (1995). *Antisocial behavior in school: Strategies and best practices.* Pacific Grove, CA: Brooks/Cole.

Walker, H. M., Severson, H. H., Todis, B. J., & Block-Pedego, A. E. (1990). Systematic Screening for Behavior Disorders (SSBD): Further validation, replication, and normative data. *Remedial and Special Education, 11*, 32–46.

Wallack, L., & Dorfman, L. (1996). Media advocacy: A strategy for advancing policy and promoting health. *Health Education Quarterly, 23*(3), 293–317.

Wallack, L., Dorfman, L., Jernigan, D., & Themba, M. (1993). *Media advocacy and public health. Power for prevention.* Newbury Park, CA: Sage.

Walsh, A. (1995). Parental attachment, drug use, and facultative sexual strategies. *Social Biology, 42*(1–2), 95–107.

Wang, L. Y., Davis, M., Robin, L., Collins, J., Coyle, K., & Baumler, E. (2000). Economic evaluation of Safer Choices: A school-based human immunodeficiency virus, other sexually transmitted diseases, and pregnancy prevention program. *Archives of Pediatric and Adolescent Medicine, 154*, 1017–1024.

Wasserman, J., Manning, W. G., Newhouse, J. P., & Winkler, J. D. (1991). The effects of excise taxes and regulations on cigarette smoking. *Journal of Health Economics, 10*, 43–64.

Webster-Stratton, C. (1981). Modification of mothers' behaviors and attitudes through a videotape modeling group discussion program. *Behavior Therapy, 12*(5), 634–642.

Webster-Stratton, C. (1982). The long-term effects of a video tape modeling parent-training program: Comparison of immediate and 1-year follow-up results. *Behavior Therapy, 13*(5), 702–714.

Weimer, D., & Vining, A. (1989). *Policy analysis: Concepts and practice.* Englewood Cliffs, NJ: Prentice-Hall.

Weinberg, B. (2001). An incentive model of the effect of parental income on children. *Journal of Political Economy, 109*(2), 266–280.

Weinberg, N. Z., Rahdert, E., Colliver, J. D., & Glantz, M. D. (1998). Adolescent substance abuse: A review of the past 10 years. *Journal of the American Academy of Child and Adolescent Psychiatry, 37*, 252–261.

Weissman, M. M., Warner, V., Wickramaratne, P. J., & Kandel, D. B. (1999). Maternal smoking during pregnancy and psychopathology in offspring followed to adulthood. *Journal of the American Academy of Child and Adolescent Psychiatry, 38*(7), 892–899.

Werner, E. E., & Smith, R. S. (1982). *Vulnerable but invincible: A longitudinal study of resilient children and youth.* New York: McGraw-Hill.

Whitbeck, L. B., Simons, R. L., Conger, R. D., Wickrama, K. A. S., Ackley, K. A., & Elder, G. H. (1997). The effects of parents' working conditions and family economic hardship on parenting behaviors and children's self-efficacy. *Social Psychology Quarterly, 60*, 291–303.

White, H. R. (1992). Early problem behavior and later drug problems. *Journal of Research in Crime and Delinquency, 29,* 412–429.

White, H. R., Brick, J., & Hansell, S. (1993, September). A longitudinal investigation of alcohol use and aggression in adolescence. *Journal of Studies on Alcohol,* (Suppl. 11), 62–77.

White, H. R., & Hansell, S. (1998). Acute and long-term effects of drug use on aggression from adolescence into adulthood. *Journal of Drug Issues, 28*(4), 837–858.

White, H. R., Hansell, S., & Brick, J. (1993). Alcohol use and aggression among youth. *Alcohol Health and Research World, 17*(2), 151–156.

White, H. R., & Labouvie, E. W. (1994). Generality versus specificity of problem behavior: Psychological and functional differences. *Journal of Drug Issues, 24*(1–2), 55–74.

White, H. R., Loeber, R., Stouthamer-Loeber, M., & Farrington, D. P. (1999). Developmental associations between substance use and violence. *Development and Psychopathology, 11*(4), 785–803.

White, W. A. T. (1988). A meta-analysis of the effects of direct instruction in special education. *Education and Treatment of Children, 11*(4), 364–374.

Wildey, M. B., Woodruff, S. I., Pampalone, S. Z., & Conway, T. L. (1995). Self-service sale of tobacco: How it contributes to youth access. *Tobacco Control, 4,* 355–361.

Willard, J. C., & Schoenborn, C. A. (1995). Relationship between cigarette smoking and other unhealthy behaviors among our nation's youth: US 1992. *Advance data from vital health statistics, 263.* Hyattsville, MD: National Center for Health Statistics.

Williams, C. L., Perry, C. L., Dudovitz, B., Veblen-Mortenson, S., Anstine, P. S., Komro, K. A., et al. (1995). A home-based prevention program for sixth-grade alcohol use: Results from Project Northland. *Journal of Primary Prevention, 16*(2), 125–147.

Williams, J. H., Ayers, C. D., Abbott, R. D., Hawkins, J. D., & Catalano, R. F. (1999). Racial differences in risk factors for delinquency and substance use among adolescents. *Social Work Research, 23*(4), 241–256.

Windle, M. (2000). Parental, sibling, and peer influences on adolescent substance use and alcohol problems. *Applied Developmental Science, 4,* 98–110.

Wolfson, M., Toomey, T. L., Forster, J. L., Wagenaar, A. C., McGovern, P. G., & Perry, C. L. (1996). Characteristics, policies, and practices of alcohol outlets and sales to underage persons. *Journal of Studies on Alcohol, 57*(6), 670–674.

Wolfson, M., Toomey, T. L., Murray, D. M., Forster, J. L., Short, B. J., & Wagenaar, A. C. (1996). Alcohol outlet policies and practices concerning sales to underage people. *Addiction, 91*(4), 589–602.

Wong, M. M., Zucker, R. A., Puttler, L. I., & Fitzgerald, H. E. (1999). Heterogeneity of risk aggregation for alcohol problems between early and middle childhood: nesting structure variations. *Development and Psychopathology, 11*(4), 727–744.

Woodward, L. J., & Fergusson, D. M. (1999). Early conduct problems and later risk of teenage pregnancy in girls. *Development and Psychopathology, 11*(1), 127–141.

Worden, J. K., Geller, B. A., Chen, M., Shelton, L. G., Secker-Walker, R. H., Solomon, D. S., et al. (1988). Development of a smoking prevention mass media program using diagnostic and formative research. *Preventive Medicine, 17,* 531–558.

World Health Organization. (2001). *Health behavior in school-aged children, 1996: United States.* Ann Arbor, MI: Inter-university Consortium for Political and Social Research.

Wyllie, A., Zhang, J. F., & Casswell, S. (1998). Positive responses to televised beer advertisements associated with drinking and problems reported by 18 to 29–year-olds. *Addiction, 93*(5), 749–760.

Yoshikawa, H. (1995). Long-term effects of early childhood programs on social outcomes and delinquency. *The Future of Children, 5*(3), 51–75.

Zador, P., Lund, A., Fields, M., & Weinberg, K. (1989). Fatal crash involvement and laws against alcohol-impaired driving. *Journal of Public Health Policy, 10,* 467–485.

Zhang, L., Wieczorek, W. F., & Welte, J. W. (1997). The nexus between alcohol and violent crime. *Alcoholism: Clinical and Experimental Research, 21*(7), 1264–1271.

Zigler, E., & Styfco, S. (2001). *The Head Start debates (friendly and otherwise).* New Haven, CT: Yale University Press.

Zimmerman, M. A., & Maton, K. I. (1992). Life-style and substance use among male African-American urban adolescents: A cluster analytic approach. *American Journal of Community Psychology, 20*(1), 121–138.

Zucker, R. A., Ellis, D. A., Bingham, C. R., & Fitzgerald, H. E. (1996). The development of alcoholic subtypes: Risk variation among alcoholic families during the early childhood years. *Alcohol Health and Research World, 20,* 46–54.

Zucker, R. A., Ellis, D. A., Bingham, C. R., Fitzgerald, H. E., & Sanford, K. (1996). Other evidence for at least two alcoholisms, II: Life course variation in antisociality and heterogeneity of alcoholic outcome. *Development and Psychopathology, 8,* 831–848.

Zucker, R. A., Fitzgerald, H. E., & Moses, H. D. (1995). Emergence of alcohol problems and the several alcoholisms: A developmental perspective on etiologic theory and life course trajectory. In D. Cicchetti & D. J. Cohen (Eds.), *Developmental psychopathology: Vol. 2. Risk, disorder, and adaptation* (pp. 677–711). New York: Wiley.

Zwerling, C., & Jones, M. P. (1999). Evaluation of the effectiveness of low blood alcohol concentration laws for younger drivers. *American Journal of Preventive Medicine, 16*(S1), 76–80.

Author Index

Aarons, S. J., 140
Abbott, R. D., 93, 117
Abernathy, T., 154
Acierno, R., 78
Adams, E. K., 38, 43
Ainsworth, M. S., 70
Aisquith, B. F., 155
Albrecht, H. T., 81
Alexander, J. F., 175, 176
Algina, J., 110
Alleyne, E., 198
Allred, C. G., 119
Altman, D. G., 154
Amdur, R. L., 188
Andrews, D. W., 187, 191, 192, 193, 218
Anes, M. D., 154
Anisman, H., 17
Anthony, J. C., 76, 112
Aos, S., 107, 108, 118, 123, 177, 179,
    181, 184, 185, 186
Arluck, G. M., 151
Armbruster, P., 124
Arnett, J. J., 80
Arthur, W. B., 36
Ary, D. V., 22, 24, 25, 90, 91, 131, 144,
    148, 191, 202, 208, 216, 218,
    247
Asbridge, M., 154
Aseltine, R. H., 13
Ashman, S. B., 68
Atkinson, D. R., 124, 159
Ayers, C. D., 117

B

Bachman, J. G., 5, 7, 11, 23, 30, 45
Baer, K., 178

Baker, E., 135, 136, 137
Baker, J., 164
Baker, T. K., 38, 159
Baltes, P. B., 14, 60
Barber, B. K., 84
Barber, J. G., 146, 163
Barkley, R. A., 183
Barnes, H. V., 107
Barnett, W. S., 73, 108, 109
Barnoski, R., 107, 123
Barone, C., 24
Barrera, M., Jr., 24, 90
Barrish, H. H., 111
Barth, R., 139
Bartholomae, S., 131
Barton, C., 176
Bartosch, W. J., 38
Bass, D., 120
Bates, J. E., 71, 82
Baugh, E. F., 68
Bauman, K. E., 143
Becker, D., 194
Beel, A., 160
Berglund, M. L., 235
Bergman, L. R., 24
Berk, M., 165
Berrueta-Clement, J. R., 73
Berry, C. C., 80
Biener, L., 80
Biglan, A., 17, 19, 22, 24, 25, 85, 86, 90,
    91, 94, 121, 131, 133, 144, 145,
    146, 147, 148, 155, 163, 166,
    167, 191, 201, 202, 208, 216,
    218, 227, 229, 240, 243, 246,
    247, 250
Bingham, C. R., 62

Birkhead, S. H., 154
Black, C., 208
Blehar, M. C., 70
Block-Pedego, A. E., 218
Blood, D. J., 142
Blose, J. O., 16
Blowers, P. A., 164
Blum, R. W., 10
Bogenschneider, M., 145
Boggess, S., 23
Boggs, S. R., 110
Bor, W., 119
Borduin, C. M., 177
Botvin, E. M., 135, 137
Botvin, G. J., 135, 136, 137
Bourbon, D., 159
Box, P., 111
Bransfield, S., 69
Brasfield, T. L., 198, 199
Brechman-Toussaint, M. L., 145, 218
Brennan, P. A., 67, 68
Brennan, P., 15
Breslau, N., 77
Brestan, E. V., 99, 101, 102, 103
Brewer, D. D., 161, 191
Brick, J., 22, 25
Briggs, X. S., 88
Brinkley, G., 89
Brody, G. H., 84
Brody, J. L., 176
Brondino, M. J., 125, 178, 179
Bronfenbrenner, U., 177
Brook, J. S., 75, 85
Brooks-Gunn, J., 80, 87
Brown, B., 66, 75
Brown, C. H., 15, 75, 100, 101, 102
Brown, J. D., 143
Brown, R. A., 75
Brown, S. A., 23, 191
Bukowski, W. M., 78
Bullock, B. M., 193
Bumbarger, B., 100
Burton, D., 134
Bushway, S. D., 100
Busner, J., 183
Buss, K. A., 69
Butterworth, T., 132

C

Cadoret, R. J., 67, 83
Cagampang, H., 139
Cain, C. A., 67
Calhoun, C., 36
Cameron, M., 163
Campbell, F. A., 73, 107, 109
Campbell, M., 182
Campos, J. J., 69

Capaldi, D., 85
Carmona, M., 147
Carnine, D. W., 244, 246
Carver, L. J., 68
Cash, R., 84
Caspi, A., 60, 70, 72, 81
Casswell, S., 146, 168
Casteel, C., 162
Catalano, R. F., Jr., 61, 93, 116, 117,
    161, 191, 225, 228, 235
Cater, J., 182
Caulkins, J., 161
Cavallo, A., 163
Celebucki, C., 167
Chabune, N., 197
Chaiken, J. M., 23
Chaiken, M. R., 23
Chaloupka, F. J., 88, 149, 150, 151, 152,
    168, 215
Chamberlain, P., 179, 180, 181, 225
Chambless, D. L., 99, 101, 102, 103
Champagne, F. A., 68
Cheng, Y.-T., 24
Chessare, J. B., 68
Chestnut, L. G., 36
Chilcoat, H. D., 77
Chisholm, K., 68, 74
Choi, W. S., 4, 80
Chou, C., 214
Chrousos, G. P., 81
Chung, P. J., 167
Cibelli, C. D., 70
Clark, S. J., 182
Clarke, S. H., 107, 109
Claxton, A. J., 16
Cloninger, C. R., 67
Coate, D., 149, 150, 151
Cohen, M. A., 34, 37, 38, 39, 42, 43, 44,
    107
Cohen, P., 75
Coleman, T., 70
Coles, C. M., 162
Colliver, J. D., 22, 197
Colon, I., 158
Colten, M. E., 13
Colvin, G., 76
Compton, W. M., 24
Comstock, G., 79
Conger, R. D., 84
Connolly, G. M., 168
Connolly, G. N., 167
Connor, D. F., 77, 183
Constantino, J. N., 182
Conway, T. L., 154
Cook, P. J., 151, 152
Costa, F. M., 24
Cottler, L. B., 24

Coultes, B., 163
Cox, A. D., 89
Cox, K. C., 31, 39, 42
Coyle, E. M., 111
Coyle, K., 140
Craft, C. A., 178
Cranston, K., 42, 4129
Crawford, G., 161
Crick, N. R., 78
Crockett, S. J., 145
Cromwell, J., 38, 44
Crouch, J. L., 179
Cueva, J. E., 182
Cummings, K. M., 150, 154
Cunningham, P. B., 177

D

Dadds, M. R., 84, 119, 217
Dahlberg, L. L., 178
Dakof, G. A., 194, 196
Danish, S. J., 24
Darroch, J. E., 38
Davidson, W. S., II, 167, 184, 188
Davies, M., 68
Davis, H. T., 183
Dawson, D. A., 75
Dawson, G., 68
Day, S. X., 130
De Mersseman, L. M., 111
DeCicca, P., 88
Deckel, A. W., 77
Dee, T. S., 88, 151
DeFries, J. C., 69
Delaney, M. A., 182
Dembo, R., 23
Dennis, M. L., 195, 196, 197
Dent, C. W., 17, 134, 143
Derzon, J. H., 75, 142, 145
DeWolff, M., 70
Diamantopolou, K., 163
Diaz, T., 135
Diekstra, R. F., W., 24
DiFranceisco, W. J., 42
DiFranza, J. R., 5, 154, 155
DiNardo, J., 160
Dishion, T. J., 71, 84, 85, 187, 188, 191,
    192, 193, 218
Disney, E. R., 77
Dodge, K. A., 71, 78, 82
Dolan, L. J., 112
Domitrovich, C. E., 100
Donohew, L., 144
Donovan, J. E., 24, 25
Dorfman, L., 141
Dorn, L. D., 81
Douglass, J. B., 38
Dresser, J., 159

Drotar, D., 125
Drummond, A. E., 163
Drummond, D. C., 159
Duffy, M., 168
Dufour, M., 22
Duncan, G. J., 87
Duncan, S. C., 24, 25, 84
Duncan, T. E., 24, 25, 84, 91, 208, 218
DuRant, R. H., 78
Dusenbury, L., 135, 136, 137
Dyte, D., 163

E

Earls, F., 87
Easterbrook, M. A., 70
Eccles, J. S., 86
Eck, J., 100
Eddy, J. M., 114, 180
Edelbrock, C. S., 183
Eiden, R. D., 70
Eisen, M., 140
Elder, G. H., 60, 166
Elder, J. P., 166
Elkins, I. J., 77
Ellickson, P., 25
Elliott, D. S., 2, 22, 23
Ellis, B. J., 82
Ellis, D. A., 62, 63
Emans, S. J., 78
Embry, D. D., 111, 156, 225
Emshoff, J., 134
Ennett, S. T., 138
Ensminger, M. E., 24, 25, 75
Epstein, A. S., 73
Evans, W. N., 150
Everingham, S. S., 153
Eyberg, S. M., 99, 101, 102, 103, 110

F

Fabian, R., 44
Fagan, J., 24
Fallon, T., 124
Farkas, A. J., 80
Farrell, A. D., 24, 25
Farrelly, M. C., 150
Farrington, D. P., 23, 59
Faulkner, A. H., 42, 4129
Fawcett, S. B., 225, 226, 227, 228, 229
Feighery, E. C., 154
Fell, J., 164
Ferdinand, R. F., 24
Ferguson, S. A., 165
Fergusson, D. M., 13, 23, 24, 25, 68, 75,
    78, 90
Fetrow, R. A., 114
Fichtenberg, C. M., 156

Fick, A. C., 87
Fields, M., 163, 165
Filazzola, A. D., 137
Findling, R. L., 183
Fiore, M. C., 38
Fisher, A., 36
Fisher, D. A., 34, 37, 42
Fitzgerald, H. E., 60, 62, 63, 71
Flay, B. R., 17, 79, 119, 121, 134, 143,
    167, 225
Flewelling, R. L., 138
Flynn, B. S., 142
Flynn, K., 142, 143, 167
Fong, G. T., 139
Foo, H.-H., 144
Foote, R. C., 110
Forehand, R. L., 84, 110
Forgatch, M. S., 75
Forrester, K. K., 86
Forster, J. L., 16, 89, 154, 155, 156, 158,
    160, 210
Foster, S. L., 62, 121, 240
Fountain, D., 34
Fountain, G., 34
Francis, D. D., 68
Francisco, V. T., 226, 229
Freed, G. L., 182
Freeman, R., 89
French, D., 84, 113
Friedman, A. S., 69
Friend, K., 147
Friese, B., 168
Fulker, D. W., 69
Funk, J. B., 79
Futterman, D. D., 144

G

Gantzer, S., 163
Garnefski, N., 24
Gensheimer, L. K., 167, 184
George, T. P., 78
Gibson, C. L., 67
Giesbrecht, N., 141, 142
Gilliam, W. S., 109
Gillmore, M. R., 25, 117
Gilpin, E. A., 4, 80, 167
Gim, R. H., 124
Giovino, G., 11, 79, 167
Glantz, M. D., 22, 77, 197
Glantz, S. A., 44, 156
Gleghorn, A., 23
Gliksman, L., 159, 160
Goeders, N. E., 82, 85
Gold, M. R., 33, 34, 35
Goldman, M. S., 81
Goldsmith, H. H., 69

Gomez, C., 140
Gordon, A. S., 75, 85
Gore, S., 13
Gorman-Smith, D., 87
Gottesman, I. I., 67
Gottfredson, D. C., 100
Gottlieb, G., 66
Gottschalk, R., 167, 184
Graham, J. W., 30
Grandy, G. S., 111
Granic, I., 193
Granick, S., 69
Grant, B. F., 75
Gray, B., 43
Gray, D., 159
Gregg, S., 189
Gregorich, S., 140
Grekin, E. R., 67, 68
Greenberg, M. T., 100, 101, 102
Grichting, W. L., 146
Griesler, P. C., 68
Grimes, J. D., 165
Grindel, C., 40
Grossman, M., 88, 149, 150, 151, 152
Grove, W. M., 67
Groves, W. B., 88
Grube, J. W., 141, 142, 158, 160, 164,
    168, 212
Gruber, J., 88
Gruenewald, P. J., 89, 151, 158, 159, 212
Grunbaum, J., 188
Gunnar, M. R., 68, 74
Gustan, S., 201
Guyll, M., 130

H

Haefele, W. F., 84
Haggerty, R. J., 100, 101, 102
Halberstam, D., 250
Haley, J., 177
Hanks, C., 106
Hanley, J. H., 179
Hanna, E. Z., 22
Hansell, S., 22, 25
Hansen, W. B., 30, 214
Hanson, C. L., 84
Harris, J. R., 82
Harris, V. W., 111
Hartmann, D. P., 78
Harwood, H. J., 34
Hasselblad, V., 38
Hatziandreu, E., 11
Haviland, M. B., 66
Hawkins, J. D., 61, 93, 116, 117, 118,
    161, 191, 225, 228, 235
He, J., 44

Heeren, T., 39, 164, 165
Henderson, C. E., 106, 194, 196
Henggeler, S. W., 84, 177, 178, 179, 191
Hennessy, M., 159
Henry, B., 70
Hesselbrock, V., 77
Hetherington, E. M., 82
Heywood, E., 83
Hill, K. G., 117
Hinds, M. W., 155
Hingson, R. W., 39, 163, 164, 165
Hogan, C., 224, 225
Hogue, A. T., 194, 195
Holder, H. D., 16, 18, 146, 147, 151,
        158, 160, 211, 212
Holder, W., 145
Hollis, J. F., 201
Hollon, S., 99, 101, 102
Holtgrave, D. R., 42, 412
Homel, R., 163
Hood, D., 218
Hops, H., 25, 84
Horner, R. H., 133
Horowitz, H. A., 70
Horwood, L. J., 13, 23, 24, 25, 68, 90
Houck, G. M., 69
Hourigan, M. E., 154, 155, 156
Howard, C. W., 24
Howard, M. O., 24
Howes, C., 73
Howland, J., 39, 163
Hoyle, R. H., 14
Huang, L. X., 150
Huber, H., 111
Huesmann, L. R., 79
Huizinga, D., 2, 23, 80
Huttunen, M. O., 68
Hyland, M., 150, 154

I

Iacono, W. G., 77, 83
Ialongo, N., 15
Inoff-Germain, G., 81
Irvine, A. B., 191, 192, 193
Isohanni, M., 68

J

Jacob, T., 62
Jamanka, A., 39
James, L. E., 208, 243
James-Ortiz, S., 136
Jason, L. A., 154, 155, 165
Jefferson, K. W., 198
Jemmott, J. B., 139
Jemmott, L. S., 139

Jensen, A. F., 37
Jernigan, D., 141
Jessor, R., 1, 24, 25
Jessor, S. L., 1
Ji, P. Y., 154
Joffe, J., 208
Johnson, B. M., 84
Johnson, C. A., 214
Johnson, M. B., 159
Johnson-Leckrone, J., 194
Johnston, L. D., 5, 7, 11, 22, 23, 26, 30,
        45, 152
Jones, M. P., 164
Jones, R. K., 164
Jorner, U., 151

K

Kamboukos, D., 87
Kandel, D. B., 68, 208
Kann, L., 165
Kaplan, S. L., 183
Karkowski, L. M., 67
Katz, A., 240
Kaufman, N., 193
Kavanagh, K., 193
Kazdin, A. E., 120
Keeler, E. B., 38
Kelder, S. H., 145, 156
Kellam, S. G., 15, 60, 74, 75, 76, 78, 93,
        111, 112, 120
Kelling, G. L., 162
Kelly, J. A., 42
Kelly, J. G., 229
Kendler, K. S., 67
Kenkel, D. S., 44, 88, 151
Kerner, J., 136
Kerrebrock, N., 150
Khalsa, J., 69
Kilpatrick, D. G., 78
Kincaid, M., 182
King, C. I., 167
King, J. A., 68
Kirby, D., 100, 101, 102, 131, 139, 140,
        162, 197, 199, 200
Kitzman, H., 105, 106, 109
Klebanov, P. K., 87
Klein, N. C., 176
Klonoff, E. A., 155
Klorman, R., 182
Koch, G. G., 143
Koehn, V., 155
Koenig, J., 38
Korpi, M., 139
Korte, S. M., 68
Kosterman, R., 93, 117
Kotsaftis, A., 183

Kowaleski-Jones, L., 85
Kracke, B., 81
Kracker, R., 144
Kreisher, C., 69
Kruk, M. R., 68
Ku, L., 87
Kupietz, S., 183

L

Labouvie, E. W., 23, 25
Lacey, J. H., 164
LaChance, P., 208
Ladd, G. W., 78
LaFond, C., 164
Laixuthai, A., 151
Landrine, H., 155
Landsburg, S. E., 17
Lang, E., 160
Lange, J. E., 159
Lantz, P. M., 201
LaPrelle, J., 143
Larson, R., 82
Laub, J. H., 87, 186
Lawrence, B. M., 37
Leboye, M., 197
Leffert, N., 61
Legrand, L. N., 83
Lemery, K. S., 69
Leonard, K. E., 62, 70
Lepper, H., 127
Leshner, A. I., 77
Lestina, D. C., 53
Levenson, S., 163
Levitsky, D. A., 66
Levitt, A., 145
Levy, D. T., 31, 39, 42, 147, 151
Lewinsohn, P. M., 75
Lewis-Palmer, T., 133
Lewit, E. M., 149, 150
Li, F., 24, 85, 90
Liberman, M., 182
Lichtenstein, E., 201, 202
Lichtman, K., 202
Liddle, H. A., 194, 196, 197
Lindberg, L. D., 23, 25
Lindenmayer, J. P., 183
Ling, X., 15, 78, 111
Lipsey, M. W., 75, 142, 145, 172, 174, 175, 184
Lipsitt, L. P., 14
Liu, D., 68
Livermore, G., 34
Loeber, R., 2, 13, 23, 25, 59, 77, 92
Lonczak, H. S., 93, 117, 235
Long, N., 110
Lorch, E. P., 144

Luebbert, J. F., 182
Luepker, R. V., 145
Lund, A., 163
Lynam, D. R., 77, 81
Lynch, B. S., 178
Lynch, M., 185
Lynn, W. R., 154
Lynskey, M. T., 13, 23, 24, 25, 78, 90
Lyons-Ruth, K., 70

M

MacKenzie, D. L., 100
MacKinnon, D. P., 142, 214, 225
Madden, P. A., 168
Madsen, C. H., 111
Magnusson, D., 24
Maibach, E., 145
Malmquist, S., 151
Malone, R. P., 182
Malow, R., 201
Manning, W. G., 38, 44, 149, 150
Marcus, S. M., 109
Marin, B., 140
Markie-Dadds, C., 119, 217
Markowitz, S., 152
Martin, S. E., 154, 164
Martinez, C. R., 62
Masse, L. C., 113
Matheny, A. P., Jr., 69
Mathios, A., 88
Maton, K. I., 24
Matson, J. L., 111
Mayer, G. R., 132, 133, 190
Mayer, J. P., 167, 184
Maynard, A., 4129
McAlister, A. L., 140
McCartney, K., 73
McCord, J., 187
McEvoy, L., 22, 75
McFadyen-Ketchum, S., 82
McGee, L., 23, 25
McGovern, P. G., 154, 155, 165, 211
McGue, M., 77, 83
McGuigan, K. A., 25
McLean, J., 163
McLoyd, V. C., 74, 87
McMahon, R. J., 110
McMurray, M. B., 183
Meaney, M. J., 68
Mednick, S. A., 15, 67, 68
Meinhardt, G., 145
Melton, G. B., 179
Melvin, C. L., 38, 43
Menard, S., 2
Merali, Z., 17
Mercer, G. W., 163

Merisca, R., 15
Meschke, L. L., 131
Metzler, C. W., 22, 85, 90, 91, 131, 133, 190, 191, 225
Midgley, C., 86
Millar, A., 89
Miller, J., 191
Miller, L. S., 87
Miller, P. M., 81
Miller, T. R., 31, 34, 35, 36, 37, 38, 39, 40, 42, 44, 53
Miller-Johnson, S., 73
Miner, L. L., 22
Minuchin, S., 177
Mitchell, C. M., 188
Moberg, D. P., 140
Modzeleski, W., 165
Moeti, R., 134
Moffitt, T. E., 69, 70, 77, 81
Moilanen, I., 68
Moise, J. F., 79
Monaghan, T. M., 184
Montgomery, D. T., 145, 218
Moore, V., 163, 181
Moran, J. R., 168
Morishima, J. K., 124
Mortensen, E. L., 68
Moschis, G. P., 89
Moses, H. D., 60
Moskowitz, J. M., 143
Mott, F. L., 85
Mott, M. A., 23
Mouren-Simeoni, M. C., 197
Moynihan, D. P., 236, 237
Mrazek, P., 100, 101, 102, 225, 246
Mullan, N., 163
Mullis, R., 145
Murray, D. M., 16, 143, 147, 158, 160, 183, 210, 211
Myers, M. G., 23

N

Nafpaktitis, M., 132
Nansel, T. R., 86
Neale, M. C., 67
Neckerman, H. J., 161
Neiderhiser, J. M., 82
Nelson, C., 145
Nelson, J. P., 168
Nelson, S., 193
Neugebauer, R., 87
Newcomb, A. F., 78
Newcomb, M. D., 23, 25
Newhouse, J. P., 38, 149, 150
Nichter, M., 79, 167
Niskanen, P., 68

Noack, P., 80
Noell, J. W., 22, 91, 131
Nottelmann, E. D., 81

O

O'Brien, C. P., 197
Ochs, L., 131
O'Connor, P., 77
Oden, S., 109, 110, 122
O'Donnell, C. R., 188
O'Donnell, J., 116
O'Grady, B., 154
O'Keefe, Z., 144
Olds, D. L., 20, 105, 106, 107, 109, 225
O'Malley, P. M., 5, 7, 11, 23, 30, 45, 152, 164
Ordway, N., 119
Orlandi, M., 154
Ornstein, S. I., 151
Osgood, D. W., 23, 24, 25
Ozechowski, T., 197

P

Pacula, R. L., 149, 152
Padgett, C. A., 143
Pagani-Kurtz, L., 113
Paik, H., 79
Paikoff, R. L., 80
Paine-Andrews, A., 226, 229
Pallonen, U. E., 202
Palmgreen, P., 144
Pampalone, S. Z., 154
Parmley, W. W., 44
Parsons, B. V., 176
Pascoe, M., 68
Patsdaughter, C. A., 40
Pattee, L., 78
Patterson, G. R., 71, 75, 76, 84, 85, 166, 187, 190
Pechacek, T. F., 154
Peek-Asa, C., 162
Peisner-Feinberg, E. S., 73
Pentz, M. A., 142, 165, 213, 214
Perla, J., 154
Perrin, E. C., 125
Perry, C. L., 107, 108, 109, 123, 145, 209, 210
Petersen, A. C., 81
Peterson, J. B., 77
Peterson, M., 70
Peterson, T. R., 176
Pettit, G. S., 71, 82
Phelps, C., 106
Phillips, D. A., 70, 72, 73
Phipps, P., 107, 123

Pickrel, S. G., 178, 179
Pierce, J. P., 4, 11, 80, 167
Pierre, N., 78
Pihl, R. O., 77, 113
Pindus, N. M., 38
Pinkerton, S. D., 42, 4129
Piper, D. L., 140
Piquero, A. R., 67
Pirie, P. L., 145
Pleck, J. H., 87
Plomin, R., 69, 82
Podolski, C. L., 79
Ponicki, W. R., 89, 151
Poon, E., 63
Portnoy, S., 77
Poulin, F., 187
Prescott, C. A., 67
Preusser, D. F., 158
Pungello, E., 73
Puttler, L. I., 71

R

Radziszewska, B., 17
Rahdert, E., 197
Raine, A., 15, 69
Ramey, C. T., 73
Ramsey, E., 76
Rantakallio, P., 68
Rappaport, J., 229
Raudenbush, S. W., 63, 87
Rebok, G. W., 60
Redmond, C., 127, 129, 130, 131
Redner, R., 188
Reese, H. W., 14
Reid, J. B., 71, 114, 180, 190
Reilly, B. A., 152
Reilly, S. L., 66
Reina-Patton, A., 155
Reiss, D., 82, 83
Renick, N. L., 136, 137
Reuter, P., 100, 161
Reynolds, C. J., 111
Richards, M. H., 82
Richardson, J. L., 17, 95
Ridge, B., 71
Rigotti, N. A., 155
Riley, D., 145
Rind, B., 79
Ringwalt, C. L., 138
Ritta, A., 202
Robbins, K., 183
Roberts, R. E., 124
Roberts, S. J., 40
Robins, L. N., 22, 75
Rodgers, G. B., 37
Rodnick, J. D., 84
Rohde, P., 75

Romano, E. O., 40, 44
Ross, H. L., 163, 165
Rossman, S. B., 38
Rotheram-Borus, M. J., 144, 162, 163,
　　197, 198, 200
Rots, N. Y., 68
Roussos, S. T., 226, 227, 228
Rowe, C., 194
Rowland, M. D., 177, 179
Rubin, B., 75
Rueter, M. A., 84
Ruhm, C. J., 151
Rusby, J. C., 86, 133
Rushton, J. L., 182
Russell, L. B., 33
Rutter, M., 63, 91
Ryan, A., 163
Ryan, J. A. M., 235
Rydell, C. P., 153
Rydon, P., 160

S

Saffer, H., 88, 151, 152, 168
Saggers, S., 159
Saigh, P. A., 111
Salend, S. J., 111
Salisbury, M., 145
Saltz, R. F., 159, 160
Sameroff, A. J., 63
Sampson, R. J., 63, 87, 88, 186, 190, 226
Sanders, M. R., 84, 119, 145, 217, 218
Saner, H., 25
Sanford, K., 62
Sargent, J. D., 80
Saudino, K. J., 69
Saunders, M., 111
Saunders-Martin, A., 154
Savageau, J. A., 155
Scales, P. C., 61
Scarr, S., 73
Schaal, B., 75
Schenzler, C., 152
Scherer, D. G., 179
Schiavo, R. S., 176
Schillo, B. A., 184
Schmitz, S., 69
Schneiger, A., 193
Schnopp-Wyatt, D. L., 165
Schoenborn, C. A., 22, 25
Schoenwald, S. K., 177, 225
Schonfeld, I. S., 77
Schuckit, M. A., 23
Schuhmann, E. M., 110
Schultz, J. A., 226, 229
Schweinhart, L. J., 73, 107, 109
Sciandra, R., 154
Scovill, L. C., 80, 81

Sealand, N., 87
Segal, B., 183
Seifer, R., 71
Severson, H. H., 218
Shaffer, D., 77
Shaffer, G., 154
Sheflin, N., 151
Sherman, J. A., 111
Sherman, L. W., 100, 101, 102
Shin, C. J. S., 129, 130, 131
Shonkoff, J. P., 70, 72
Shopland, D., 11
Shrier, L. A., 78
Sickmund, M., 4, 10
Siegel, A. W., 80, 81
Siegel, J. E., 33
Siegel, M., 80, 167
Siegel, T. C., 120
Silbereisen, R. K., 80, 81
Silva, P. A., 70, 77, 81, 168
Sing, C. F., 66
Singh, S., 87
Slesnick, N., 176
Sloan, F. A., 152
Sloss, E. M. S., 38
Slovic, P., 5
Small, M. L., 165
Smith, D. I., 159
Smith, G. T., 81
Smith, R. G., 164
Smith, R. S., 74
Smith, S. V., 37
Smolkowski, K., 22, 85, 91, 191, 208
Snyder, H. N., 4, 10
Snyder, L. B., 142
Sonenstein, F. L., 87
Sorensen, L., 40
Sparling, J., 73
Spicer, R. S., 39, 40, 44, 53
Spoth, R. L., 127, 129, 130, 131, 225
Spracklen, K. M., 85, 187
Sprague, J. R., 133
Sputore, B., 159
Stacy, A. W., 134, 142
Stark, M. J., 124
Stein, R. E., K., 125
Stephenson, M. T., 144
Stevens, V. J., 201
Stevenson, L. Y., 42
Stewart, F., 38
Stewart, L., 146
Stice, E., 23
Stockwell, T., 160
Stoddard, J. J., 43
Stone, M., 145
Stoolmiller, M., 75, 114
Stouthamer-Loeber, M., 13, 23, 59, 77

Strupp, B. J., 66
Stuster, J. W., 164
Styfco, S., 109
Sue, S., 124
Sugai, G., 133
Sullivan, G., 163
Sulzer-Azaroff, B., 132
Susman, E. J., 81
Sussman, S. Y., 134, 202
Swiezy, N. B., 111
Swisher, J. D., 165

T

Talbot, B., 165
Tarnowski, K. J., 125
Tarter, R., 69
Tauchen, G., 151
Tauras, J. A., 88, 149, 150
Taylor, T. K., 146, 227
Taylor-Greene, S., 133
Templeton, A. R., 66
Themba, M., 141
Thomas, S. M., 87
Thornberry, T. P., 2
Thornton, T. N., 178
Tibbetts, S. G., 67
Tippetts, A. S., 164
Tobler, N. S., 131, 133, 134, 135, 138
Todd, A. W., 133
Todis, B. J., 218
Tolan, P., 87
Tolley, G., 44
Tonry, M., 185
Toomey, T. L., 89, 147, 157, 160
Tortu, S., 137
Trebow, E. A., 214
Tremblay, R. E., 75, 113
Treno, A. J., 146
Tromovitch, P., 79
Troughton, E., 83
Trussell, J., 38, 40, 42, 4129
Tully, L. A., 119
Turner, C. W., 176
Tye, J. B., 154

U

Umar, A. M., 111

V

Valli, R., 158
Van Horn, Y. V., 15
van IJzendoorn, M. H., 70
Van Kammen, W. B., 23, 59
Veblen-Mortenson, S., 209
Verhulst, F. C., 24
Vernon, S. W., 124

Vingilis, E., 163
Vining, A., 31
Violette, D. M., 36
Viscusi, W. K., 36, 37
Vitaro, F., 113
Voas, R. B., 159, 164, 165, 212
Vogt, T. M., 201, 202
von Cleve, E., 116, 117

W

Wachs, T. D., 59, 62, 74, 80, 93
Wagenaar, A. C., 16, 89, 144, 147, 148,
        157, 158, 160, 164, 210, 216,
        225, 247
Wakefield, M., 79, 167, 215
Wakschlag, L. S., 67
Waldron, H. B., 176, 188
Walker, H. M., 76, 218
Walker, P. S., 24
Walker, R. D., 24
Wall, S., 70
Wallack, L., 141, 145, 168
Walsh, A., 70
Wang, L. Y., 38
Warburton, J., 176
Warner, V., 68
Wasserman, G. A., 87
Wasserman, J., 38, 149, 150
Wassermann, E., 183
Waters, E., 70
Webster-Stratton, C., 119
Wechsler, H., 150
Weikart, D. P., 73, 107, 109
Weimer, D., 31
Weinberg, B., 74
Weinberg, K., 163
Weinberg, N. Z., 22, 197
Weinstein, M. C., 33
Weis, J. G., 24
Weissman, M. M., 68
Wells, E. A., 191
Welte, J. W., 23
Werner, E. E., 74
Whitbeck, L. B., 74
White, H. R., 13, 22, 23, 24, 25
White, W. A. T., 120

Whiteman, M., 75, 85
Wickramaratne, P. J., 68 Wieczorek, W.
        F., 23
Wiersema, B., 37
Wildey, M. B., 154
Willard, J. C., 22, 25
Williams, A. F., 158
Williams, C. L., 145
Williams, J. H., 117
Williams, S., 23
Wilson, D. B., 172, 174
Windle, M., 85
Winkler, J. D., 149, 150
Winnett, T., 145
Winter, M., 164, 165
Wold, M. M., 111
Wolfson, M., 16, 158, 160, 210
Wong, M. M., 71
Woodruff, S. I., 154
Woodward, L. J., 68, 75
Worden, J. K., 142, 145
Wyllie, A., 168

X

Xie, Y., 109

Y

Yoerger, K., 75, 85
Yoshikawa, H., 107
Yudelson, H., 145, 218

Z

Zador, P., 163
Zamula, W. F., 37
Zellman, G. L., 140
Zentall, S. R., 131
Zerba, K. E., 66
Zhang, J. F., 168
Zhang, L., 23
Zigler, E. F., 109
Zimmerman, M. A., 24
Ziskind, D., 201
Zoref, L., 208
Zucker, R. A., 60, 62, 63, 69, 71
Zwerling, C., 164

Subject Index

"*f*" following a page number indicates a figure; "*t*" following a page number indicates a table.

Abortions, costs to society and, 40–42. *see also* Sexual behavior
Academic failure. *see also* School
  early aggression and, 76
  in middle childhood, 77–78
ADHD, pharmacotherapy and, 182–183
Adolescent development, 80–89. *see also* Development
Adolescent Transitions Program. *see also* Intervention
  description, 187, 191–193
  substance use and, 191
Advertising, 167–168. *see also* Media
Advocacy. *see also* Policy
  community-based, 240–241
  media-based interventions as, 145–147
Aggressive behavior. *see also* Antisocial behavior; Violence
  Good Behavior Game and, 111–112
  Iowa Strengthening Families Program and, 128–130
  in middle childhood, 75–76*t*
  pharmacotherapy for treatment of, 181–183
  questionable interventions for, 185–186
  school-based interventions regarding, 132–133
  television viewing and, 79–80
Alcohol use. *see also* Multiproblem youth
  in alternative schools, 189*t*
  Communities Mobilizing for Change on Alcohol program and, 210–211

community-based interventions and, 219
Community Trials Project and, 211–213
description, 5–6*f*
differences in, 10–12, 11*t*
economy and, 88–89
interventions for, 190–191, 202–206
Iowa Strengthening Families Program and, 128–130
media-based interventions and, 141–147
methods used to estimate the costs of, 39
in middle childhood, 75–76*t*
Midwestern Prevention Program and, 213–214
peer influences on, 85
perceived benefits of, 80–81
policy regarding, 151–152, 156–160, 163–165, 168
Project Northland and, 209–210
Project SixTeen and, 208
relationship to other problem behaviors, 23–25, 27–29, 28*f*
Saving Lives Project and, 211
school-based interventions regarding, 133–139
statewide policy regarding, 215
Antisocial behavior. *see also* Aggressive behavior; Criminal acts; Delinquency; Multiproblem youth; Violence

Antisocial behavior (*continued*)
    community-based interventions and,
        216–217, 219
    description, 3–4
    differences in, 10–12, 11*t*
    drug use and, 85
    genetic influences of development and,
        82–83
    interventions for, 173–175, 202–206
    juvenile justice interventions and, 183–
        185
    methods used to estimate the costs of,
        42–43
    in middle childhood, 75–76*t*
    Multidimensional Family Therapy and,
        194–196
    Multidimensional Treatment Foster
        Care and, 179–181
    Multisystemic Therapy and, 177–179
    questionable interventions for, 185–186
    relationship to other problem
        behaviors, 23–25, 27–29, 28*f*
Assessment
    of interventions, 248–249
    ongoing within the community, 231–
        238, 237*f*
Attachment
    infancy and early childhood
        development and, 70
    stress and, 74
Automobile accidents. *see also* Drunk
        driving
    alcohol use and, 22, 163–165
    Community Trials Project and, 211–
        213
    costs of, 34–35
    policy regarding availability and
        opportunity of alcohol and, 156–
        157
    policy regarding the price of alcohol
        and, 151–152
    Saving Lives Project and, 211
Awareness of behaviors, 18–19

B

Becoming a Responsible Teen program,
    198–200. *see also* Intervention
Behavior. *see also* Aggressive behavior;
        Antisocial behavior
    consequences and, 17
    policy and, 147
Behavior management, in schools, 132–
    133
Behavioral scientist, role in collaborative
        partnerships, 229–230
Binge drinking. *see also* Alcohol use
    drug use and, 22

methods used to estimate the costs of,
    39
rates of, 6
Biopsychosocial characteristics, 15–16*t*
Birth complications, 15. *see also* Prenatal
        development
Birth control, 162–163. *see also*
        Condoms; Sexual behavior
Boot camps, 185. *see also* Intervention
Bullying, within schools, 86

C

Cambridge–Somerville Youth Study, 187–
    188
Childcare, infancy and early childhood
        development and, 72–73
Christchurch study, 90–92
Cigarette smoking. *see also* Multiproblem
        youth
    Adolescent Transitions Program and,
        192–193
    in alternative schools, 189*t*
    community-based interventions and,
        219
    description, 4–5*f*
    differences in, 10–12, 11*t*
    economy and, 88–89
    interventions and, 187–190, 189*t*, 201–
        202, 202–206
    Iowa Strengthening Families Program
        and, 128–130
    likelihood of other behaviors and, 22
    media-based interventions and, 141–
        147
    media representation and, 79–80
    methods used to estimate the costs of,
        43–44
    in middle childhood, 75–76*t*
    Midwestern Prevention Program and,
        213–214
    Multidimensional Treatment Foster
        Care and, 181
    policy regarding, 149–150*t*, 154–156,
        165–166, 167
    during pregnancy, 67–69
    Project SixTeen and, 208
    relationship to other problem
        behaviors, 23–25, 27–29, 28*f*
    school-based interventions regarding,
        133–139
    shared vision and, 227
    statewide policy regarding, 215
Cocaine abuse, costs to society and, 39–
    40. *see also* Drug use
Coercive family processes. *see also*
        Family; Parenting
    description, 110–111

early aggression and, 76
as a risk factor, 71–72
Collaborative partnerships. *see also*
    Community
recommendations from, 249–250
shared vision of, 226–231
Communication
    within the family, 84–85
    Functional Family Therapy and, 175–177
    Project Northland and, 209–210
    sexual behavior and, 131–132
Communities Mobilizing for Change on
    Alcohol program, 210–211. *see
    also* Intervention
Communities That Care, 228–229. *see
    also* Collaborative partnerships
Community
    adolescent development and, 86–87
    collaborative partnerships and, 226–231
    developmental interventions and, 238–243, 244t–245t, 246–247
    focusing on, 19
    ideal, 223–226
    innovations and, 247–250
    interventions based in, 208–214, 215–221
    Multisystemic Therapy and, 177–179
    ongoing assessment within, 231–238, 237f
    Pittsburgh Youth Study on, 92
    policing within, 166–167
Community Trials Project, 211–213. *see
    also* Intervention
Condoms. *see also* Sexual behavior
    access to, 162–163
    following Becoming a Responsible Teen
    program, 199
Consequences
    effect on behavior, 17
    Functional Family Therapy and, 175–177
    of incarceration, 186
    Multidimensional Treatment Foster
    Care and, 179–181
    of multiple problem behavior, 27–29, 28f
    policy regarding, 163–167
    punishment as, 190
Costs to society. *see also individual
    intervention programs*
    concepts of evaluating, 33–38
    description, 12, 55–56
    imposed by multiproblem youth, 44–46, 45t, 47t–51t, 52t–53, 54t, 55t
    interventions and, 106–107, 108

Iowa Strengthening Families Program
    and, 130
methods used to estimate, 38–44
reasons to assess, 31–33
youth diversion programs and, 184
Criminal acts. *see also* Antisocial behavior
    definitions of, 3–4
    drug use and, 22
    Functional Family Therapy and, 175–177
    incarceration and, 186
    interventions and, 173–175, 187–190, 189t, 202–206
    juvenile justice interventions and, 183–185
    methods used to estimate the costs of, 42–43
    Multidimensional Treatment Foster
    Care and, 179–181
    Multisystemic Therapy and, 177–179
    policy regarding, 152, 161, 166–167
    prevention efforts in, 161–162
    questionable interventions for, 185–186
Cumulative continuity, 60. *see also*
    Development

D

DARE, 138–139. *see also* Intervention
Daycare, infancy and early childhood
    development and, 72–73
Decision making, influences on, 14
Delinquency. *see also* Antisocial behavior;
    Criminal acts
    Adolescent Transitions Program and, 191–193
    Functional Family Therapy and, 175–177
    incarceration and, 186
    interventions for, 173–175, 202–206
    interventions that promote, 187–190, 189t
    juvenile justice interventions and, 183–185
    Multidimensional Treatment Foster
    Care and, 179–181
    Multisystemic Therapy and, 177–179
    pharmacotherapy for treatment of, 181–183
    questionable interventions for, 185–186
Depression
    during adolescence, 80
    alcohol use and, 22
    SSRIs and, 182
Development. *see also* Life course
    developmental perspective
    adolescence, 80–89

Development (*continued*)
    implications for prevention and
        interventions, 92–95, 218–219,
        238–243, 244*t*–245*t*, 246–247
    infancy and early childhood, 69–74
    middle childhood, 74–80, 76*t*
    prenatal and perinatal, 63, 66–69
    risk factors throughout, 63, 64*t*–65*t*
Diversion programs, 183–184. *see also*
        Criminal acts; Intervention
Drug abuse. *see also* Drug use
    description, 7–9*f*, 8*f*
    differences in, 10–12, 11*t*
Drug Abuse Resistance Education, 138–
        139. *see also* Intervention
Drug dependence. *see also* Drug use
    description, 7–9*f*, 8*f*
    differences in, 10–12, 11*t*
Drug use. *see also* Multiproblem youth
    Adolescent Transitions Program and,
        191–193
    in alternative schools, 189*t*
    binge drinking and, 22
    compared to abuse or dependence of
        drugs, 7–8
    description, 7–9*f*, 8*f*
    differences in, 10–12, 11*t*
    economy and, 88–89
    Functional Family Therapy and, 176–
        177
    interventions for, 190–191, 196–197,
        202–206
    Iowa Strengthening Families Program
        and, 128–130
    media-based interventions and, 141–147
    methods used to estimate the costs of,
        39–40
    Midwestern Prevention Program and,
        213–214
    Multidimensional Family Therapy and,
        194–196
    Multidimensional Treatment Foster
        Care and, 181
    Multisystemic Therapy and, 177–179
    peer influences on, 85
    pharmacotherapy for treatment of,
        181–183
    policy regarding, 152–153, 160–161
    Project SixTeen and, 208
    relationship to other problem
        behaviors, 23–25, 27–29, 28*f*
    school-based interventions regarding,
        133–139
    violence and, 42
Drunk driving. *see also* Alcohol use;
        Automobile accidents
    Community Trials Project and, 211–213

policy regarding the consequences of,
        163–165
    Saving Lives Project and, 211

E

Early childhood development. *see also*
        Development
    description, 69–74
    interventions during, 104–110, 218
Economy. *see also* Costs to society
    adolescent development and, 87–89
    assessment and, 236, 237*f*
    infancy and early childhood
        development and, 73–74
Environment
    design, 161–162
    genetic influences of development and,
        66–67
    relationship to future problem
        behaviors, 15–16*t*
    supportive, 94–95
    temperament and, 69
Environmental design, 161–162
Estrogen, 81–82
Ethnic differences
    description, 10–12, 11*t*, 61–62
    interventions and, 124–126
    multiproblem youth and, 24–25
Executive functioning deficits, in middle
        childhood, 77–78
Experimental evaluation, 19

F

Failure, academic. *see also* School
    early aggression and, 76
    in middle childhood, 77–78
Family
    adolescent development and, 83–85
    Adolescent Transitions Program and,
        191–193
    Christchurch study on, 90–92
    coercive family processes and, 71–72,
        76, 110–111
    early aggression and, 76
    Functional Family Therapy and, 175–177
    genetic influences of development and,
        82–83
    infancy and early childhood
        development and, 70–72
    interventions and, 124–125, 128–132
    Linking Interests of Families and
        Teachers program and, 114–115
    media-based interventions and, 144–
        145
    Montreal Longitudinal Experimental
        Study and, 112–114

Multidimensional Treatment Foster
Care and, 179–181
Multisystemic Therapy and, 177–179
Pittsburgh Youth Study on, 92
Project Northland and, 209–210
puberty and, 81–82
punishment within, 190
Seattle Social Development Program
and, 115–118
Fast Track, 120. see also Intervention
Functional Family Therapy. see also
Intervention
description, 175–177
substance use and, 191

G

Gender differences
description, 10–12, 11t, 61–62
multiproblem youth and, 24–25
in puberty, 81–82
Genetic influences
during adolescent development, 82–83
interventions and, 93–94
during prenatal and perinatal
development, 66–67
Good Behavior Game, 111–112. see also
Intervention
Government response. see Policy
Group norms, effect on behavior, 19
Group treatment, that promotes
delinquency, 187–190, 189t. see
also Intervention

H

Head Start, 109–110. see also
Intervention
Health-related problems
access to health care and condoms and,
162–163
alcohol use and, 22
policy regarding availability and
opportunity of alcohol and, 157–
158
quality of life and, 35–37
Heroin abuse, costs of, 39–40. see also
Drug use
High school dropouts, costs of, 44
HIV/AIDS. see also Sexual behavior
access to health care and condoms and,
162–163
Becoming a Responsible Teen program
and, 198–200
drug use and, 7
interventions and, 200–201
methods used to estimate the costs of,
40–42

rates of, 10, 11–12
school-based interventions regarding,
139–140
Homicide. see Murder
Hormones, 81–82. see also Adolescent
development

I

Identity development, during adolescence,
80
Incarceration. see also Intervention
description, 186
interventions and, 174–175
as punishment, 190
Incidence-based costs, 34. see also Costs
to society
Indicated interventions, 172. see also
Intervention
Infancy development. see also
Development
description, 69–74
interventions during, 218
Informed consent, in community
assessment, 233–234
Innovations, 247–250
Institutionalization. see also Criminal acts
description, 186
interventions and, 174–175
as punishment, 190
Intellectual deficits, in middle childhood,
77–78
Interactional continuity, 60. see also
Development
Intervention. see also Prevention
Adolescent Transitions Program, 191–
193
Becoming a Responsible Teen program,
198–200
community-based, 208–214, 215–221
costs of, 34
for delinquency and antisocial behavior,
173–175
description, 20, 30, 121–126, 172–
173
developmental implications for, 92–95,
238–243, 244t–245t, 246–247
effective, 98, 99t–103t, 104
family-focused, 128–132
Functional Family Therapy, 175–177
incarceration as, 186
juvenile justice, 183–185
Multidimensional Family Therapy,
194–196
Multidimensional Treatment Foster
Care, 179–181
Multisystemic Therapy, 177–179
pharmacotherapy as, 181–183

Intervention (*continued*)
   during prenatal, perinatal and early
      childhood, 104–110
   punishment as, 190
   questionable, 185–186
   research needed to implement, 243,
      246–247
   for school-age children, 110–120
   school-based, 132–140, 141
   for sexual behavior, 197–198, 200–201
   statewide, 215
   for substance misuse, 190–191, 196–
      197
   that promote delinquency, 187–190,
      189*t*
   that target cigarette smoking, 201–202
   via the media, 140–147
Iowa Strengthening Families Program,
      128–130. *see also* Intervention

J

Job Training Partnership Act, 185–186.
      see also Intervention
Juvenile justice interventions, 183–185.
      see also Intervention

K

Kids Count report card system, 235–236.
      see also Assessment

L

Law. *see* Policy
Life course developmental perspective. *see
      also* Development
   description, 14–19, 16*t*
   of multiple problem behavior, 60–63
Life Skills Training program, 135–137.
      see also Intervention
Linking Interests of Families and Teachers
      program, 114–115. *see also*
      Intervention
Lithium, 182

M

Marijuana use. *see* Drug use
Media
   Communities Mobilizing for Change on
      Alcohol program and, 210–211
   Community Trials Project and, 211–
      213
   effect in middle childhood, 79–80
   effect on behavior, 19
   intervention campaigns via, 140–147,
      230–231, 240–241
   policy regarding advertising, 167–
      168

Medical costs. *see also* Costs to society
   description, 34
   imposed by multiproblem youth, 44–
      46, 45*t*, 47*t*–51*t*, 52*t*–53, 54*t*, 55*t*
Medications, 181–183
Middle childhood development. *see also*
      Development
   description, 74–80, 76*t*
   interventions during, 110–120, 218–219
Midwestern Prevention Program, 213–
      214. *see also* Intervention
Montreal Longitudinal Experimental
      Study, 112–114. *see also*
      Intervention
Multidimensional Family Therapy, 194–
      196. *see also* Intervention
Multidimensional Treatment Foster Care,
      179–181
Multiproblem youth. *see also* Alcohol use;
      Antisocial behavior; Cigarette
      smoking; Drug use; Sexual
      behavior
   consequences and, 27–29, 28*f*
   costs imposed by, 44–46, 45*t*, 47*t*–51*t*,
      52*t*–53, 54*t*, 55*t*–56
   description, 3, 23–25, 30
   interventions and, 204–206, 204–206
   life course developmental perspective
      of, 60–63
   public health perspective's focus on, 14
   rates of, 22–23
   research regarding, 89–92, 91*f*
   serious levels of, 23
Multisystemic Therapy. *see also*
      Intervention
   description, 177–179
   substance use and, 191
Murder. *see also* Antisocial behavior;
      Criminal acts
   alcohol use and, 22
   youth rates of, 4

N

National assessment system, 234–238,
      237*f*. *see also* Assessment
Norms, group, effect on behavior, 19

O

Olds Nurse Visitation Program, 105–107,
      108–109. *see also* Intervention

P

Parenting
   adolescent development and, 83–85
   Adolescent Transitions Program and,
      191–193

coercive family processes and, 71–72,
    76, 110–111
early aggression and, 76
Functional Family Therapy and, 175–
    177
genetic influences of development and,
    82–83
infancy and early childhood
    development and, 70–72, 73–74
interventions and, 124–125, 128–132
Linking Interests of Families and
    Teachers program and, 114–115
media-based interventions and, 144–
    145
Montreal Longitudinal Experimental
    Study and, 112–114
Multidimensional Treatment Foster
    Care and, 179–181
Multisystemic Therapy and, 177–179
Project Northland and, 209–210
puberty and, 81–82
punishment and, 190
Seattle Social Development Program
    and, 115–118
training programs targeting, 119–120
Triple-P program, 119–120, 217–218
Partnerships, collaborative. see also
    Community
recommendations from, 249–250
shared vision of, 226–231
Peer relationships
adolescent development and, 85
interventions that promote delinquency
    and, 187–189t
in middle childhood, 78
Montreal Longitudinal Experimental
    Study and, 112–114
Multidimensional Family Therapy and,
    194–196
Multidimensional Treatment Foster
    Care and, 179–181
Multisystemic Therapy and, 177–179
victimization and, 86
Perinatal development. see also
    Development
description, 63, 66–69
interventions during, 104–110
Perry Preschool Project, 107–108, 108–
    109. see also Intervention
Persuasion
effect on behavior, 19
Project Northland's utilization of, 209–
    210
sexual behavior and, 131–132
via the media, 141–147
Pharmacotherapy, 181–183
Pittsburgh Youth Study, 92

Policy
assuring detection and consequences,
    163–167
Communities Mobilizing for Change on
    Alcohol program and, 210–211
community-based, 219
description, 147–148
media-based interventions and, 145–147
recommendations, 203
regarding advertising, 167–168
regarding availability and opportunity,
    154–163
regarding effective practices, 241–242
regarding the price of substances, 149,
    150t, 151–154
statewide, 215
value of, 168–170
Positive Action Program, 118–119. see
    also Intervention
Positive reinforcement, effect on behavior,
    17
Pregnancy. see also Sexual behavior
access to health care and condoms and,
    162–163
interventions and, 200–201, 218
methods used to estimate the costs of,
    40–42
prenatal and perinatal development
    and, 66–69, 104–110
relationship to other problem
    behaviors, 29
risk factors throughout, 63, 66–69
smoking during, 43
Prenatal development. see also
    Development
birth complications and, 15
description, 63, 66–69
interventions during, 104–110, 218
Preparing for the Drug-Free Years
    program, 130–131. see also
    Intervention
Prevalence-based costs, 33–34. see also
    Costs to society
Prevention. see also Intervention
of crime, 161–162
description, 20, 30
developmental implications for, 92–95
research regarding, 121–126
universal, 127–128
Privacy, in community assessment, 234
Project Northland, 209–210. see also
    Intervention
Project SixTeen, 208. see also Intervention
Protective factors
life course developmental perspective
    of, 60–63
for multiple problems, 59

Puberty, 81–82. *see also* Adolescent
    development
Public health perspective, 13–14
Public policy
    assuring detection and consequences,
        163–167
    Communities Mobilizing for Change on
        Alcohol program and, 210–
        211
    community-based, 219
    description, 147–148
    media-based interventions and, 145–
        147
    recommendations, 203
    regarding advertising, 167–168
    regarding availability and opportunity,
        154–163
    regarding effective practices, 241–242
    regarding the price of substances, 149,
        150*t*, 151–154
    statewide, 215
    value of, 168–170
Punishment, 190

Q

Quality of life. *see also* Costs to society
    cigarette smoking and, 44
    description, 35–37
    imposed by multiproblem youth, 44–
        46, 45*t*, 47*t*–51*t*, 52*t*–53, 54*t*, 55*t*
    sexual behavior and, 41

R

Racial differences
    in cigarette smoking, 88
    description, 10–12, 11*t*
    multiproblem youth and, 24–25
Random breath testing, 163–164. *see also*
    Alcohol use; Drunk driving
Recidivism
    following Functional Family Therapy,
        176–177
    interventions and, 173–175
    Multidimensional Treatment Foster
        Care and, 179–181
    youth diversion programs and, 183–184
Relationships, peer
    adolescent development and, 85
    interventions that promote delinquency
        and, 187–189*t*
    in middle childhood, 78
    Montreal Longitudinal Experimental
        Study and, 112–114
    Multidimensional Family Therapy and,
        194–196

Multidimensional Treatment Foster
    Care and, 179–181
Multisystemic Therapy and, 177–
    179
victimization and, 86
Research. *see also* Intervention; *specific
    intervention programs*
    disseminating information from, 242–
        243, 244*t*–245*t*, 246–247
    establishing a universal assessment
        model and, 238
    innovations and, 247–250
    on interventions, 121–126
    on multiproblem youth, 89–92, 91*f*
    needed, 231, 250
    needed to implement intervention, 243,
        246–247
    recommendations, 220
    regarding policy, 147–148
Resource costs. *see also* Costs to society
    description, 34
    imposed by multiproblem youth, 44–
        46, 45*t*, 47*t*–51*t*, 52*t*–53, 54*t*,
        55*t*
Rights, individual, in community
    assessment, 233–234
Risk factors
    of the community, 86–87
    intellectual deficits as, 77–78
    life course developmental perspective
        of, 60–63
    for multiple problems, 59
    during prenatal and perinatal
        development, 63, 66–69
    research regarding, 122
    throughout development, 64*t*–65*t*
Risperidone, 183
Ritalin, 182–183

S

Saving Lives Project, 211. *see also*
    Intervention
Scared Straight interventions, 185. *see
    also* Intervention
School
    access to condoms in, 162–163
    adolescent development and, 86
    alcohol policy within, 165
    alternative, 188–189*t*
    failure, 76, 77–78
    Good Behavior Game and, 111–112
    interventions and, 124–125, 132–140,
        141
    Linking Interests of Families and
        Teachers program and, 114–
        115

Montreal Longitudinal Experimental
    Study and, 112–114
Seattle Social Development Program
    and, 115–118
smoking policy within, 165–166
Seattle Social Development Program, 115–
    118. see also Intervention
Selected interventions, 172. see also
    Intervention
Selective serotonin reuptake inhibitors,
    182
Sex education, 140. see also Intervention;
    Sexual behavior
Sexual abuse, as a risk factor, 78–79
Sexual behavior. see also Multiproblem
    youth
    access to health care and condoms and,
        162–163
    in alternative schools, 189t
    Becoming a Responsible Teen program
        and, 198–200
    community-based interventions and,
        217
    description, 9–10
    differences in, 10–12, 11t
    family-focused programs regarding,
        131–132
    interventions for, 197–198, 200–201,
        202–206
    methods used to estimate the costs of,
        40–42
    relationship to other problem
        behaviors, 22–25, 27–29, 28f
    school-based interventions regarding,
        139–140
Sexually transmitted diseases. see also
    HIV/AIDS; Sexual behavior
    Becoming a Responsible Teen program
        and, 198–200
    interventions and, 200–201
    methods used to estimate the costs of,
        40–42
    rates of, 9–10
    school-based interventions regarding,
        139–140
Shared vision. see also Community
    collaborative partnerships and, 226–
        231
    features of, 232
Skill training
    description, 119–120
    effect on behavior, 19
    Montreal Longitudinal Experimental
        Study and, 112–114
    Multidimensional Family Therapy and,
        194–196

school-based interventions and, 133–
    139
Smoking. see Cigarette smoking
SSRIs, 182
Stress
    effect on behavior, 17
    infancy and early childhood exposure
        to, 74
    prenatal exposure to, 67–69
    puberty and, 81–82
Substance use. see Alcohol use; Cigarette
    smoking; Drug use
Suicide
    alcohol use and, 22
    methods used to estimate the costs of,
        44
    policy regarding availability and
        opportunity of alcohol and, 157–
        158
Synar Amendment, 169–170, 242. see
    also Policy

T

Television viewing. see Media
Temperament
    in infancy and early childhood, 69
    as a risk factor, 70–72
Teratogens, prenatal exposure to, 67–69
Testosterone, 81–82
Tobacco use. see Cigarette smoking
Trauma, exposure to in middle childhood,
    78–79
Treatment. see Intervention
Triple-P program, 119–120, 217–218. see
    also Intervention; Parenting

U

Universal prevention, 127–128. see also
    Prevention

V

Valproate, 183
Victimization, within schools, 86
Violence
    in alternative schools, 189t
    Community Trials Project and, 211–
        213
    methods used to estimate the costs of,
        42–43
    policy regarding access to weapons
        and, 161
    policy regarding the price of alcohol
        and, 152
Vital Signs system, 234–238, 237f. see
    also Assessment

W

Work loss costs. *see also* Costs to
    society
  description, 35
  imposed by multiproblem youth, 44–
    46, 45*t*, 47*t*–51*t*, 52*t*–53, 54*t*,
    55*t*

Y

Youth diversion programs, 183–184. *see
    also* Intervention

Z

Zero-tolerance laws, regarding drunk
    driving, 164–165